Cardiovascular Development and Congenital Malformations

Molecular & Genetic Mechanisms

EDITED BY

Michael Artman, MD

Chairman of Pediatrics
University of Iowa

D. Woodrow Benson, MD, PhD

Professor of Pediatrics
Director, Cardiovascular Genetics
Division of Cardiology, Cincinnati Children's Hospital Medical Center

Deepak Srivastava, MD

Pogue Distinguished Chair in Research on Cardiac Birth Defects
Joel B. Steinberg, M.D. Chair in Pediatrics
Professor, Departments of Pediatrics and Molecular Biology
University of Texas Southwestern Medical Center at Dallas

Makoto Nakazawa, MD

Professor and Head, Pediatric Cardiology
The Heart Institute of Japan, Tokyo Women's Medical University

FOREWORD BY

Atsuyoshi Takao
Edward B. Clark

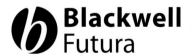

© 2005 by Blackwell Publishing

Blackwell Futura is an imprint of Blackwell Publishing
Blackwell Publishing, Inc., 350 Main Street, Malden, Massachusetts 02148-5020, USA
Blackwell Publishing Ltd, 9600 Garsington Road, Oxford OX4 2DQ, UK
Blackwell Publishing Asia Pty Ltd, 550 Swanston Street, Carlton, Victoria 3053, Australia

First published 2005
Reprinted 2006

ISBN-13: 978-1-4051-3128-5
ISBN-10: 1-4051-3128-4

Library of Congress Cataloging-in-Publication Data

Cardiovascular development and congenital malformations: molecular and genetic machanisms (sic] / edited by Michael Artman ... [et al.] ; foreword by Atsuyoshi Takao, Edward B. Clark.
        p.   ;   cm.
    Includes bibliographical references and index.
    ISBN 1-4051-3128-4 (alk. paper)
    1. Heart–Abnormalities.   2. Heart–Growth.
    [DNLM: 1. Cardiovascular Abnormalities–genetics.   2 Heart Defects,
        Congenital–genetics. WG 220 C267 2005] I. Artman, Michael, 1952–
    RC687.C36 2005
    616.1'2043—dc22

                                                            2004029172

Acquisitions: Steven Korn
Development Editor: Vicki Donald
Set in Minion 9.5/12pt by SNP Best-set Typesetter Ltd, Hong Kong
Printed and bound by Replika Press Pvt. Ltd, India

For further information on Blackwell Publishing, visit our website:
www.blackwellcardiology.com

Contents

Foreword

Scientific advances depend on the intersection of talent, tools and ideas. Some of these elements can be designed. Others depend upon fortuitous events, the vision of clinical leaders and the resources that bring together a critical mass of individuals. Such has been the parallel histories of clinical pediatric cardiology and cardiac development.

Pediatric cardiology has evolved from despair and autopsy to fetal diagnosis and early surgical intervention, and infant survival has increased from 50% to more than 95%. As senior cardiologists, we now care for patients in their fifth and sixth decades of life, but still the question remains: what caused my child's heart defect?

The modern era of cardiovascular development arose in the 1970s simultaneously in centers of excellent clinical care. Clinicians recognized that understanding normal development would eventually lead to defining etiology and prevention. So, in Japan, the Netherlands, Switzerland and the USA, scientists focused the tools of modern biology on the problem of heart development.

This new generation of scientists was in many ways isolated because there was no established venue to meet and share ideas and respond to the constructive criticism of colleagues. Enter the catalyst: Atsuyoshi Takao MD.

Dr Takao assembled the leaders of science and pathology for 4 days of intensive interaction. The meetings were nearly magical in the stimulating atmosphere of science happening in real time. The published proceedings became standard references for collaborators and scientific techniques. The Takao Conference is now the longest running venue bringing together senior scientists who focus on cardiovascular development.

This volume is a worthy successor to the tradition of the Takao Meeting publications. For the neophyte and the senior scientist, the range of topics from situs and looping to exploratory genetic analysis covers the field comprehensively.

Evolution rewards success with longevity. For those of us long-of-tooth, gratification lies in the geometric growth of the field, a complexity of analysis and the early success in prevention. Cardiovascular development is now a well-established and highly valued scientific discipline attracting new generations who will be our successors. We trust that you the reader will join us in the appreciation of this dedicated work that advances understanding of normal and abnormal heart development.

Atsuyoshi Takao
Edward B. Clark

Contributors

Katsumi Ando, DVM
Department of Anatomy
Saitama Medical School
Saitama, Japan

Masahiko Ando
Heart Institute of Japan
Tokyo Women's Medical University
Tokyo, Japan

Hiroshi Akazawa
Department of Cardiovascular Science and Medicine
Chiba University Graduate School of Medicine
Inohana, Chuo-ku,
Chiba, Japan

Kaoru Akimoto
Department of Pediatric Cardiology
Division of Genomic Medicine
Tokyo Women's Medical University
Tokyo, Japan

Stephen L. Archer, MD
Vascular Biology Group
Alberta Heart and Stroke Research Centre
University of Alberta
Edmonton, Canada

Michael Artman, MD
Departments of Pediatrics
University of Iowa
Iowa City, IA

Yoshihito Atsumi, MD
Division of Internal Medicine
Saiseikai Central Hospital
Tokyo, Japan

Antonio Baldini
Department of Pediatrics (Cardiology)
Baylor College of Medicine
Houston, TX

H. Scott Baldwin, MD
Department of Pediatrics (Cardiology)
Vanderbilt University Medical Center
Nashville, TN

Lance F. Barker
Department of Pediatrics
University of Utah
Salt Lake City, UT

Joey V. Barnett
Department of Pharmacology
Vanderbilt University Medical Center
Nashville, TN

Craig T. Basson
Molecular Cardiology Laboratory
Cardiology Division
Department of Medicine
Weill Medical College of Cornell University
New York, NY

Nico A. Blom
Department of Pediatrics
Leiden University Medical Center
Leiden, The Netherlands

Damien Bonnet
INSERM 0016
Hôpital Necker Enfants Malades
Paris, France

Marit J. Boot
Department of Anatomy and Embryology
Leiden University Medical Center
Leiden, The Netherlands

Thomas K. Borg
Department of Cell and Developmental Biology and Anatomy
University of South Carolina
Columbia, SC

Karla R. Bowles
Department of Molecular and Human Genetics
Baylor College of Medicine
Texas Children's Hospital
Houston, TX

Neil E. Bowles
Department of Molecular and Human Genetics
Baylor College of Medicine
Texas Children's Hospital
Houston, TX

Thomas Brand
Department of Cell and Molecular Biology
Technical University of Braunschweig
Braunschweig, Germany

Philip R. Brauer
Department of Biomedical Sciences
Creighton University
Omaha, NB

Nigel A. Brown
Anatomy & Developmental Biology
Basic Medical Sciences
St George's Hospital Medical School
Cranmer Terrace
University of London, SW17 0RE

Benoit G. Bruneau
Cardiovascular Research
The Hospital for Sick Children
Toronto
ON, Canada

Margaret Buckingham
CNRS URA 1947
Department of Developmental Biology
Pasteur Institute
Paris, France

James Buggy
Department of Physiology, Pharmacology and Neurosciences
University of South Carolina
Columbia, SC

John B. E. Burch
Department of Cell and Developmental Biology
Fox Chase Cancer Center
Philadelphia, PA

Rossella Capolino
Medical Genetics
Bambino Gesù Hospital
Rome, Italy

Wayne Carver
Department of Cell and Developmental Biology and Anatomy
University of South Carolina
Columbia, SC

YiPing Chen
Department of Cell and Molecular Biology
Tulane University
New Orleans, LA

Jung Yun Choi
Seoul National University
Seoul, Korea

Vincent M. Christoffels
Experimental and Molecular Cardiology Group
Academic Medical Centre
University of Amsterdam
The Netherlands

Mon-Li Chu
Jefferson Institute of Molecular Medicine
Department of Dermatology and Cutaneous Biology
Thomas Jefferson University
Jefferson Medical College
Philadelphia, PA

Edward B. Clark
Department of Pediatrics
Primary Children's Medical Center
University of Utah
Salt Lake City, UT

William A. Coetzee
Departments of Pediatrics
Physiology and Neuroscience and Pharmacology
New York University School of Medicine
New York, NY

Simon J. Conway
Institute of Molecular Medicine and Genetics
Medical College of Georgia
Augusta, GA

Emanuela Conti
Medical Genetics
University 'La Sapienza' and Mendel-CSS Institute
Rome, Italy

Tony Creazzo
Department of Pediatrics
Duke University Medical Center
Durham, NC

Rodney Dale
Department of Medicine
Section of Cardiology
University of Chicago
Chicago, IL

Bruno Dallapiccola
Medical Genetics
University 'La Sapienza' and Mendel-CSS Institute
Rome, Italy

Piet A. J. De Boer
Experimental and Molecular Cardiology Group
Academic Medical Centre
University of Amsterdam
The Netherlands

Huub J. M. de Groot
Leiden Institute of Chemistry
Leiden University
Leiden, The Netherlands

Marco C. DeRuiter
Department of Anatomy and Embryology
Leiden University Medical Center
Leiden, The Netherlands

Jay S. Desgrosellier
Department of Pharmacology
Vanderbilt University Medical Center
Nashville, TN

Maria Cristina Digilio
Medical Genetics
Bambino Gesù Hospital
Rome, Italy

Nata Diman
Molecular Cardiology Laboratory
Cardiology Division
Department of Medicine
Weill Medical College of Cornell University
New York, NY

Thomas Doetschman
Department of Cell Biology
University of Cincinnati
Cincinnati, OH

Angela V. Edwards
Department of Cell and Developmental Biology
Fox Chase Cancer Center
Philadelphia, PA

Fumio Endo
Department of Pediatrics
Kumamoto University School of Medicine
Japan

Jonathan A. Epstein
Cardiovascular Division
University of Pennsylvania
Philadelphia, PA

Kees Erkelens
Leiden Institute of Chemistry
Leiden University
Leiden, The Netherlands

John F. Fallon
Department of Anatomy
University of Wisconsin Medical School
Madison, WI

Glenn I. Fishman
Division of Cardiology
New York University School of Medicine
New York, NY

Hidetoshi Fujino
Department of Pediatrics
Shiga University of Medical Science
Otsu, Shiga, Japan

Maya Fujiwara
Department of Pediatric Cardiology
Division of Genomic Medicine
Tokyo Women's Medical University
Tokyo, Japan

Michiko Furutani, BS
Department of Pediatric Cardiology
Division of Genomic Medicine
Tokyo Women's Medical University
Tokyo, Japan

Jason B. Garrison
Department of Pediatrics
Cardiovascular Development Research Program
Children's Hospital of Pittsburgh
University of Pittsburgh,
Rangos Research Center
Pittsburgh, PA

Bruce D. Gelb, MD
Departments of Pediatrics and Human Genetics
Mount Sinai School of Medicine
New York, NY

Adriana C. Gittenberger-de Groot
Department of Anatomy & Embryology
Leiden University Medical Center
Leiden, The Netherlands

Anita Go
Departments of Pediatrics
Physiology and Neuroscience and Pharmacology
New York University School of Medicine
New York, NY

Elizabeth Goldmuntz, MD
Division of Cardiology
The Children's Hospital of Philadelphia
Department of Pediatrics
The University of Pennsylvania School of Medicine
Philadelphia, PA

Marsha M. Goldstein
Impath, Inc.
New York NY and University of Medicine and Dentistry New Jersey
Newark, NJ

Robert G. Gourdie
Department of Cell Biology and Anatomy
Medical University of South Carolina
Charleston, SC

Bianca C. W. Groenendijk
Department of Anatomy and Embryology
Leiden University Medical Center
Leiden, The Netherlands

Dieter Gross
Brüker Analytische Messtechnik GmbH
Rheinstetten
Germany

Paul Grossfeld, MD
Division of Pediatric Cardiology
University of California
San Diego/Children's Hospital of San Diego
San Diego, CA

Christopher Hall
Department of Cell Biology
Cornell University Medical College
New York, NY

Yuji Hamamichi
Department of Pediatrics
Toyama Medical & Pharmaceutical University
Toyama, Japan

Kenji Hamaoka
Department of Pediatric Cardiology and Nephrology
Kyoto Prefectural University of Medicine
Graduate School of Medical Science
Kyoto, Japan

Takashi Hanato, MD
Department of Pediatrics
Shiga University of Medical Science
Otsu, Shiga, Japan

Noriyuki Haneda
Department of Pediatrics
Shimane Medical University
Shimane, Japan

Ming-Da Han
Department of Cell Biology
University of Medicine & Dentistry
NJ-SOM, Stratford, NJ

Takashi Hanato
Department of Pediatrics
Shiga University of Medical Science
Otsu, Shiga, Japan

Mari Hara
Department of Pathology
Faculty of Medicine
Mie University
Tsu, Mie, Japan

Gwyneth Harry, MSc
Vascular Biology Group
Alberta Heart and Stroke Research Centre
University of Alberta
Edmonton, Canada

Ikuo Hashimoto
Department of Pediatrics
Toyama Medical & Pharmaceutical University1
Toyama, Japan

Kyoko Hashimoto
Vascular Biology Group
Alberta Heart and Stroke Research Centre
University of Alberta
Edmonton, Canada

Cathy J. Hatcher
Molecular Cardiology Laboratory
Cardiology Division
Department of Medicine
Weill Medical College of Cornell University
New York, NY

Deborah J. Henderson
Institute of Human Genetics
University of Newcastle upon Tyne
International Centre for Life
Newcastle upon Tyne
UK

Kenneth W. Hewett
Department of Cell Biology and Anatomy
Medical University of South Carolina
Charleston, SC

Beerend P. Hierck
Department of Anatomy and Embryology
Leiden University Medical Center
Leiden, The Netherlands

Kayoko Hirayama-Yamada
Heart Institute of Japan
Tokyo Women's Medical University
Tokyo, Japan

Keiichi Hirono
Department of Pediatrics
Toyama Medical & Pharmaceutical University1
Toyama, Japan

Stan Hoffman
Medical University of South Carolina
Charleston, SC

Bianca Hogers
Department of Anatomy and Embryology
Leiden University Medical Center
Leiden, The Netherlands

Kazuhiro Hosokawa, MD
Division of Internal Medicine
Saiseikai Central Hospital
Tokyo, Japan

Norman Hu
Department of Pediatrics
University of Utah
Salt Lake City, UT

June Huh
Samsung Medical Center
Seoul, Korea

Romulo Hurtado
Department of Cell Biology
Cornell University Medical College
New York, NY

Fukiko Ichida, MD
Department of Pediatrics
Toyama Medical & Pharmaceutical University1
Toyama, Japan

Shinichiro Imamura, DVM, PhD
Department of Pediatric Cardiology
The Heart Institute of Japan
Tokyo Women's Medical University
Tokyo, Japan

Kyoko Imanaka-Yoshida
Department of Pathology
Faculty of Medicine
Mie University
Tsu, Mie, Japan

Naoki Ito
Department of Cell Biology and Anatomy
Cornell University Medical College
New York, NY

Louisa M. Jones
Anatomy & Developmental Biology
Basic Medical Sciences
St George's Hospital Medical School
Cranmer Terrace
University of London
UK

Kunitaka Joo
Kyushu Welfare Pension Hospital
Fukuoka, Japan

Amy L. Juraszek
Department of Cell Biology and Anatomy
Cardiovascular Development Biology Center
Medical University of South Carolina
Charleston, SC

Chip Justus
Department of Cell Biology and Anatomy
Medical University of South Carolina
Charleston, SC

Mitsuhiro Kamisago
Heart Institute of Japan
Tokyo Women's Medical University
Tokyo, Japan

Nobuyuki Kanzawa
Department of Cell Biology
Cornell University Medical College
New York, NY

Hiroshi Kasanuki, MD
The Heart Institute of Japan
Tokyo Women's Medical University
Tokyo, Japan

Taichi Kato
Heart Institute of Japan
Tokyo Women's Medical University
Tokyo, Japan

Bradley B. Keller, MD
Department of Pediatrics
Cardiovascular Development Research Program
Children's Hospital of Pittsburgh
University of Pittsburgh,
Rangos Research Center
Pittsburgh, PA

Robert G. Kelly
CNRS URA 1947
Department of Developmental Biology
Pasteur Institute
Paris, France

Hong Ryang Kil
Chungnan National University
Seoul, Korea

Min-Su Kim
Molecular Cardiology Laboratory
Cardiology Division
Department of Medicine
Weill Medical College of Cornell University
New York, NY

Soo Jin Kim
Sejong General Hospital
Seoul, Korea

Young Hwue Kim
University of Ulsan
College of Medicine and Asan Medical Center
Seoul, Korea

Mitsuru Kimura, MD
Division of Internal Medicine
Saiseikai Central Hospital
Tokyo, Japan

Jae Kon Ko
University of Ulsan
College of Medicine and Asan Medical Center
Seoul, Korea

Lazaros Kochilas
Cardiovascular Division
University of Pennsylvania
Philadelphia, PA

Frantisek Kolar
Center for Experimental Cardiovascular Research
Institute of Physiology
Academy of Sciences of the Czech Republic
Prague, Czech Republic

Issei Komuro
Department of Cardiovascular Science and Medicine
Chiba University Graduate School of Medicine
Inohana, Chuo-ku,
Chiba, Japan

Jan Kopecky
Center for Integrated Genomics
Institute of Physiology
Academy of Sciences of the Czech Republic
Prague, Czech Republic

Srinagesh V. Koushik
Institute of Molecular Medicine and Genetics
Medical College of Georgia
Augusta, GA

Paul A. Krieg
Department of Cell Biology and Anatomy
University of Arizona College of Medicine
Tucson, AZ

Edward L. Krug
Medical University of South Carolina
Charleston, SC

Boudewijn P. T. Kruithof
Experimental and Molecular Cardiology Group
Cardiovascular Research Institute Amsterdam
Academic Medical Center, Amsterdam
The Netherlands

Pavel Kucera
Institute of Physiology
University of Lausanne
Switzerland

Raju Kucherlapati
Center for Genetics and Genomics
Harvard Medical School
Boston, MA

Heung Jae Lee
Samsung Medical Center
Seoul, Korea

Sang Bum Lee
Kyungpook National University
Seoul, Korea

Volker Lehmann
Brüker Analytische Messtechnik GmbH
Rheinstetten
Germany

Jun Liao
Department of Molecular Genetics
Albert Einstein College of Medicine
Bronx, NY

Kersti K. Linask
Department of Cell Biology
University of Medicine & Dentistry
NJ-SOM, Stratford, NJ

Andrew Lindsley
Institute of Molecular Medicine and Genetics
Medical College of Georgia
Augusta, GA

Chengyu Liu
Alkek Institute of Bioscience & Technology
Texas A&M Health Sciences Center
Houston, TX

Wei Liu
Alkek Institute of Bioscience & Technology
Texas A&M Health Sciences Center
Houston, TX

Christopher A. Loffredo, PhD
Lombardi Cancer Center
Georgetown University School of Medicine
Washington, DC

Mei Fang Lu
Alkek Institute of Bioscience & Technology
Texas A&M Health Sciences Center
Houston, TX

Oliver A. T. Lyons
Anatomy & Developmental Biology
Basic Medical Sciences
St George's Hospital Medical School
Cranmer Terrace
University of London
UK

Jae Sook Ma
Chonnam National University
Seoul, Korea

Manabu Maeda
Institute of Molecular Medicine and Genetics
Medical College of Georgia
Augusta, GA

Salvatore Mancarella
Departments of Pediatrics
Physiology and Neuroscience and Pharmacology
New York University School of Medicine
New York, NY

Bruno Marino
Pediatric Cardiology
Institute of Pediatrics
University 'La Sapienza'
Rome, Italy

Roger R. Markwald
Medical University of South Carolina
Department of Cell Biology and Anatomy
Cardiovascular Developmental Biology Center
Charleston, SC

James F. Martin
Alkek Institute of Bioscience & Technology
Texas A&M Health Sciences Center
Houston, TX

Kempei Matsuoka, MD
Division of Internal Medicine
Saiseikai Central Hospital
Tokyo, Japan

Rumiko Matsuoka, MD
Department of Pediatric Cardiology
Tokyo Women's Medical University
Tokyo, Japan

Marek Michalak
Canadian Institute of Health Research Group in Molecular
  Biology of Membrane Proteins and Department of
  Biochemistry
University of Alberta
Edmonton, Canada

Evangelos D. Michelakis
Vascular Biology Group
Alberta Heart and Stroke Research Centre
University of Alberta
Edmonton, Canada

Takashi Mikawa
Department of Cell & Developmental Biology
Weill Medical College of Cornell University
New York, NY

Federica Mileto
Pediatric Cardiology
Institute of Pediatrics
University 'La Sapienza'
Rome, Italy

Susumu Minamisawa
Department of Pediatric Cardiology
Tokyo Women's Medical University
Tokyo, Japan

Keiichi Miyamoto
Department of Chemistry for Materials Faculty of
Engineering
Mie University
Tsu, Mie, Japan

Toshio Miyawaki
Department of Pediatrics
Toyama Medical & Pharmaceutical University1
Toyama, Japan

Corey H. Mjaatvedt
Medical University of South Carolina
Department of Cell Biology and Anatomy
Cardiovascular Developmental Biology Center
Charleston, SC

Melinda Modrell
Department of Medicine
Section of Cardiology
University of Chicago
Chicago, IL

Daniel G. M. Molin
Department of Anatomy and Embryology
Leiden University Medical Center
Leiden, The Netherlands

Yukihiko Momiyama, MD
First Department of Internal Medicine
National Defense Medical College
Saitama, Japan

Kazuo Momma
Pediatric Cardiology
The Heart Institute of Japan
Tokyo Women's Medical University
Tokyo, Japan

Antoon F. M. Moorman
Experimental and Molecular Cardiology Group
Cardiovascular Research Institute Amsterdam
Academic Medical Center, Amsterdam
The Netherlands

Ricardo Moreno-Rodriguez
Hospital Infantil 'Federico Gomez' Mexico City
Mexico City
Mexico

Masae Morishima
Department of Pediatrics (Cardiology)
Baylor College of Medicine
Houston, TX

Bernice Morrow
Department of Molecular Genetics
Albert Einstein College of Medicine
Bronx, NY

Rohit Moudgil, MSc
Vascular Biology Group
Alberta Heart and Stroke Research Centre
University of Alberta
Edmonton, Canada

Masao Nakagawa
Department of Pediatrics
Shiga University of Medical Science
Otsu, Shiga, Japan

Yuji Nakajima, MD
Department of Anatomy
Graduate School of Medicine
Osaka City University
Osaka, Japan

Hiroaki Nakamura, PhD
Department of Anatomy
Saitama Medical School
Saitama, Japan

Kimitoshi Nakamura
Department of Pediatrics
Kumamoto University School of Medicine
Japan

Toshio Nakanishi
The Heart Institute
Tokyo Women's Medical University
Tokyo, Japan

T. Nakaoka
Department of Advanced Medical Science
Institute of medical Science
University of Tokyo
Tokyo

Tomotaka Nakayama
First Department of Pediatrics
Toho University
Tokyo, Japan

Makoto Nakazawa
Department of Pediatric Cardiology
Division of Genomic Medicine
Tokyo Women's Medical University
Tokyo, Japan

Miyuki Namikata
Department of Pathology
Faculty of Medicine
Mie University
Tsu, Mie, Japan

Tsutomu Narita
Department of Pediatrics
Shiga University of Medical Science
Otsu, Shiga, Japan

Frans T. M. Nieuwstadt
Department of Aero and Hydrodynamics
Technical University Delft
Delft, The Netherlands

Setsuko Nishijima
Department of Pediatrics
Shiga University of Medical Science
Otsu, Shiga, Japan

Toshihiko Ogura, MD, PhD
Graduate School of Biological Sciences
Nara Institute of Science and Technology
Takayama, Ikoma
Nara, Japan

Fumitaka Ohsuzu, MD
First Department of Internal Medicine
National Defense Medical College
Saitama, Japan

Nobuhiko Okamoto
Department of Pediatrics
Shiga University of Medical Science
Otsu, Shiga, Japan

Bohuslav Ostadal
Center for Experimental Cardiovascular Research and
Institute of Physiology
Academy of Sciences of the Czech Republic
Prague, Czech Republic

Ivana Ostadalova
Center for Experimental Cardiovascular Research and
Institute of Physiology
Academy of Sciences of the Czech Republic
Prague, Czech Republic

In Sook Park
University of Ulsan
College of Medicine and Asan Medical Center
Seoul, Korea

Jennifer Palie
Alkek Institute of Bioscience & Technology
Texas A&M Health Sciences Center
Houston, TX

David Pennisi
Department of Cell and Developmental Biology
Weill Medical College of Cornell University
New York, NY

Helen M. Phillips
Institute of Human Genetics
University of Newcastle upon Tyne
International Centre for Life
Newcastle upon Tyne
UK

Robert E. Poelmann
Department of Anatomy & Embryology
Leiden University Medical Center
Leiden, The Netherlands

Clifton P. Poma
Department of Cell Biology
Cornell University Medical College
New York, NY

Mathieu J. B. M. Pourquie
Department of Aero and Hydrodynamics
Technical University Delft
Delft, The Netherlands

Robert L. Price
Department of Cell and Developmental Biology and Anatomy
University of South Carolina
Columbia, SC

Ivan M. Rebeyka, MD
Vascular Biology Group
Alberta Heart and Stroke Research Centre
University of Alberta
Edmonton, Canada

Maria Reckova
Department of Cell Biology and Anatomy
Medical University of South Carolina
Charleston, SC

Rhonda Rogers
Institute of Molecular Medicine and Genetics
Medical College of Georgia
Augusta, GA

Chen Rui
Department of Pediatrics
Toyama Medical & Pharmaceutical University1
Toyama, Japan

Tsutomu Saji
First Department of Pediatrics
Toho University
Tokyo, Japan

Nurul H. Sarker
Institute of Molecular Medicine and Genetics
Medical College of Georgia
Augusta, GA

Anna Sarkozy
Medical Genetics University La Sapienza
Rome, Italy

Mariko Sato
Huntsman Cancer Institute Center for Children
Departments of Oncological Sciences and Pediatrics
University of Utah
Salt Lake City, UT

Eul Ju Seo
University of Ulsan
College of Medicine and Asan Medical Center
Seoul, Korea

David Sedmera
Department of Cell Biology and Anatomy
Medical University of South Carolina
Charleston, SC

Isao Shiraishi, MD
Department of Pediatric Cardiology and Nephrology
Kyoto Prefectural University of Medicine
Graduate School of Medical Science
Kyoto, Japan

Maxim Shulimovich
Department of Cell Biology
Cornell University Medical College
New York, NY

Milan Šamánek
Kardiocentrum
University Hospital Motol
Prague, Czech Republic

Libor Skarka
Center for Experimental Cardiovascular Research and
Institute of Physiology
Academy of Sciences of the Czech Republic
Prague, Czech Republic

Eric M. Small
Department of Cell Biology and Anatomy
University of Arizona College of Medicine
Arizona

Yan Song
Molecular Cardiology Laboratory
Cardiology Division
Department of Medicine
Weill Medical College of Cornell University
New York, NY

Deepak Srivastava
Departments of Pediatrics and Molecular Biology
University of Texas Southwestern Medical Center
Dallas, TX

Shekhar Srivastava
Departments of Pediatrics
Physiology and Neuroscience and Pharmacology
New York University School of Medicine
New York, NY

Paul Steendijk
Department of Cardiology
Leiden University Medical Center
Leiden, The Netherlands

Sandra Stekelenburg-de Vos
Department of Obstetrics and Gynecology
Erasmus Medical Center
Rotterdam, The Netherlands

Henry M. Sucov
Department of Cell and Neurobiology
Institute for Genetic Medicine
University of Southern California
Los Angeles, CA

Yukiko Sugi
Department of Cell Biology and Anatomy and Cardiovascular
Developmental Biology Center
Medical University of South Carolina
Charleston, SC

Yoshihiko Suzuki, MD
Division of Internal Medicine
Saiseikai Central Hospital
Tokyo, Japan

Eric C. Svensson
Department of Medicine
Section of Cardiology
University of Chicago
Chicago, IL

Gyorgyi Szebenyi
Department of Anatomy
University of Wisconsin Medical School
Madison, WI

Tetsuro Takamatsu
Department of Pathology and Cell Regulation
Kyoto Prefectural University of Medicine
Graduate School of Medical Science
Kyoto, Japan

Takeshi Takami
Pediatric Cardiology
The Heart Institute of Japan
Tokyo Women's Medical University
Tokyo, Japan

Atsuyoshi Takao
Department of Pediatric Cardiology
Division of Genomic Medicine
Tokyo Women's Medical University
Tokyo, Japan

Kimiko Takebayashi-Suzuki
Department of Cell Biology
Cornell University Medical College
New York, NY

Atsuhito Takeda
Department of Pediatric Cardiology
The Heart Institute of Japan
Tokyo Women's Medical University
Tokyo, Japan

Yoshihiro Takeuchi, MD
Department of Pediatrics
Shiga University of Medical Science
Otsu, Shiga, Japan

Marco Tartaglia
Department of Pediatrics
Mount Sinai School of Medicine
New York, NY

Bernard Thébaud, MD
Vascular Biology Group
Alberta Heart and Stroke Research Centre
University of Alberta
Edmonton, Canada

Robert P. Thompson
Cell Biology and Anatomy
Medical University of South Carolina
Charleston, SC

Kimimasa Tobita, MD
Department of Pediatrics
Cardiovascular Development Research Program
Children's Hospital of Pittsburgh
University of Pittsburgh,
Rangos Research Center
Pittsburgh, PA

Jeffrey A. Towbin
Department of Molecular and Human Genetics
Baylor College of Medicine
Texas Children's Hospital
Houston, TX

Katsuaki Toyoshima
Department of Pediatric Cardiology
The Heart Institute of Japan
Tokyo Women's Medical University
Tokyo, Japan

Shinichi Tsubata
Department of Pediatrics
Toyama Medical & Pharmaceutical University1
Toyama, Japan

Takeshi Tsuda
Jefferson Institute of Molecular Medicine
Department of Dermatology and Cutaneous Biology
Thomas Jefferson University
Jefferson Medical College
Philadelphia, PA

Tohru Tsuji
Department of Pediatrics
Southern Tohoku General Hospital
Kohriyama, Japan

Keiichiro Uese
Department of Pediatrics
Toyama Medical & Pharmaceutical University1
Toyama, Japan

Nicolette T. C. Ursem
Department of Obstetrics and Gynecology
Erasmus Medical Center
Rotterdam, The Netherlands

Maurice J. B. van den Hoff
Experimental and Molecular Cardiology Group
Cardiovascular Research Institute Amsterdam
Academic Medical Center, Amsterdam
The Netherlands

Laura Villavicencio
Hospital Infantil 'Federico Gomez' Mexico City
Mexico City
Mexico

Jian Wang
Institute of Molecular Medicine and Genetics
Medical College of Georgia
Augusta, GA

Noriko Watanabe
Department of Pediatrics
Shiga University of Medical Science
Shiga, Japan

Sayaka Watanabe
Department of Pediatrics
Toyama Medical & Pharmaceutical University1
Toyama, Japan

Andy Wessels
Medical University of South Carolina
Department of Cell Biology and Anatomy
Cardiovascular Developmental Biology Center
Charleston, SC

Jeannine Wilk
Department of Medicine
Section of Cardiology
University of Chicago
Chicago, IL

Jury W. Wladimiroff
Department of Obstetrics and Gynecology
Erasmus Medical Center
Rotterdam, The Netherlands

D. Woodrow Benson, MD, PhD
Cardiovascular Genetics
Division of Cardiology
Children's Hospital Medical Center
Cincinnati, OH

Xi-Chen Wu, PhD
Vascular Biology Group
Alberta Heart and Stroke Research Centre
University of Alberta
Edmonton, Canada

Huansheng Xu
Department of Pediatrics (Cardiology)
Baylor College of Medicine
Houston, TX

Hiroyuki Yamagishi
Division of Pediatric Cardiology
Department of Pediatrics
Keio University School of Medicine
Tokyo, Japan

Toshiyuki Yamagishi, PhD
Department of Anatomy
Saitama Medical School
Saitama, Japan

Sadamu Yamamoto, PhD
Junior College
Saitama Prefectural University
Koshigayashi
Saitama, Japan

N. Yamashita
Department of Advanced Medical Science
Institute of Medical Science
University of Tokyo
Tokyo, Japan

Yukuto Yasuhiko
Department of Biological Sciences
Graduate School of Science
University of Tokyo, Japan

Takahiko Yokoyama
The Second Department of Anatomy
Kyoto Prefecture University of Medicine
465 Kajii-cho, Kawaramachi-dori
Hirokoji-agaru, Kamikyo-ku
Kyoto 602–0842, Japan

Han Wook Yoo
University of Ulsan
College of Medicine and Asan Medical Center
Seoul, Korea

Toshimichi Yoshida
Department of Pathology
Faculty of Medicine
Mie University
Tsu, Mie, Japan

Kyoko Yoshida-Imanaka
Department of Pathology
Mie University
School of Medicine
Tsu, Mie, Japan

Masaaki Yoshigi
Department of Pediatrics
University of Utah
Salt Lake City, UT

H. Joseph Yost, PhD
Huntsman Cancer Institute Center for Children
Departments of Oncological Sciences and Pediatrics
University of Utah
Salt Lake City, UT

Stephane Zaffran
CNRS URA 1947
Department of Developmental Biology
Pasteur Institute
Paris, France

X. Zhang
Department of Advanced Medical Science
Institute of Medical Science
University of Tokyo
Tokyo, Japan

Bin Zhou, PhD
Department of Pediatrics (Cardiology)
Vanderbilt University Medical Center
Nashville, TN

Ying-Ying Zhou
Departments of Pediatrics
Physiology and Neuroscience and Pharmacology
New York University School of Medicine
New York, NY

PART 1

Establishing left–right patterning and cardiac looping

Editorial perspective

Deepak Srivastava

A wide variety of congenital cardiovascular malformations can be attributed to abnormalities in the process of cardiac looping that leads to proper alignment of inflow and outflow tracts. This essential step of morphogenesis is intimately related to signaling pathways that establish the proper direction of cardiac looping and general embryonic left–right asymmetry. Work from multiple investigators has begun to reveal the basic underpinnings of left–right determination and its interpretation by the heart. The chapters here describe the role of vortical, unidirectional nodal flow established by beating cilia on the surface of the embryonic node. While the exact mechanism through which unidirectional nodal flow establishes left–right asymmetry remains controversial, evidence is presented to support the presence for a second non-motile form of cilia in the node that bends in response to the nodal flow. Upon bending, these "sensory" cilia trigger a calcium-dependent signaling cascade within nodal cells, which somehow may result in the asymmetric left–right gene expression. In a subsequent chapter a potential link to a calcium-dependent pathway is provided by the observation that the *inv* gene product can interact with calmodulin. A transcriptional link between the left–right signaling pathways and the events of morphogenesis at the organ level is described by analysis of mice lacking isoforms of Pitx2, a transcription factor that is left–right asymmetric and subsequently is expressed in distinct regions of the forming heart. Finally, evidence for an even earlier event in *Xenopus* involving differential phosphorylation events in individual left and right-sided cells is provided suggesting that left–right determination may occur prior to ciliary-mediated nodal events. Through diverse approaches using multiple model organisms, remarkable progress has been made in understanding the events linking early embryonic left–right decisions to signaling and transcriptional pathways that impinge on normal cardiac morphogenesis.

CHAPTER 1

Microenvironment provides left–right instructions to migrating precardiac mesoderm

H. Joseph Yost

Construction of the vertebrate heart requires cell migration and cell invasion from several regions in the embryo. Precardiac mesoderm cells migrate extensive distances during gastrulation to reach the heart-forming region at the ventral midline,[1] where they begin expression of cardiac-specific genes. Cardiac neural crest cells arrive from the dorsal neural tube to invade the outflow tract and, in the case of zebrafish, to form cardiomyocytes in the atrium and ventricle.[2] Proepicardial cells migrate across the surface of the forming heart to participate in the development and patterning of coronary arteries and conduction system.[3] Epithelial to mesoderm transformation causes cells to migrate and to invade extracellular matrix in order to form cardiac cushions and valves.[4] In all of these examples, the nature of these cells after migration, including their gene expression patterns, cell shapes, and cellular physiology, are remarkably distinct from their premigratory states. This suggests that migrating cells receive patterning information during the process of migration. It is possible that patterning information is encoded in molecules embedded in the "microenvironment," the extracellular matrix and surfaces of other cells that are contacted by migrating cells. Because the interactions of migrating cells with microenvironments are fleeting, in most cases it is technically challenging to study cell decisions during the act of migration, or to delineate the information-bearing molecules that are embedded in the path of cell migration. Often the best alternative is to manipulate these interactions

and assess the downstream developmental defects.

Embryos from the amphibian *Xenopus laevis* are uniquely suited for experimental manipulations of cell–cell and cell–matrix interactions. We can assess the interactions of mesoderm cells that migrate during gastrulation, including lateral plate and precardiac mesoderm, with microenvironments that are established on the surface of embryonic ectoderm cells (Fig. 1.1). Results from ectoderm cell transplantation experiments suggest that the basal surface of ectoderm, or matrix deposited by ectoderm, is necessary for normal left–right patterning of mesoderm that contacts the ectoderm during migration in gastrula stages.[5] These transplantations cause a localized perturbation of extracellular matrix, so that fibronectin matrix on the surface of transplanted cells is disrupted while matrix in the surrounding field of cells is normal. Fate-mapping indicates that mesoderm cells that migrate across the transplanted cells and the denuded matrix are deficient in left–right patterning, whereas neighboring mesoderm cells that migrate across adjacent untransplanted ectoderm have normal patterning. These results suggest that the microenvironment established by ectoderm cells is necessary for transmitting left–right patterning to migrating mesoderm.[5] Perturbation of the entire ectoderm matrix, by inhibiting fibronectin deposition or by heparinase digestion of cell-surface and extracellular heparin sulfate proteoglycans (HSPGs), results in randomization of left–right patterning in all migrating mesoderm[5].

Inhibition of HSGP synthesis before and during mesoderm cell migration blocks subsequent cardiac tube looping, but inhibition of HSPG synthesis after mesoderm migration had no effect on heart looping.[6] Together, these results suggest that HSPGs are involved in the transmission of left–right information from ectoderm to migrating mesoderm.

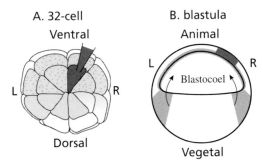

A. 32-cell
Ventral

L   R

Dorsal

B. blastula
Animal

L   R

Blastocoel

Vegetal

Fig. 1.1 Migrating mesoderm contacts microenvironment on ectoderm surface. (A) 32-cell embryos can be injected into specific left or right side cell lineages with molecules that alter gene expression in that lineage. (B) At the blastula stage, the embryo is a ball of cells with an internal extracellular space (blastocoel). The animal cap ectoderm cells express syndecan-1 and syndecan-2 and form a fibronectin extracellular matrix on the basal surface. Mesoderm cells at the equator invade the blastocoel and migrate on the basal surface of ectoderm cells during gastrulation. The dark patch is representative of a clone of ectoderm cells injected at the 32-cell stage (as in A). Targeted alterations of gene expression in clones of ectoderm cells, or injections of reagents into the blastocoel which modify cell surface or extracellular matrix, are used to alter the microenviroment of the migrating mesoderm cells. Similarly, mesoderm cells can be injected to alter downstream signaling pathways in migrating cells. Adapted from ref. 5.

The next challenge was to identify which family of HSPGs is involved in left–right patterning. Syndecans are single-pass transmembrane HSPGs that have multiple glycosaminoglycan (GAG) attachment sites on the extracellular surface and highly conserved serine-phosphorylation sites and a PDZ-protein binding domain on the intracellular side. The observation by Amy Teel that syndecan-1 and syndecan-2 mRNAs are sequestered during oogenesis to the side of the egg that gives rise to ectoderm, and that syndecans are expressed exclusively in ectoderm cells during gastrulation, made them likely candidates.[7] Ken Kramer then took on the challenge to test the functions of syndecans in early development.

Using the ability to microinject specific lineages in the ectoderm or mesoderm, including exclusively left or right sides, either RNA that encodes dominant negative syndecans or antisense morpholinos to block translation of endogenous syndecan RNA, we found that ectodermal syndecan-2 is essential for the transmission of left–right information from ectoderm to migrating mesoderm (Fig. 1.2).[8] Syndecan-2 is phosphorylated on in right ectoderm and not in left ectoderm.[9] Strikingly, a phospho-mimetic mutant form of syndecan-2 acts as a dominant negative when expressed on the left side, where endogenous syndecan is not phosphorylated, and has no effect when expressed on the right side, where endogenous syndecan is normally phosphorylated. Conversely, a syndecan-2 mutant that cannot be phosphorylated has a dominant-negative effect when expressed in right, but no effect when expressed in left ectoderm, where endogenous

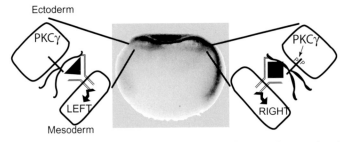

Ectoderm

PKCγ   PKCγ

LEFT   RIGHT

Mesoderm

Fig. 1.2 PKC-gamma and syndecan-2 in left–right development. Syndecan-2 is asymmetrically phosphorylated in gastrula, as revealed by a phosphospecific anti-syndecan-2 antibody. This phosphorylation is dependent on PKC-gamma and drives inside-out transmission of left–right information from ectoderm to migrating mesoderm during gastrulation. The LR information transduced through syndecan-2 leads to asymmetric patterning of the mesoderm. Adapted from refs 8 and 9.

syndecan-2 is not phosphoryl-ated.[9] This indicates that both "phospho-states" of syndecan-2, phosphorylated on the right and not on the left, are essential for normal left–right development. Injection of activated receptors in mesoderm identified downstream signaling pathways that function in migrating mesoderm. Results with pharmacological inhibitors, morpholinos and dominant-negative constructs against several PKCs indicate that PKC-gamma is necessary for the phosphorylation of syndecan-2 in right-sided ectoderm.[9]

The next question is what initiates the asymmetric activity of PKC-gamma activity? PKC-gamma RNA and protein seem to be symmetrically distributed along the left–right axis. Members of this conventional family of PKCs (alpha, beta, and gamma) are sensitive to diacylglycerol (DAG) and intracellular calcium pathways.[10] There is a barrier in gap-junctional communication between the left and right side of the animal cap during blastula stages,[11] and experimentally enhancing junctional connections between these cells can perturb left–right development.[12] Right animal cap blastomeres have a higher transient level of H^+/K^+ ATPase maternal RNA, which might establish a transient membrane voltage potential that is asymmetric between left and right cells.[13] This suggests that a transient spike in membrane voltage in right blastomeres is shared through junctional connections on the right but cannot be transmitted to the left side. From these observations, we propose that a transient spike in activity that is dependent on junctional communication, such as intracellular calcium or components of the DAG pathways, drives the asymmetric activity of PKC-gamma.[14] One of the next steps will be to assess whether these events in blastula-stage embryos, or pathways initiated as early as fertilization,[15,16] are linked to the asymmetric phosphorylation of syndecan-2 by PKC-gamma. An understanding of the genetic and embryological mechanisms of left–right development in vertebrate models systems is leading to new classifications of laterality phenotypes, which will be instrumental in the discovery of the genetic basis of complex congenital heart defects in humans.

References

1 Stalsberg H, DeHaan RL. The precardiac areas and formation of the tubular heart in the chick embryo. *Dev Biol* 1969; **19(2)**: 128–59.

2 Sato M, Yost HJ. Cardiac neural crest contributes to cardiomyogenesis in zebrafish. *Dev Biol* 2003; **257(1)**: 127–39.

3 Mikawa T, Gourdie RG. Pericardial mesoderm generates a population of coronary smooth muscle cells migrating into the heart along with ingrowth of the epicardial organ. *Dev Biol* 1996; **174(2)**: 221–32.

4 Sugi Y, Markwald RR. Formation and early morphogenesis of endocardial endothelial precursor cells and the role of endoderm. *Dev Biol* 1996; **175(1)**: 66–83.

5 Yost HJ. Regulation of vertebrate left–right asymmetries by extracellular matrix. *Nature* 1992; **357(6374)**: 158–61.

6 Yost HJ. Inhibition of proteoglycan synthesis eliminates left–right asymmetry in Xenopus laevis cardiac looping. *Development* 1990; **110(3)**: 865–74.

7 Teel AL, Yost HJ. Embryonic expression patterns of Xenopus syndecans. *Mech Dev* 1996; **59(2)**: 115–27.

8 Kramer KL, Yost HJ. Ectodermal syndecan-2 mediates left–right axis formation in migrating mesoderm as a cell-nonautonomous Vg1 cofactor. *Dev Cell* 2002; **2(1)**: 115–24.

9 Kramer KL, Barnette JE, Yost HJ. PKCgamma regulates syndecan-2 inside-out signaling during xenopus left–right development. *Cell* 2002; **111(7)**: 981–90.

10 Parekh DB, Ziegler W, Parker PJ. Multiple pathways control protein kinase C phosphorylation. *Embo J* 2000; **19(4)**: 496–503.

11 Olson DJ, Moon RT. Distinct effects of ectopic expression of Wnt-1, activin B, and bFGF on gap junctional permeability in 32-cell Xenopus embryos. *Dev Biol* 1992; **151(1)**: 204–12.

12 Levin M, Mercola M. Gap junctions are involved in the early generation of left–right asymmetry. *Dev Biol* 1998; **203(1)**: 90–105.

13 Levin M *et al.* Asymmetries in H+/K+-ATPase and cell membrane potentials comprise a very early step in left–right patterning. *Cell* 2002; **111(1)**: 77–89.

14 Kramer KL, Yost HJ. Cardiac left–right development: are the early steps conserved? *Cold Spring Harb Symp Quant Biol* 2002; **67**: 37–43.

15 Yost HJ. Development of the left–right axis in amphibians. *Ciba Found Symp* 1991; **162**: 165–76; discussion 176–81.

16 Yost HJ. Vertebrate left–right development. *Cell* 1995; **82(5)**: 689–92.

CHAPTER 2

Calmodulin–inv protein interaction and left–right determination

Takahiko Yokoyama, Yukuto Yasuhiko

Mouse *inv* (inversion of embryonic turning) mutation was discovered in a family of transgenic mice carrying tyrosinase minigenes.[1] This mouse is unique since most of homozygous mice show a consistent reversal of the left–right asymmetry. The left-side expressions of *nodal, lefty* and *PitX2* genes are reversed in the *inv* mutant, indicating that *inv* acts upstream of these genes.[2,3]

Integration of tyrosinase minigenes in the *inv* mutant accompanies a large genomic deletion that removes an internal portion of a novel gene,[4] which encodes 1062 amino acids containing 15 tandem repeats of the ankyrin motif and two nuclear localization signals.[4,5] The deletion abrogates all but the first 91 amino acids of the encoded protein.[4] Introduction of the gene can rescue all the phenotypes associated with the *inv* mutant, demonstrating that the disrupted gene is the *inv* gene.[4]

Vortical movement of node cilia creates an extracellular flow directing from right to left.[6] This flow is proposed to create the left–right gradient of a hypothetical molecule, which in turn activates downstream cascades to establish the left–right asymmetry. Mutants lacking node cilia cannot produce this flow and thus show randomization of the body situs.[6] Although node cilia are present in the *inv* mutant, the nodal flow is turbulent. Because of this abnormal slow flow in the *inv* mutant, the hypothetical molecule is speculated to activate at the right side before it reaches the left side.[7] However, a recent report shows that slow node flow does not affect body situs. What is critical for determining body situs is the direction of the node flow.[8] Thus, it remains to be elucidated why body situs is inverted in the *inv* mutant.

As a first step to understand the function of the inv protein in the establishment of the left–right asymmetry, we searched molecules interacting with inv protein using a yeast two-hybrid assay. A clone that potentially binds inv protein is calmodulin.[9] A search in the inv protein sequence found two IQ motifs lying at amino acids 554–576 (named IQ1) and 913–935 (named IQ2). To confirm that inv protein binds calmodulin at these sites, we generated several GST–inv fusion proteins. We examined interaction between GST–inv fusion proteins and calmodulin by a gel overlay assay. GST–inv fusion proteins that contained either the IQ1 or IQ2 site could bind calmodulin, but a fusion protein lacking the IQ motif could no longer bind calmodulin. Calmodulin is a Ca^{2+} binding protein conserved among species and involved in a variety of cellular calcium-dependent signaling pathways.[10] Calcium regulates interaction between calmodulin and target proteins, and so calmodulin acts as a calcium sensor.

Our next step was to find out whether calcium regulated calmodulin–inv protein interaction. We focused on the IQ2 site, since *inv* mRNA injection into *Xenopus* embryos showed that the IQ2 site is critical for its function, as described below. We undertook two experiments. The first was a gel overlay assay. Membranes, onto which GST–inv fusion proteins were transferred, were incubated with biotinylated calmodulin in a buffer containing or excluding calcium, and then incubated with avidin-conjugated peroxidase. The complex was visualized with an enhanced chemiluminescence (ECL) system. The second experiment was precipitation of the calmodulin–inv protein complex using magnet beads. Partially purified GST–inv fusion protein was digested with PreScission protease and mixed with biotinylated calmodulin. The inv protein–calmodulin complex was mixed with avidin-conjugated magnetic beads and collected with a magnet, electrophoresed, and then transferred onto PVDF membranes. Membranes were hybridized with anti-inv antibody and visualized with an ECL system. Both assays demonstrated that interaction between calmodulin and the IQ2 site was facilitated in a low calcium concentration, whereas interaction was somewhat inhibited in a high calcium concentration.

To know if *inv* has a role in the establishment of left–right asymmetry in *Xenopus*, we injected mouse *inv* mRNA into the right blastomere in two-cell stage *Xenopus* embryos, which showed high percentages of reversed cardiac orientation. Contrarily, injection of mouse *inv* mRNA into the left blastomere had no significant effect. Expression patterns of *nodal* and *PitX2* were altered when *inv* mRNA was injected into the right blastomere, suggesting that the randomiza-tion of the cardiac situs induced by the injection could have resulted from the altered expression of the *nodal* and *PitX2* genes.

Using this system, we examined the functional significance of the interaction of *inv* with calmodulin. We made mouse *inv* constructs that lacked a region(s) encoding the IQ motif or various lengths of the C-terminus. These constructs were used as templates to generate mRNA for injections into two-cell stage *Xenopus* embryos. All mRNA lacking the region encoding the IQ2 site failed to randomize cardiac orientation.

Since the IQ2 site is the target site for inv protein to bind calmodulin, it is most likely that inv protein lacking the IQ2 site failed to bind with calmodulin, which led to the loss of its ability to randomize the left–right asymmetry. These results indicate that inv protein requires calmodulin-binding for its function in the *Xenopus* system, and implies that the calmodulin-binding form of mouse inv protein is an active form. Further, the present biochemical

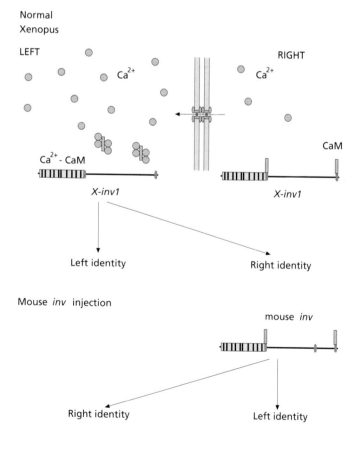

Fig. 2.1 A model explaining the inv–calmodulin pathway determining left–right asymmetry in *Xenopus* embryos. The model assumes that *Xenopus inv* is uniformly distributed in an embryo, and that calcium concentration is high in the left side and low in the right. *Xenopus* inv (X-inv1) protein is active when it interacts with calmodulin, and inactive when it detaches from calmodulin. Contrarily, mouse inv protein is active when it interacts with calmodulin. Interaction between calmodulin and mouse inv protein occurs at low Ca^{2+} concentrations. Mouse inv protein that binds calmodulin activates a cascade to establish the left-side identity.

analysis showed that Ca^{2+} controls calmodulin–inv binding, suggesting that Ca^{2+} is also likely to control *inv* activity.

There was a marked difference between the right and left blastomeres in their response to injected *inv* mRNA. Randomization of left–right asymmetry was induced only when *inv* mRNA was injected into the right blastomere, whereas injection into the left blastomere had no effect.

Figure 2.1 depicts a model explaining these results. This model hypothesizes that *Xenopus inv* is expressed symmetrically and that endogenous *Xenopus* inv protein is normally active in the left blastomere and inactive in the right. An injection of mouse *inv* mRNA in the right blastomere induced aberrant activation of an *inv* pathway to determine the left side identity in the right side. In mice, the *inv* gene expresses symmetrically (as so far examined). If *Xenopus inv* is expressed symmetrically, our results suggest that a calcium calmodulin system may also be involved in the establishment of left–right asymmetry in *Xenopus*.

The kidneys of *inv* mice show not only situs inversus but also cysts.[1] Polycystin-1 and polycystin-2 are the products of *PKD1* and *PKD2*, respectively,[10,11] genes that are mutated in most cases of autosomal dominant polycystic kidney disease. Polycystin-2 functions as a calcium channel.[11–13] Since Ca^{2+} regulates calmodulin–inv protein interaction, we have pointed out a possible connection between polycystins and *inv* via calcium for cyst formation in kidneys and establishment of left–right asymmetry. As we predicted, mice lacking the *PKD2* gene are reported to show randomization of left–right asymmetry.[14] This result strengthens our hypothesis that polycystins and *inv* might have the same cascade to establish left–right asymmetry and cyst formation in kidneys.

Evidence that the primary cilia are involved in cyst formation in kidneys has accumulated.[15,16] Polycystin-2 localizes in the primary cilium of kidney cells. Polaris protein localizes in the primary cilium of kidney epithelial cells. Mice with polaris mutations lack cilia not only in kidney cells but also in nodes, and show defective left–right asymmetry in addition to cysts of the kidneys.[17]

It is possible that polycystins regulate calcium transition in cilia, which then control inv protein function. We are presently attempting to elucidate

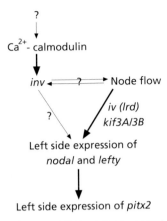

Fig. 2.2 A pathway establishing left-side expression of *nodal, lefty* and *PitX2* genes. Vortical movement of node cilia induces left side expression of *lefty, nodal*, then *PitX2*. The present study suggested that Ca^{2+}-calmodulin signaling controls the *inv* function that induces the left side expression of *nodal* and *lefty*. It remains to be elucidated how node cilia and the *inv* pathway are related in the establishment of left–right asymmetry.

how inv protein and calcium transition in cilia are related (Fig. 2.2).

References

1 Yokoyama T, Copeland NG, Jenkins NA *et al.* Reversal of left–right asymmetry: a situs inversus mutation. *Science* 1993; **263**: 679–82.

2 Meno C, Saijoh Y, Fujii H *et al.* Left–right asymmetric expression of the TGF beta-family member lefty in mouse embryos. *Nature* 1996; **38**: 151–5.

3 Lowe LA, Supp DM, Sampath K *et al.* Conserved left–right asymmetry of nodal expression and alterations in murine situs inversus. *Nature* 1996; **381**: 158–61.

4 Mochizuki T, Saijoh Y, Tsuchiya K *et al.* Cloning of *inv*, a gene that controls left/right asymmetry and kidney development. *Nature* 1998; **395**: 177–81.

5 Morgan D, Turnpenny L, Goodship J *et al. Inversin*, a novel gene in the vertebrate left–right axis pathway, is partially deleted in the inv mouse. *Nat Genet* 1998; **20**: 149–56.

6 Nonaka S, Tanaka Y, Okada Y *et al.* Randomization of left–right asymmetry due to loss of nodal cilia generating leftward flow of extraembryonic fluid in mice lacking KIF3B motor protein. *Cell* 1998; **95**: 829–37.

7 Okada Y, Nonaka S, Tanaka Y *et al.* Abnormal nodal flow precedes situs inversus in iv and inv mice. *Mol Cell* 1999; **4**: 459–68.

8 Nonaka S, Shiratori H, Saijoh Y, Hamada H. Determination of left–right patterning of the mouse embryo by artificial nodal flow. *Nature* 2002; **418**: 96–9.

9 Yasuhiko Y, Imai F, Ookubo K *et al.* Calmodulin binds to inv protein: implication for regulation of inv function. *Dev Growth Diff* 2001; **43**: 671–81.

10 The European Polycystic Kidney Disease Consortium. The polycystic kidney disease 1 gene encodes a 14 kb transcript and lies within a duplicated region on chromosome 16. *Cell* 1994; **77**: 881–94.

11 Mochizuki T, Wu G, Hayashi T *et al.* PKD2, a gene for polycystic kidney disease that encodes an integral membrane protein. *Science* 1996; **272**: 1339–42.

12 Hanaoka K, Qian F, Boletta A *et al.* Co-assembly of polycystin-1 and -2 produces unique cation-permeable currents. *Nature* 2000; **408**: 990–4.

13 Koulen P, Cai Y, Geng L *et al.* Polycystin-2 is an intracellular calcium release channel. *Nat Cell Biol* 2002; **4**: 191–7.

14 Pennekamp P, Karcher C, Fischer A *et al.* The ion channel polycystin-2 is required for left–right axis determination in mice. *Curr Biol* 2002; **12**; 938–43.

15 Yoder BK, Hou X, Guay-Woodford LM. The polycystic kidney disease proteins, polycystin-1, polycystin-2, polaris, and cystin, are co-localized in renal cilia. *J Am Soc Nephrol* 2002; **13**: 2508–16.

16 Yoder BK, Tousson A, Millican L *et al.* Polaris, a protein disrupted in orpk mutant mice, is required for assembly of renal cilium. *Am J Physiol Renal Physiol* 2002; **282**: F541–52.

17 Murcia NS, Richards WG, Yoder BK *et al.* The oak ridge polycystic kidney (orpk) disease gene is required for left–right axis determination. *Development* 2000; **127**: 2347–55.

CHAPTER 3

Misexpression of upstream laterality genes on downstream mechanisms of heart looping: a flectin perspective

Kersti K. Linask, Ming-Da Han, YiPing Chen,
Thomas Brand, Philip R. Brauer

A critical step during early vertebrate cardiogenesis is that the straight heart tube bends to the right. For future modeling of the heart, precision of this bending is essential for correct orientation of the four presumptive cardiac chambers, septa, valves, and for the establishment of connections to the vascular system. This rightward bend at the beginning of cardiac looping is the first detectable morphologic break in embryonic symmetry. For this reason, looping direction provides a benchmark for misexpression analyses of laterality genes in left–right axis determination.[1] These studies, however, have provided no information as to the mechanistic basis of why looping direction downstream is altered.

Our studies were undertaken to gain a morphologic, mechanistic understanding of heart looping. We have consistently observed a strong correlation between the asymmetric expression of protein flectin in the extracellular matrix and the direction of looping. Flectin, as we previously reported, is expressed at higher levels in the left dorsal mesocardium and adjacent myocardial wall than on the right side during the looping stages.[2] We suspected that the protein may help to elucidate the mechanistic basis of cardiac bending directionality. With this objective misexpression analyses of *Pitx2c* and *CFC* that result in randomization of heart looping direction were carried out and embryonic hearts were assayed for flectin expression. Based upon these experiments, we conclude that the sidedness of flectin protein expression primarily in the dorsal mesocardium serves as a better indicator of looping direction than sidedness of *Pitx2c* gene expression in the heart.

Flectin was first isolated from the interphotoreceptor matrix of the developing chick eye.[3] The 6.9 kb message is translated into a protein with a relative molecular mobility of 250 000 M_r. Flectin is first expressed in the left lateral plate mesoderm and only after a delay, in the right.[4] As a result of this left–right delay in the timing of its expression, a left-sided dominance of flectin protein arises in the dorsal mesocardial fold and myocardial wall of the heart.[2] When laterality genes *CFC* or *Pitx2c* are misexpressed using either retroviral or antisense approaches at stage 5 in the chick embryo, looping direction is randomized.[5,6] Misexpression of Pitx2c or CFC resulted in left-sided *Pitx2c* expression, bilateral expression, or no expression. In contrast, flectin expression provided a consistent correlation with bending direction. Regardless of *Pitx2c* message expression in the heart fields, when there is more flectin in the left myocardial wall/dorsal mesocardial (DM) fold, then the heart bends normally to the right. When more flectin is present in the right side, the heart bends abnormally to the left. When the left–right difference in flectin expression is nearly equivalent, the heart tube does not bend. This suggested that laterality genes may be modulating the *timing* of flectin synthesis in a left–right manner by modulation of a parallel pathway that leads to flectin expression in the heart and dorsal mesocardium. Mechanistically flectin seems to be critical to looping, because when we perturb flectin using antibodies, looping direction also becomes randomized, hearts remain unlooped, or cardiabifida occurs.[4] The latter experiments also highlighted the importance of the matrix asymmetry of the dorsal mesocardial folds and adjacent myocardial wall for specification of looping direction specifically in the *anterior* region of the heart (Fig. 3.1). More recent experiments indicate that directionality is determined at approximately the 7- to 8-somite stage [unpubl. obs.].

As the dorsal mesocardium (DM) seems to be a critical region for looping (see also ref. 7), we focused our analyses on this region. The dorsal mesocardial folds, as well as the fibronectin matrix-mediated attachment of the endocardium to the ventral mid-point of the foregut floor anchors the heart's position to this embryo midline structure. Flectin associates with the mid-region by fine, lateral fibrils emanating from the basement membrane underlying the myocardium from both the right and left sides. Thus, any asymmetric stress–strain differences in the folds would be transmitted to this mid-region. After looping, flectin remains detectable in the myocardium at low levels, is expressed in the vascular network, and begins to be expressed in many other developing systems.

Once looping direction is defined anteriorly, the DM folds are quickly broken down, first in the cardiac mid-portion and then spreading rapidly cephalad and caudad (Fig. 3.2). Because a number of matrix molecules colocalize to the DM region [in prep.], it was expected that possibly matrix metalloproteinases (MMPs) would be involved in the breakdown of the folds. This was found to be the case. MMPs were found localized in the dorsal mesocardial region at the time the DM folds breakdown. To

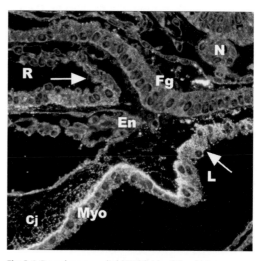

Fig. 3.1 Dorsal mesocardial (DM) folds of the chick embryonic heart at stage 12. Ventral view of a normal dextral looping heart. White arrows, DM folds. More flectin (white signal) is present in left fold and adjacent myocardial (Myo) wall, as well as within the cardiac jelly (Cj). Note endocardial (En) cells approaching ventral floor of the foregut. L, left; R, right; Fg, foregut; N, notochord. Modified from ref. 2 with permission from Elsevier Publishers.

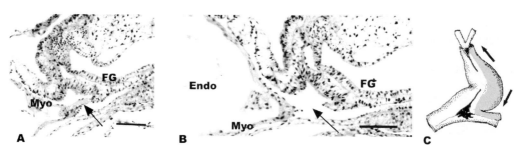

Fig. 3.2 Breakdown of the dorsal mesocardium seen in a 20-somite chick embryo. (A) Black arrow, dorsal mesocardium just before it breaks. Scale bar = 100 µm. (B) Black arrow points to the region where the folds have just broken down to release the attachment of the heart to the foregut region. Scale bar = 50 µm. (C) Dorsal view of dextral looping heart. Dark line, dorsal mesocardium with permanent attachment point shown at caudal end; arrows, direction of dorsal mesocardium breakdown. FG, foregut; Myo, myocardium; Endo, endocardium.

determine whether the MMPs are active during this period and whether the activity affects heart development, MMP activity was inhibited using a general protease inhibitor. A stage-dependent effect of the inhibitor was observed. When embryos were exposed after formation of a heart tube, the heart was no longer able to swing out to the right side away from the body wall, nor was the bending of the loop able to deepen, as was seen with control hearts in untreated embryos. When sectioned, experimental hearts revealed that MMP inhibition lead to aberrant ventral closure of both the foregut and the heart tube: both tube formation and looping direction were perturbed. The extent of perturbation depends on the timing of exposure in relation to the anterior posterior developmental progression of heart development and the stage of the embryo.

In the course of the above experiments an additional importance of the dorsal mesocardial area to the heart became apparent. A permanent, matrix-mediated, attachment region of the dorsal mesocardium remains at the caudal, sinoatrial end of the tubular heart. After looping in the human embryo, this region reportedly acts as an important midline anchor for myocardial and mesenchymal atrial structures, i.e. for the primary atrial septum, the left venous valve, and the inferior edge of the right venous valve.[8] The endocardial–endothelial cells within the permanent dorsal mesocardium are thought to serve as a conduit for the developing pulmonary vein to reach the primary atrial segment.[9] At the caudal end of the dorsal mesocardial area, MMP expression is no longer detected. Thus, this matrix-defined, metalloproteinase-protected, midline region continues throughout looping to maintain a proper alignment of the atrial compartments and serves as a connection to the pulmonary system. Thus, the caudal DM region continues as a midline reference point throughout looping during heart tube morphogenesis.

Based upon our results from the experimental manipulations of looping, the following model of chick heart morphoregulation between stage 9 and the 16- to 18-somite stage is suggested: asymmetry in the heart tube and dorsal mesocardium, as exemplified by the flectin matrix of the DM and adjacent myocardial wall, establishes a physical, differential, left–right tension. As soon as the anterior DM forms concomitant with the enclosure of the heart tube,

looping direction is specified by the left–right asymmetric properties of the DM folds. The apparently more flexible left DM fold remains extended and closely associated with the left foregut area, and the left myocardial wall begins to bulge out to form the outer curvature. Once the dextral looping direction is established in the anterior part of the heart, this is maintained owing to constraints of the extraembryonic membrane, which is closely associated with the heart. As the heart tube begins to lengthen with the addition of two new segments, the inlet area at the atrioventricular part of the heart and the outlet region from the anterior secondary heart field,[10] the bending of the heart tube deepens as metalloproteinases aid in the breakdown of the dorsal mesocardial attachment in the mid-portion of the heart tube. The detachment extends rapidly toward both ends allowing the heart tube bending to deepen. Both the cephalic attachment and the permanent caudal DM attachment areas initially serve as constraints on the tube as it is lengthening through the addition of segments. This would add stress to force further bending of the heart. Once looping seems to be nearly completed, the cephalic attachment is also broken down. The caudal attachment remains, serving to anchor the heart and to provide a critical midline reference for future modeling of the post-looped heart.

Acknowledgments

This work was supported by an American Heart Association Established Investigator Grant.

References

1 Mercola M, Levin M. Left-right asymmetry determination in vertebrates. *Annu Rev Cell Dev Biol* 2001; **17**: 779–805.

2 Tsuda T, Philp N, Zile MH, Linask KK. Left–right asymmetric localization of flectin in the extracellular matrix during heart looping. *Dev Biol* 1996; **173**: 39–50.

3 Mieziewska K, Szel A, Van Veen T, Aguirre GD, Philp N. Redistribution of insoluble interphotoreceptor matrix components during photoreceptor differentiation in the mouse retina. *J Comp Neurol* 1994; **345**: 115–24.

4 Linask KK, Yu X, Chen YP, Han MD. Directionality of heart looping: effects of *Pitx2c* misexpression on flectin asymmetry and midline structures. *Dev Biol* 2002; **246**: 407–17.

5 Schlange T, Schnipkoweit I, Andree B *et al.* Chick CFC controls *Lefty 1* expression in the embryonic midline and

nodal expression in the lateral plate. *Dev Biol* 2001; **234**: 376–89.

6 Yu X, St Amand TR, Wang S *et al.* Differential expression and functional analysis of *Pitx2* isoforms in regulation of heart looping in the chick. *Development* 2001; **128**: 1005–13.

7 Taber LA, Lin IE, Clark E. Mechanics of cardiac looping. *Dev Dynamics* 1995; **203**: 42–50.

8 Wessels A, Anderson RH, Marwald RR *et al.* Atrial development in the human heart: an immunohistochemical study with emphasis on the role of mesenchymal tissues. *Anat Rec* 2000; **259**: 288–300.

9 Webb S, Brown NA, Wessels A, Anderson RH. Development of the murine pulmonary vein and its relationship to the embryonic venous sinus. *Anat Rec* 1998; **250**: 325–34.

10 Markwald RR, Trusk T, Moreno-Rodriguez R. Formation and septation of the tubular heart: integrating the dynamics of morphology with emerging molecular concepts. In: de la Cruz MV, Markwald RR, eds. *Living Morphogenesis of the Heart*. Boston: Birkhauser, 1998: 43–84.

CHAPTER 4

Pleiotropic effects of *Pitx2* isoform c on morphogenesis in the mammalian heart

Nigel A. Brown, Louisa M. Jones, Oliver A. T. Lyons,
Chengyu Liu, Wei Liu, Jennifer Palie, Mei Fang Lu,
James F. Martin

Pitx2 is a paired-related homeobox gene that has a key role in the control of left–right asymmetric morphogenesis,[1] being the final step in a left-sided cascade of gene expression that originates at the node.[2] Identified as the gene mutated in Rieger syndrome 1, *Pitx2* also functions in eye, tooth, and abdominal wall development.[3,4] A major feature of complete loss of *Pitx2* function in mouse is right isomerism.[5–8] Detailed analysis of the role of *Pitx2* in cardiovascular development is, however, complicated by the embryonic lethality and profound body distortion of complete *Pitx2* nulls.

Pitx2 is expressed as several isoforms: *Pitx2c* is asymmetrically expressed, while *Pitx2a* and *Pitx2b* are co-expressed with *Pitx2c* in symmetrical regions of the embryo.[6,9–11] A fourth *Pitx2* isoform, *Pitx2d*, has recently been described in humans.[12] *Pitx2c* is encoded by exons 4, 5, and 6, and uses a distinct promoter from that of *Pitx2a* and *Pitx2b* (Plate 1a)[2]. Exons 5 and 6, which encode the homeodomain, are common to all isoforms in mice (Plate 1a). We have shown that asymmetric morphogenesis of different organs requires different doses of *Pitx2c*.[9] To study *Pitx2c* function free from the complication of loss of other isoforms, we generated an isoform-specific knockout. We replaced exon 4 with a PGKneomycin LoxP cassette (*Pitx2 δc neo*; Plate 1c). *Pitx2 δc neo* mice were crossed to the *CMV cre recombinase* deletor strain to generate the *Pitx2 δc* allele. Both *Pitx2 δc neo* and *Pitx2 δc–/–* mutants, obtained at Mendelian

ratios at 18.5 dpc, were born alive but soon became cyanotic and died.

We have not observed any difference in morphology between the *Pitx2 δc neo* and *Pitx2 δc* alleles, so these are not distinguished here. *Pitx2 δc* mutant hearts loop correctly to the right (Plate 1k,m,o) and have normal left located atrioventricular (AV) canals (Plate 2b), confirming that the left lateral plate pathway mediated by *Pitx2* does not control the initial asymmetries of the heart. Much of the cardiovascular system develops from bilaterally symmetrical primordia, which are subsequently remodeled. These include the aortic arches, the venous sinuses and their tributaries, and the primary atrium. All these primordia developed abnormally in *Pitx2 δc* mutants, predominantly with a symmetrical, right isomeric phenotype (atria shown in Plate 2d). In addition, however, several other regions of the heart, which do not develop from symmetrical primordia, were also affected in *Pitx2 δc* mutants, suggesting a wider role of the gene, specifically in the outflow tract (OFT), AV and atrial septums, and in the ventricles.

Pitx2 δc mutants all have abnormal OFTs, predominantly with the aortic and pulmonary trunks transposed (Plate 1e,g,i), associated with double outlet right ventricle and ventricular septal defects. At full term, the aortic and pulmonary trunks do not spiral around each other (Plate 1f,g). This seems to directly reflect lack of spiraling of the conotruncal cushions, which can be observed already at E11 (Plate 1k,m,o). Thus, *Pitx2* δ*c* patterns the spatial arrangement of the cushions, independently of the morphogenesis of the myocardial wall, which is normal. *Pitx2c* may maintain signaling between the myocardium and the underlying endothelium, analogous to its role in epithelial–mesenchymal signaling in tooth organogenesis.[7,13] We have shown that cardiac neural crest cells are not involved in OFT defects in *Pitx2* δ*c* mutants,[14] unlike other researchers, who have studied complete *Pitx2* nulls.[15]

At E18.5, *Pitx2* δ*c* mutants all display common AV junctions, with variable septation and commitment to the left ventricle (Plate 1d,e), and also atrial septal defects (ASD, Plate 2c,d). Up to E12, both the primary atrial septum and the dorsal mesocardium (from which the spina vestibuli is derived, which forms the broad base of the septum), express *Pitx2c*, despite their mid-line location (Plate 2h). The inner curve of the heart (Plate 2f), and myocardium overlaying the AV cushions (Plate 2g) also expresses *Pitx2c*. To assess the later contribution of *Pitx2c* expressing cells to these, and other, regions we generated a *Cre* knock-in allele.

Pitx2 δ*abc*^*creneo* was generated by introducing an IRES Cre Flt-flanked PGKneomycin cassette into exon 5 (removing function of all *Pitx2* isoforms), then subsequently removing neo by crossing with a FLPe deleter strain. When *Pitx2* δ*abc*^*creneo* was crossed with the *lacZ* Rosa26 reporter strain[16] and embryos were examined between E11.5 and E16.5, labeled daughter cells were found extensively in the superior AV cushion (Plate 2m) and the dorsal mesocardium (Plate 2n). As *Pitx2c* is never detected in endocardium, this fate mapping suggests a myocardial source for these *lacZ*-labeled cells. Cells have been shown to invade the AV cushion from overlaying myocardium.[17] In compound *Pitx2* δ*abc*^*creneo*/*Pitx2* δ*c* mutants, there was no staining in AV cushion mesenchyme (not shown).[14] Thus, *Pitx2c* may be required for the myocardial invasion of AV cushion mesenchyme, and lack of this contribution may explain the AV defects observed. Another population of *Pitx2c* expressing cells that may invade the AV cushions, however, originates from the dorsal mesocardium, and this will require further study.

LacZ staining was detected on both sides of the OFT tract myocardium at E11.5 (Plate 2j), whereas gene expression is restricted to the left at E9.5 and 10.5 (Plate 2e,g), suggesting that *Pitx2* daughter cells move from left to right sides. The distribution of *lacZ*-positive cells in the OFT tract in *Pitx2* δ*abc*^*creneo*/*Pitx2* δ*c* mutant embryos was similar to that of the wild type (not shown). Thus, although *Pitx2c* is expressed in the branchial precursor population for OFT myocardium,[14,18] it seems that *Pitx2* is not required for movement of these cells into the OFT.

Pitx2c is expressed in right ventricular, as well as inner curve, myocardium at E10.5 (Plate 2f).[10,19] At later stages, daughter *lacZ*-labeled cells are found mostly to the right of the interventricular boundary, and eventually populate a major portion of this region (Plate 2i–m). In compound null embryos, this stained area was much reduced (not shown).[14] The same region is affected in *Pitx2c* mutants labeled with a transgene that marks the secondary heart field, which contributes to the OFT and right ventricle (Plate 2o,p). One interpretation of these data is that *Pitx2* functions in growth of the right ventricular myocardium. Further experiments are needed to distinguish between defective movement of precursors into the right ventricle and reduced proliferation, as has been suggested for other *Pitx2* mutant cells.[15]

Acknowledgments
Supported by grants from the British Heart Foundation (RG/98004), Harry S. and Isabel C. Cameron Foundation, NIDCR (R29 DE12324 and R01DE013509) and March of Dimes (5-FY00–135).

References

1 Capdevila J, Vogan KJ, Tabin CJ, Izpisua Belmonte JC. Mechanisms of left–right determination in vertebrates. *Cell* 2000; **101**: 9–21.

2 Shiratori H, Sakuma R, Watanabe M *et al.* Two-step regulation of left–right asymmetric expression of *Pitx2*, initiation by nodal signaling and maintenance by *Nkx2*. *Mol Cell* 2001; **7**: 137–49.

3 Semina EV, Reiter R, Leysens NJ *et al.* Cloning and characterization of a novel bicoid-related homeobox transcription factor gene, RIEG, involved in Rieger syndrome. *Nat Genet* 1996; **14**: 392–9.

4 Alward WL. Axenfeld–Rieger syndrome in the age of molecular genetics. *Am J Ophthalmol* 2000; **130**: 107–15.

5 Gage PJ, Suh H, Camper SA. Dosage requirement of *Pitx2* for development of multiple organs. *Development* 1999; **126**: 4643–51.

6 Kitamura K, Miura H, Miyagawa-Tomita S *et al.* Mouse Pitx2 deficiency leads to anomalies of the ventral body wall, heart, extra- and periocular mesoderm and right pulmonary isomerism. *Development* 1999; **126**: 5749–58.

7 Lin CR, Kioussi C, O'Connell S *et al. Pitx2* regulates lung asymmetry, cardiac positioning and pituitary and tooth morphogenesis. *Nature* 1999; **401**: 279–82.

8 Lu MF, Pressman C, Dyer R, Johnson RL, Martin JF. Function of Rieger syndrome gene in left–right asymmetry and craniofacial development. *Nature* 1999; **401**: 276–8.

9 Liu C, Liu W, Lu MF, Brown NA, Martin JF. Regulation of left–right asymmetry by thresholds of *Pitx2c* activity. *Development* 2001; **128**: 2039–48.

10 Schweickert A, Campione M, Steinbeisser H, Blum M *Pitx2* isoforms: involvement of *Pitx2c* but not *Pitx2a* or *Pitx2b* in vertebrate left–right asymmetry. *Mech Dev* 2000; **90**: 41–51.

11 Yu X, St Amand TR, Wang S *et al.* Differential expression and functional analysis of *Pitx2* isoforms in regulation of heart looping in the chick. *Development* 2001; **128**: 1005–13.

12 Cox CJ, Espinoza HM, McWilliams B *et al.* Differential regulation of gene expression by PITX2 isoforms. *J Biol Chem* 2002; **277**: 25001–10.

13 Lu MF, Cheng HT, Kern MJ *et al. Prx-1* functions cooperatively with another paired-related homeobox gene, *Prx-2*, to maintain cell fates within the craniofacial mesenchyme. *Development* 1999; **126**; 495–504.

14 Liu C, Liu W, Palie J *et al. Pitx2c* patterns anterior myocardium and aortic arch vessels and is required for local cell movement into atrioventricular cushions. *Development* 2002; **129**: 5081–91.

15 Kioussi C, Briata P, Baek SH *et al.* Identification of a Wnt/Dvl/Beta-Catenin–*Pitx2* pathway mediating cell-type-specific proliferation during development. *Cell* 2002; **111**: 673–85.

16 Soriano P. Generalized *lacZ* expression with the *ROSA26* Cre reporter strain. *Nat Genet* 1999; **21**: 70–1.

17 van den Hoff MJB, Kruithof BPT, Moorman AFM, Markwald RR, Wessels A. Formation of myocardium after the initial development of the linear heart tube. *Dev Biol* 2001; **240**: 61–76.

18 Kelly RG, Brown NA, Buckingham ME. The arterial pole of the mouse heart forms from *Fgf10*-expressing cells in pharyngeal mesoderm. *Dev Cell* 2001; **1**: 435–40.

19 Campione M, Ros MA, Icardo JM *et al. Pitx2* expression defines a left cardiac lineage of cells: evidence for atrial and ventricular molecular isomerism in the iv/iv mice. *Dev Biol* 2001; **231**: 252–64.

CHAPTER 5

Signal transduction during cardiac myofibrillogenesis and looping

Isao Shiraishi, Tetsuro Takamatsu, Kenji Hamaoka

Looping and myofibrillogenesis

Cardiac looping is the earliest and the most critical morphogenetic event in the embryonic heart that determines the shape of the heart. This is also the first embryonic process that develops the left–right asymmetry of the body. A couple of decades ago, various mechanisms were proposed for the looping process using conventional morphological techniques such as electron microscopy, autoradiography, or cell fate mapping. These included differential regional cell proliferation, asymmetrical myofibril differentiation and contractility, and differential cell aggregation patterns.[1] Recent advances in developmental biology have explored the molecular mechanisms of early cardiac development. Especially, many transcription factors have been identified that are essential for the early development of the heart as well as for determination of the left–right body axis. Nkx2.5 is regarded as the most upstream cardiac-specific transcription factor for cardiac cell lineage,[2–4] GATA4 and MEF2C are working in cooperation with Nkx2.5.[3] dHAND and eHAND are important for right and left ventricular chamber formation.[5] Pitx2, lefty, nodal, and left–right dynein play important roles during the determination of the left–right body axis.[6] In spite of the accumulating evidence of the molecular hierarchies of the transcription factors, the precise mechanism of the normal cardiac looping process still remains uncertain.

Cytoskeletons, extracellular matrix, and cell adhesion molecules have been implicated in the direct regulation of cellular structure and function such as cell shape, spreading, polarity, and migration *in vitro.* These components also play crucial roles in the morphogenesis of the multicellular organs. To understand the mechanism of cardiac looping, it is essential to investigate what kind of cytoskeletal changes are taking place during the looping process and how these changes influence neighboring cells and gross morphogenesis. The most drastic cytoskeletal change that occurs simultaneously during looping is myofibrillogenesis. Because myofibrils are highly organized and contractile cytoskeleton, we speculated that arrangement of myofibrils determines the shape of each cardiomyocyte and eventually influences the looping process as a whole. Using confocal scanning laser microscopy and optical tomographic technique, we have performed 3D observations of myofibril formation, cell–cell and cell–matrix adhesions of whole-mounted chick or mouse embryonic heart tube without making histological serial sections. We found that:

1 from the earliest stages of myofibrillogenesis, myofibrils in neighboring myocytes interconnected with one another and constituted network structure in the outer cells and circumferential alignments at the bottom of the inner myocardial cell layer;[7]

2 the alignment of myofibrils developed in association with changing cell–cell[8] and cell–matrix[9,10] adhesions and phosphorylation of tyrosine residue at the adhesion sites;[11]

3 inhibition of focal adhesion kinase, which is a main substrate of tyrosine phosphorylation at the bottom of the inner cell layer, results in disruption of the normal looping process [in prep.].

These results indicate that myofibril formation and organization are dynamically regulated by cell–cell and cell–matrix adhesions during the looping process and that the circumferential alignments of developing myofibrils are crucial for the normal cardiac looping process.

Since the looping process simultaneously progresses with the formation and organization of developing myofibrils, it seems that various kinds of signaling molecules are working as a linkage between nuclear transcription factors and cytoplasmic myofibrils and cell adhesion molecules. We summarize the proposed signaling mechanisms during cardiac myofibrillogenesis and looping (Plate 3) and also discuss the possible link between the formation of myofibrils and transcription regulation.

Specialized structures and signaling molecules

Focal adhesions and costameres

Focal adhesion is a specialized region of cell–substrate contact formed by clusters of integrins and is observed during the early stages of myofibrillogenesis *in vitro*[10,12,13] and *in vivo*.[9,11] Focal adhesion is responsible for the activation of multiple signal-transduction systems, providing a mechanism for the cell–matrix adhesion-dependent regulation of gene expression for cell growth, migration, survival, and apoptosis. Clustering of integrins results in activation of focal adhesion kinase (FAK) and subsequent phosphorylation of Src, Cas, and paxillin. Activation of FAK also, directly or indirectly, promotes mitogen activated protein (MAP) kinases including extracellular signal-regulated kinase (ERK), PI3-kinase and Akt pathway, and small G proteins Rho, Rac, and Ras.[14] Rho has been implicated in actin polymerization, stress fiber formation, focal adhesion formation, and myosin light kinase phosphorylation.[15] Rho has profound effects on myofibril organization and hypertrophic responses in cardiac myocytes.[16] Inhibition of Rho kinase results in GATA4 inhibition and cardiac bifida in chick embryo.[17] Rho seems to play crucial roles during myofibrillogenesis and development of embryonic heart.

In cardiac myocytes, focal adhesions form a part of costameres, which are band-like structures linking the Z-band to the sarcolemmal membranes. Costameres are the primary conduits of the externally applied or intrinsically generated mechanical load, and are important sites for signal transduction between the inside and outside of cells.

Z-bands

Cardiac myocytes rely on Z-bands for the assembly and maintenance of sarcomeres.[18] Z-bands are also the major sites for subcellular localization of signaling molecules[14] such as muscle LIM proteins (zyxin, alpha-actinin associated LIM proteins). These Z-band-associated proteins have a dynamic distribution in cells, suggesting that Z-band is not a part of sarcomeric structure but an important site for signaling molecules. Muscle LIM proteins (MLPs) are striated muscle-specific cysteine-rich cytoskeletal proteins and localize at Z-bands, costameres, and intercalated disks. MLPs play a primary role in the mechanical integrity of the muscle cytoarchitecture because null mutant mice developed dilated cardiomyopathy and heart failure. Another interesting feature of MLPs is that they exhibit a dual subcellular localization, with protein accumulation in the nucleus at the beginning of muscle differentiation and later in the cytoplasm as differentiation proceeds. The ability of skeletal MLPs to interact with a transcription factor MyoD[19] has lead to a speculation that MLPs play a direct role in transcription regulation with Nkx2.5.

Intercalated disks

In cardiac myocytes, intercalated disks are specialized structures for cell–cell adhesions. Intercalated disks consist of clusters of N-cadherin-based adhesion complex including β-catenine.[20] Cytosolic β-catenine also works as a signaling molecule of the Wnt pathway, which plays an important role during the early differentiation and survival of cardiomyocytes.[21] Since looping and myofibrillogenesis progress in association with dynamic changes of N-cadherin-based cell–cell adhesions, β-catenine might play a significant role as a signaling molecule and as a part of the cytoskeleton.

Conclusions

Many transcription factors that are essential for early cardiac development have been identified and the molecular hierarchy of these proteins is being established. In contrast, factors that practically determine cell shape and movement are cytoskeletons, cell adhesion molecules, and extracellular matrix. Elucidating the interactions between the upstream transcription factors and downstream targets of cytoskeletal and structural proteins will be a next step of cardiac embryology.

References

1 Manasek FJ. Control of early embryonic heart morphogenesis: a hypothesis. *Ciba Found Symp* 1983; **100**: 4–19.

2 Komuro I, Izumo S. *Csx*: a murine homeobox-containing gene specifically expressed in the developing heart. *Proc Natl Acad Sci USA* 1993; **90**: 8145–9.

3 Tanaka M, Chen Z, Bartunkova S, Yamasaki N, Izumo S. The cardiac homeobox gene *Csx/Nkx2.5* lies genetically upstream of multiple genes essential for heart development. *Development* 1999; **126**: 1269–80.

4 Lints TJ, Parsons LM, Hartley L, Lyons I, Harvey RP. *Nkx-2.5*: a novel murine homeobox gene expressed in early heart progenitor cells and their myogenic descendants. *Development* 1993; **119**: 419–31.

5 Srivastava D, Cserjesi P, Olson EN. A subclass of bHLH proteins required for cardiac morphogenesis. *Science* 1995; **270**: 1995–9.

6 Yost HJ. Establishment of left–right asymmetry. *Int Rev Cytol* 2001; **203**: 357–81.

7 Shiraishi I, Takamatsu T, Minamikawa T, Fujita S. 3-D observation of actin filaments during cardiac myofibrinogenesis in chick embryo using a confocal laser scanning microscope. *Anat Embryol (Berl)* 1992; **185**: 401–8.

8 Shiraishi I, Takamatsu T, Fujita S. 3-D observation of N-cadherin expression during cardiac myofibrillogenesis of the chick embryo using a confocal laser scanning microscope. *Anat Embryol (Berl)* 1993; **187**: 115–20.

9 Shiraishi I, Takamatsu T, Fujita S. Three-dimensional observation with a confocal scanning laser microscope of fibronectin immunolabeling during cardiac looping in the chick embryo. *Anat Embryol (Berl)* 1995; **191**: 183–9.

10 Shiraishi I, Simpson DG, Carver W *et al.* Vinculin is an essential component for normal myofibrillar arrangement in fetal mouse cardiac myocytes. *J Mol Cell Cardiol* 1997; **29**: 2041–52.

11 Shiraishi I, Takamatsu T, Price RL, Fujita S. Temporal and spatial patterns of phosphotyrosine immunolocalization during cardiac myofibrillogenesis of the chicken embryo. *Anat Embryol (Berl)* 1997; **196**: 81–9.

12 Heidkamp MC, Bayer AL, Kalina JA, Eble DM, Samarel AM. GFP-FRNK disrupts focal adhesions and induces anoikis in neonatal rat ventricular myocytes. *Circ Res* 2002; **90**: 1282–9.

13 Kovacic-Milivojevic B, Roediger F, Almeida EA *et al.* Focal adhesion kinase and p130Cas mediate both sarcomeric organization and activation of genes associated with cardiac myocyte hypertrophy. *Mol Biol Cell* 2001; **12**: 2290–307.

14 Ross RS, Borg TK. Integrins and the myocardium. *Circ Res* 2001; **88**: 1112–9.

15 Etienne-Manneville S, Hall A. Rho GTPases in cell biology. *Nature* 2002; **420**: 629–35.

16 Hoshijima M, Sah VP, Wang Y, Chien KR, Brown JH. The low molecular weight GTPase Rho regulates myofibril formation and organization in neonatal rat ventricular myocytes. Involvement of Rho kinase. *J Biol Chem* 1998; **273**: 7725–30.

17 Wei L, Roberts W, Wang L *et al.* Rho kinases play an obligatory role in vertebrate embryonic organogenesis. *Development* 2001; **128**: 2953–62.

18 Borg TK *et al.* Specialization at the Z line of cardiac myocytes. *Cardiovasc Res* 2000; **46**: 277–85.

19 Kong Y, Flick MJ, Kudla AJ, Konieczny SF. Muscle LIM protein promotes myogenesis by enhancing the activity of MyoD. *Mol Cell Biol* 1997; **17**: 4750–60.

20 Linask KK, Knudsen KA, Gui YH. N-cadherin-catenin interaction: necessary component of cardiac cell compartmentalization during early vertebrate heart development. *Dev Biol* 1997; **185**: 148–64.

21 Nakamura T, Sano M, Songyang Z, Schneider MD. A Wnt- and beta-catenin-dependent pathway for mammalian cardiac myogenesis. *Proc Natl Acad Sci USA* 2003; **100**: 5834–9.

CHAPTER 6

Biological role of fibulin-2 in cardiovascular development

Takeshi Tsuda, Mon-Li Chu

Introduction

The extracellular matrix (ECM) interacts with cells and promotes and regulates cellular functions such as adhesion, migration, proliferation, and differentiation. The fibulins are an emerging family of ECM proteins characterized by tandem arrays of calcium-binding epidermal growth factor (EGF)-like modules and a common C-terminal globular domain (Fig. 6.1). Five members have been identified to date, and all, except fibulin-3, have been implicated to play a role in cardiovascular development.[1–7]

Fibulin-1 and -2 are more related to each other because they contain an additional anaphyla-toxin-like domain, and there is some overlap in spatiotemporal expression during cardiovascular development, especially during the development of endocardial cushion tissue.[8,9] Our recent study indicated that, in addition to cardiac valvuloseptal development, fibulin-2 is synthesized by the smooth muscle precursor cells of the developing aortic arch vessels and the coronary endothelial cells during coronary vascular development, suggesting its role in cell transformation and differentiation.[7] Targeted inactivation of fibulin-1 in mice revealed that fibulin-1 is critical for the structural integrity of the walls of small blood vessels.[10] The biological role of fibulin-2 is currently under intensive investigation in our laboratory using a gene targeting technique to create fibulin-2 null mutant mice. In the following, the possible biological roles of fibulin-2 are discussed.

Fibulin-2 and endocardial cushion tissue

During the development of endocardial cushion tissue in mice, fibulin-2 begins to be synthesized by the transformed mesenchymal cells upon their exposure to the preexisting cardiac ECM.[7] Robust upregulation of fibulin-2 in the endocardial cushion tissue is only seen after the presence of mesenchymal cells. The fibulin-2 protein within the endocardial cushion tissue appears as a fibrillar network structure connecting proliferating mesenchymal cells and endocardial cells, suggesting its possible role in facilitating optimal migration, proliferation, and differentiation of the transformed mesenchymal cells. Although it has been known that fibulin-2 is a prominent component of cardiac valves in an adult heart,[9] it is not certain whether fibulin-2 contributes to the integrity of the valve tissue to any extent.

Fibulin-2 and coronary vascular development

Coronary vascular formation involves the following four processes: (1) migration of endothelial precursors; (2) formation of the endothelial plexus; (3) remodeling of the endothelial plexus; (4) growth and maturation of the coronary vessels.[11] Coronary vasculogenesis begins in the subepicardial ECM, which is composed of vitronectin,[12] fibronectin, elastin, and laminin, followed by the deposition of collagens, first type IV and then types III and I.[13] Fibulin-

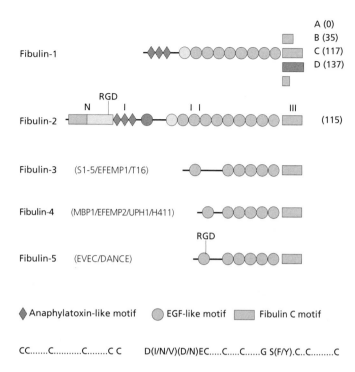

Anaphylatoxin-like motif   ⬤ EGF-like motif   ▭ Fibulin C motif

Fig. 6.1 Molecular structure of fibulin family (fibulin-1 to -5).

CC.......C...........C........C C   D(I/N/V)(D/N)EC.....C.....C......G S(F/Y).C..C.........C

2 begins to be synthesized by the epicardial cells as they migrate over the heart, and continues to be expressed throughout coronary vascular development (Fig. 6.2). Even in the adult heart, fibulin-2 is actively produced by the coronary arterial and venous endothelial cells, and, to a lesser extent, by the fibroblasts in the perivascular interstitial tissue, suggesting its role in maintaining vascular homeostasis.

Fibulin-5, recently shown to be essential for elastic fiber formation in skin, lungs, and aorta,[14,15] has a similar spatiotemporal expression pattern to fibulin-2 during cardiac development in mouse embryo after the heart looping stages (after embryonic day 9.5),[5–7] suggesting a common role in stabilizing elastic tissue during vascular development. Unlike fibulin-5, however, expression of fibulin-2 protein is more restricted to cardiac valves and blood vessels; fibulin-2 is only expressed in the blood vessels in the lung or skin tissue.

Fibulin-2 and development of the aorta

Fibulin-2 specifically marks the transformed mesenchymal cells after their settlement in the basement membrane of the endothelial tube.[7] Robust upregu-

lation of fibulin-2 synthesis takes place immediately after the attachment of mesenchymal cells onto the basement membrane of the aortic vessels, which seems to trigger the rapid proliferation of the migrated mesenchymal cells and gradual differentiation into the smooth muscle cells.[7] It is speculated that the first task facing the precursor cells of vascular smooth muscle is to produce ECM to assemble the specific scaffolding to establish a baseline frame of the future vascular structure.[16] The formation of an alternating structure of elastin layers and smooth muscle layers in the aortic medical is a complex process in which fibulin-2 is involved as one important element.

Fibulin-2 and wound healing: blood vessel formation

Fibulin-2 was reported to be highly sensitive to various matrix metalloproteinases[17] and to be upregulated during wound repair,[18] indicating a strong involvement in tissue remodeling. It has been reported that fibulin-2 is a strong ligand for tropoelastin and fibrillin-1, and is localized in the interface between elastin cores and microfibrils.[19,20] This suggests that fibulin-2 plays a role in facilitating tropo-

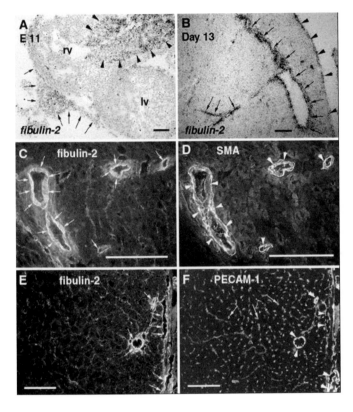

Fig. 6.2 (A), (B) *In situ* hybridization of fibulin-2 in E11 mouse embryo (A) and in postnatal day 13 mouse heart (B). (A) Fibulin-2 is mainly expressed in the mesenchymal cells in the outflow tract cushion tissue (arrowheads) and in the epicardial cells (arrows). (B) Postnatally, fibulin-2 mRNA expression is predominantly seen in the coronary endothelial cells (arrows) and in the epicardial cells (arrowheads). (C)–(F) Double-staining immunohistochemistry in the adult mouse myocardium (3 months old). (C) Fibulin-2 protein localization outlines the coronary arterial endothelial cells (arrows), but not capillary vessels. (D) α smooth muscle actin (SMA) localization indicates the presence of arterial smooth muscle (arrowheads). (E) Fibulin-2 protein is predominantly seen in the arterial endothelial cells (arrows), not in the capillary vessels. (F) PECAM-1 expression indicates the presence of endothelial cells, both arterial (arrowheads) and capillary (arrows). Scale bars = 100 μm.

elastin deposition on the microfibril scaffold mainly during vascular development. New blood vessel formation is a critical step in the wound healing process.

Possible biological role of fibulin-2

In addition to providing microfibrillar structure in the extracellular space, fibulin-2 seems to modulate cell transformation and differentiation during both embryonic development and the wound healing process. Fibulin-2 was shown to possess multiple binding sites to various other ECM molecules *in vitro*.[19,21] It is the combined effect of all these ECM molecules including fibulin-2 that regulates tissue development and tissue homeostasis.

References

1 Argraves WS, Tran H, Burgess WH, Dickerson K. Fibulin is an extracellular matrix and plasma glycoprotein with repeated domain structure. *J Cell Biol* 1995; **111**: 3155–64.

2 Pan T-C, Sasaki T, Zhang RZ *et al.* Structure and expression of fibulin-2, a novel extracellular matrix protein with multiple EGF-like repeats and consensus motifs for calcium binding. *J Cell Biol* 1993; **123**: 1269–77.

3 Lecka-Czernik B, Lumpkin CKJ, Goldstein S. An overexpressed gene transcript in senescent and quiescent human fibroblasts encoding a novel protein in the epidermal growth factor-like repeat family stimulates DNA synthesis. *Mol Cell Biol* 1995; **15**: 120–8.

4 Giltay R, Timpl R, Kostka G. Sequence, recombinant expression and tissue localization of two novel extracellular matrix proteins, fibulin-3 and fibulin-4. *Matrix Biol* 1999; **18**: 469–80.

5 Nakamura T, Ruiz-Lozano P, Lindner V *et al.* DANCE, a novel secreted RGD protein expressed in developing, atherosclerotic, and balloon-injured arteries. *J Biol Chem* 1999; **274**: 22476–83.

6 Kowal RC, Richardson JA, Miano JM, Olson EN. EVEC, a novel epidermal growth factor-like repeat-containing protein upregulated in embryonic and diseased adult vasculature. *Circ Res* 1999; **84**: 1166–76.

7 Tsuda T, Wang H, Timpl R, Chu ML. Fibulin-2 expression marks transformed mesenchymal cells in developing cardiac valves, aortic arch vessels, and coronary vessels. *Dev Dyn* 2001; **222**; 89–100.

8 Spence SG, Argraves WS, Walters L, Hungerford JE, Little CD. Fibulin is localized at sites of epithelial-mesenchymal transitions in the early avian embryo. *Dev Biol* 1992; **151**: 473–84.

9 Zhang HY, Chu M-L, Pan T-C *et al*. Extracellular matrix protein fibulin-2 is expressed in the embryonic endocardial cushion tissue and is a prominent component of valves in adult heart. *Dev Biol* 1995; **167**: 18–26.

10 Kostka G, Giltay R, Bloch W *et al*. Perinatal lethality and endothelial cell abnormalities in several vessel compartments of fibulin-1-deficient mice. *Mol Cell Biol* 2001; **21**: 7025–34.

11 Morabito CJ, Kattan J, Bristow J. Mechanisms of embryonic coronary artery development. *Curr Opin Cardiol* 2002; **17**: 235–41.

12 Bouchey D, Drake J D, Wunch AM, Little CD. Distribution of connective tissue proteins during development and neovascularization of the epicardium. *Cardiovas Res* 1996; **31**: E104–15.

13 Rongish BJ, Hinchman G, Doty MK, Baldwin HS, Tomanek RJ. Relationship of the extracellular matrix to coronary neovascularization during development. *J Mol Cell Cardiol* 1996; **28**: 2203–15.

14 Nakamura T, Lozano PR, Ikeda Y *et al*. Fibulin-5/DANCE is essential for elastogenesis *in vivo*. *Nature* 2002; **415**: 171–5.

15 Yanagisawa H, Davis EC, Starcher BC *et al*. Fibulin-5 is an elastin-binding protein essential for elastic fibre development in vivo. *Nature* 2002; **415**: 168–71.

16 Drake CJ, Hungerford JE, Little CD. Morphogenesis of the first blood vessels. *Ann N Y Acad Sci* 1998; **857**: 155–79.

17 Sasaki T, Mann K, Murphy G, Chu ML, Timpl R. Different susceptibilities of fibulin-1 and fibulin-2 to cleavage by matrix metalloproteinases and other tissue proteanses. *Eur J Biochem* 1996; **240**: 427–34.

18 Fässler R, Sasaki T, Timpl R, Chu M-L, Werner S. Differential regulation of fibulin, tenascin-C, and nidogen expression during wound healing of normal and glucocorticoid-treated mice. *Exp Cell Res* 1996; **222**: 111–16.

19 Reinhardt DP, Sasaki T, Dzamba BJ *et al*. Fibrillin-1 and fibulin-2 interact and are colocalized in some tissues. *J Biol Chem* 1996; **27**: 19489–96.

20 Sasaki T, Göhring W, Miosge N *et al*. Tropoelastin binding to fibulins, nidogen-2 and other extracellular matrix proteins. *FEBS Lett* 1999; **460**: 280–4.

21 Sasaki T, Göhring W, Pan T-C, Chu M-L, Timpl R. Binding of mouse and human fibulin-2 to extracellular matrix ligands. *J Mol Biol* 1995; **254**: 692–9.

CHAPTER 7

TBX5 regulates cardiac cell behavior during cardiogenesis

Cathy J. Hatcher, Min-Su Kim, David Pennisi, Yan Song, Nata Diman, Marsha M. Goldstein, Takashi Mikawa, Craig T. Basson

Mutations in human *TBX5* cause congenital structural abnormalities of the heart and limb in autosomal dominant Holt–Oram syndrome.[1-3] Holt–Oram syndrome presents as congenital heart disease in the setting of preaxial radial ray limb deformity. Our previous analyses have shown that TBX5 haploinsufficiency causes human atrial and ventricular defects as well as abnormalities of myocardial and trabecular structure that reflect cardiac isomerism.[2,4] Missense mutations of specific TBX5 domains have been associated with a greater predilection for more marked cardiac or limb malformations.[2]

To determine the cellular functions of TBX5 during cardiogenesis, we have used replication defective retroviruses to overexpress wild-type and mutant human TBX5 isoforms *in vitro* and *in vivo*.[5] TBX5 overexpression inhibits cell proliferation of D17 canine osteosarcoma cells and MEQC quail cardiomyocyte-like cells (Fig. 7.1). *In vivo*, we have shown that TBX5 overexpression in embryonic chick hearts inhibits myocardial growth and trabeculation (Plate 4). Echocardiographic studies of viable transgenic chick embryos *in ovo* suggest that TBX5 overexpression diminishes left ventricular function. PCNA analysis in TBX5 transgenic chick hearts demonstrates suppression of embryonic cardiomyocyte proliferation *in vivo*, and TBX5 growth arrest activities *in vitro* and *in vivo* are, at least in part, noncell autonomous. Morphologic changes of the ventricles and myocardial growth arrest as a consequence of TBX5 overexpression in the developing chick heart are not necessarily associated with abnormal chamber specification. Immunohistochemical studies to localize atrial myosin heavy chain demonstrate that its expression remains restricted to the atria in E15 TBX5 transgenic chick hearts and absent from the ventricles.[5] Similarly, despite evidence that murine TBX5 can alter mouse atrial natriuretic factor, *ANF*, and atrial myosin heavy chain, *AMHC1*, gene expression,[6-8] our RT-PCR and immunohistochemical analyses do not demonstrate any significant change in *ANF* and *AMHC1* expression, respectively, in genetically engineered chick hearts. Strikingly, high levels of TBX5 overexpression achieved with replication-competent retrovirus does alter ventricular septal morphology and cardiomyocyte differentiation of the chick (see Ogura, Chapter 18). Thus, our model dissociates cell proliferation from atrial specification. Such dissociation may be a consequence not only of the timing of TBX5 overexpression intrinsic to distinct experimental designs in the murine and our chick studies, but may also reflect differential TBX5 dosage sensitivities for cardiomyocyte proliferation and for cardiomyocyte differentiation even in the chick.

These findings are not limited to avian cardiogenesis. We have studied TBX5 expression during growth of mammalian cells as well, and these studies of nongenetically manipulated tissues suggest physiologic regulation of TBX5 during cell proliferation. For instance, the cardiac-derived rat H9c2 cell line grows as myoblasts in culture and ultimately ceases proliferation and differentiates into myotubes.

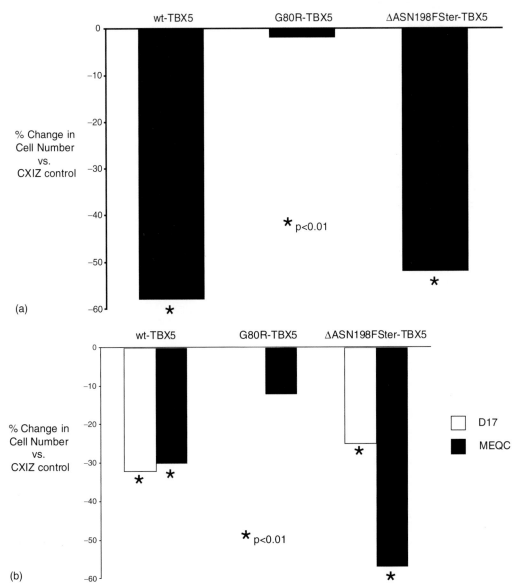

Fig. 7.1 Paracrine effect of TBX5 isoform expression on D17 osteosarcoma and MEQC 'cardiomyocyte-like' cell proliferation. (a) Change in MEQC cell number over a 3-day assay period after 48 h of infection with CXIZ retrovirus containing TBX5 expressing isoforms. Wild type TBX5 and ΔASN198FSter-TBX5 overexpression both markedly decrease cell number compared with cells infected with CXIZ retrovirus alone whereas G80R-TBX5 does not significantly alter MEQC proliferation. Similar data were obtained with D17 osteosarcoma cells. (b) Change in cell number of uninfected D17 and MEQC cells after 3 days of co-culture with cells infected with CXIZ retrovirus containing TBX5 expressing isoforms. Co-culture with wild type TBX5 and ΔASN198FSter-TBX5 overexpressing cells both markedly decrease MEQC and D17 cell number compared with cells infected with CXIZ retrovirus alone whereas co-culture G80R-TBX5 does not significantly alter cell proliferation. Thus, TBX5 growth inhibition is non-cell autonomous.

Comparison of TBX5 expression in cultures of H9c2 cells reveals that although proliferating H9c2 myoblasts do not express TBX5, nonproliferating myotubes have activated TBX5 expression (Fig. 7.2). Liberatore and colleagues[6] similarly demonstrated that transgenic TBX5 overexpression in the murine ventricle produces impaired trabeculation and thinning of the myocardium, probably a consequence of TBX5 inhibition of cell proliferation. Our findings also correlate with an inverse relationship between TBX5 expression and expression of markers of cell proliferation during human organogenesis. We have shown[5] that actively proliferating regions of the heart, thumb, and retina do not express high levels of TBX5, whereas mitotically quiescent regions of these tissues express high levels of TBX5. Thus, we concluded that TBX5 can act as a growth arrest signal during human embryogenesis.

Not all TBX5 activities, however, are mediated via its effects on cell proliferation. When we used immunohistochemistry to study TBX5 expression during human cardiogenesis, we observed that TBX5 protein is expressed not only in the myocardium but also throughout the embryonic epicardium and atrioventricular conduction tissue.[9] Interestingly, we also noted that TBX5 was expressed in the endothelium and the smooth muscle of embryonic coronary vasculature but not in other systemic vascular beds. Previous analysis of the development of

the coronary vasculature in the developing chick embryo demonstrated that the epicardial mantle originates from the proepicardial organ by migration of proepicardial cells.[10] These proepicardial progenitor cells ultimately give rise to the coronary vascular endothelial and smooth muscle cells. We, therefore, set out to test the hypothesis that chick TBX5 plays an active role in epicardial and coronary vascular development during chick cardiogenesis [in prep.]. We demonstrated that chick TBX5 is expressed in the chick proepicardial organ at Hamburger–Hamilton stage 17 prior to cell migration into the myocardium. We then used retrovirus-mediated transgenesis to augment TBX5 expression in the embryonic chick proepicardium.

Microinjection of control CXIZ retrovirus results in the incorporation of β-galactosidase-positive cells into both the epicardium and coronary vasculature in E15 transgenic chick hearts. However, when CXIZ retrovirus encoding TBX5 as well as the *lacZ* reporter gene is microinjected, no β-galactosidase-positive cells are present in either the epicardium or the coronary vasculature. *In vitro* migration studies as well as time course studies *in vivo* in the developing chick embryo, further demonstrate that wild-type TBX5 inhibits cell migration. This activity is specific for TBX5 and is obliterated by missense mutation of the TBX5 T-box. Furthermore, TBX5 inhibition of migration is independent of the effects on cell proliferation. Unlike TBX5 growth arrest activity, however, TBX5 inhibition of cell migration is cell autonomous. In addition, we demonstrated that chick proepicardial cells physiologically inactivate TBX5 expression during migration, and these findings correlate with the distribution of TBX5 in migrating and nonmigrating cells of this lineage during human embryogenesis. Therefore, we propose that TBX5 participates in development of the epicardium and coronary vasculature, and TBX5 overexpression impairs this process via altered cell migration. Recent experimental studies by others have also suggested a role for TBX5 effects on cell migration in the limb.[11]

Thus, we propose that TBX5 contributes to cardiogenesis by modifying a range of cell behaviors. These include the arrest of cardiomyocyte growth and inhibition of the migration of epicardial and vascular progenitor cells. We anticipate that the subtleties of cardiac structure are mediated via local

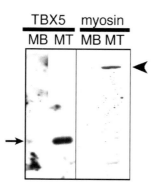

Fig. 7.2 Native Rat H9c2 regulation of TBX5 expression in coordination with cell proliferation. Western blot analysis was performed on protein lysates prepared from proliferating myoblast (MB) and nonproliferating myotubes (MT) cultures of rat H9c2 muscle cells. Proliferating myoblasts do not express TBX5. Upon cessation of proliferation, H9c2s express cardiac markers such as ß-myosin heavy chain (arrowhead) as well as TBX5 (arrow).

balances between TBX5 plus similar inhibitory factors and opposing factors that may promote growth and cell migration. Such factors may include both T-box and non-T-box genes, and elucidation of such local interplay is an important target of future investigation.

Acknowledgments

Supported by the March of Dimes Birth Defects Foundation.

References

1 Basson CT, Bachinsky DR, Lin RC *et al.* Mutations in human TBX5 cause limb and cardiac malformation in Holt–Oram syndrome. *Nat Genet* 1997; **15**: 30–5.

2 Basson CT, Huang T, Lin RC *et al.* Different TBX5 interactions in heart and limb defined by Holt–Oram syndrome mutations. *Proc Natl Acad Sci USA* 1999; **96**: 2919–24.

3 Li QY, Newbury-Ecob RA, Terret JA *et al.* Holt–Oram syndrome is caused by mutations in TBX5, a member of the Brachyury (T) gene family. *Nat Genet* 1997; **15**: 21–9.

4 Basson CT, Cowley GS, Solomon S *et al.* The clinical and genetic spectrum of the Holt–Oram syndrome (Heart-Hand syndrome). *N Engl J Med* 1994; **330**: 885–91.

5 Hatcher CJ, Kim MS, Mah CS *et al.* TBX5 transcription factor regulates cell proliferation during cardiogenesis. *Dev Biol* 2001; **230**: 177–88.

6 Liberatore CM, Searcy-Schrick RD, Yutzey KE. Ventricular expression of TBX5 inhibits normal heart chamber development. *Dev Biol* 2000; **223**: 169–80.

7 Hiroi Y, Kudoh S, Monzen K *et al.* TBX5 associates with Nkx2–5 and synergistically promotes cardiomyocyte differentiation. *Nat Genet* 2001; **28**: 276–80.

8 Bruneau BG, Nemer G, Schmitt JP *et al.* A murine model of Holt–Oram syndrome defines roles of the T-box transcription factor TBX5 in cardiogenesis and disease. *Cell* 2001; **106**: 709–21.

9 Hatcher CJ, Goldstein MM, Mah CS *et al.* Identification and localization of TBX5 transcription factor during cardiac morphogenesis. *Dev Dyn* 2000; **219**: 90–5.

10 Reese DE, Mikawa T, Bader DM. Development of the coronary vessel system. *Circ Res* 2002; **91**: 761–8.

11 Ahn DG, Kourakis MJ, Rohde LA, Silver LM, Ho RK. T-box gene TBX5 is essential for formation of the pectoral limb bud. *Nature* 2002; **417**: 754–8.

CHAPTER 8

Cardiac homeobox protein Csx/Nkx2.5 and its associated proteins

Hiroshi Akazawa, Issei Komuro

The vertebrate heart is formed as a result of coordinated myocardial cell differentiation and complex morphogenetic interactions among cells from multiple embryonic origins.[1] Recent studies have established the notion that cardiac transcription factors govern this intricate process of cardiogenesis by regulating cardiac-specific gene expression.

Csx/Nkx2.5 is an essential transcription factor involved in normal cardiac development

Csx/Nkx2.5 is a member of NK homeobox gene family that is conserved in evolution and acts as a DNA-binding transcriptional activator.[2] In *Drosophila*, *tinman* is expressed in presumptive mesoderm and is required for cell-fate specification of the dorsal vessel, the equivalent of the vertebrate heart, and visceral muscle.[3] *Csx/Nkx2.5* was isolated as a potential mammalian homolog of *tinman*.[4,5] During murine embryogenesis, *Csx/Nkx2.5* is highly expressed in the heart progenitor cells at E7.5 and continues to be expressed at a high level in the heart through adulthood. Targeted disruption of murine *Csx/Nkx2.5* resulted in embryonic lethality at E9–10 owing to the arrested looping morphogenesis of the heart tube and growth retardation.[6,7] Expression of several cardiac genes in the heart of embryos homozygous for *Csx/Nkx2.5* was compromised including *ventricular isoform of myosin light chain 2* (*MLC2v*), *atrial natriuretic peptide* (*ANP*), *brain natriuretic peptide*, *cardiac ankyrin-repeat protein* (*CARP*), *MEF2C*,

eHAND/HAND1, *N-myc*, and *Iroquois homeobox gene 4*.[6–10] These data indicate that *Csx/Nkx2.5* plays a crucial role in transcriptional regulation of several sets of cardiac-specific genes and reigns over the hierarchical cascade of cardiac transcription factors.

In search for the direct downstream target genes of Csx/Nkx2.5, we analyzed the promoters of various cardiac-specific genes. Among several genes tested, Csx/Nkx2.5 strongly transactivated the *ANP* promoter.[11] Transactivation of the *ANP* promoter was dependent on the Csx/Nkx2.5 DNA-binding site located in the *ANP* promoter. We further hypothesized that transcriptional activity of Csx/Nkx2.5 is exquisitely regulated by post-translational modification, and extended our research focusing on protein–protein interactions involving Csx/Nkx2.5 and its associated proteins. Csx/Nkx2.5 controls the cardiac gene program in concert with other cardiac transcription factors such as GATA4 and Tbx5.

Csx/Nkx2.5 and GATA4

GATA4 is a zinc finger-containing transcription factor that is required for normal process of cardiogenesis.[12,13] Co-immunoprecipitation and GST pull-down assay experiments showed that Csx/Nkx2.5 and GATA4 directly interact with each other both *in vivo* and *in vitro* (Fig. 8.1a, b) via the homeodomain of Csx/Nkx2.5 and the zinc-finger domain of GATA4.[11] Overexpression of both Csx/Nkx2.5 and GATA4 induced much stronger transactivation of the luciferase construct containing the 300-bp 5′ flanking region of the rat *ANP* gene (ANP(300)-*luc*) than that induced by expression of Csx/Nkx2.5 alone (Fig. 8.1c).[11] This result suggested that Csx/Nkx2.5 and GATA4 synergistically activate the *ANP* gene. Deletion and mutation analyses revealed that the Csx/Nkx2.5-binding site, located at −250 in the *ANP* promoter, was responsible for

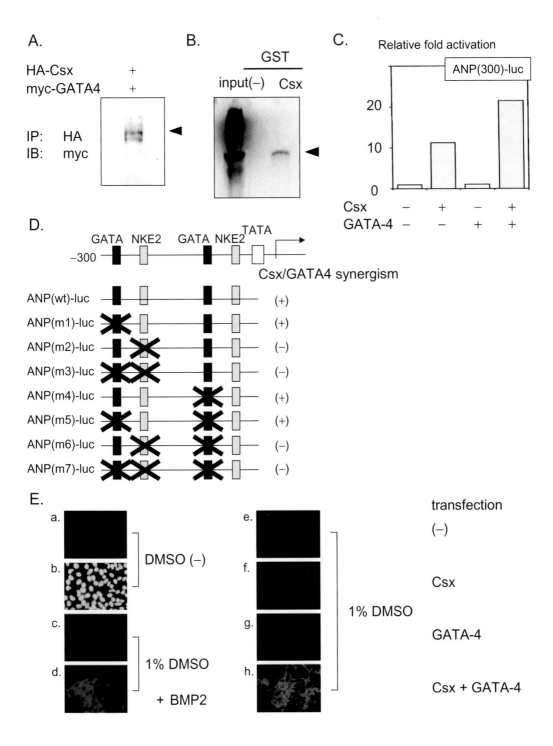

transcriptional activation by Csx/Nkx2.5. Although the GATA site was located at −280, adjacent to Csx/Nkx2.5-binding site, GATA4 alone induced no significant activation of the ANP(300)-*luc* construct. Furthermore, deletion of the GATA site at −280 had little effect on the synergistic transactivation of the *ANP* promoter between Csx/Nkx2.5 and GATA4. Based on the result that deletion of the Csx/Nkx2.5-binding site at −250 abolished the cooperative activation of the *ANP* promoter between Csx/Nkx2.5 and GATA4, this synergistic transactivation is dependent on binding of Csx/Nkx2.5 to the Csx/Nkx2.5-binding site but not on binding of GATA4 to the GATA site (Fig. 8.1d). Recent literatures have indicated transcriptional cooperativity between Csx/Nkx2.5 and GATA4 in promoter activation of *cardiac α-actin,*[14] *CARP,*[15] and *A1 adenosine receptor* genes.[16]

Consistent with several lines of evidence that bone morphogenic protein (BMP) signaling is necessary for induction of cardiac development, stable overexpression of the BMP antagonist noggin completely abrogated myocardial cell differentiation of P19CL6 cells, which are derivatives of P19 and differentiate efficiently into beating cardiomyocytes in adherent conditions in the presence of 1% DMSO.[17,18] Simultaneous overexpression of Csx/Nkx2.5 and GATA4 restored normal cardiac differentiation in this situation, although overex-

pression of Csx/Nkx2.5 or GATA4 alone did not (Fig. 8.1e).[17] Collectively, Csx/Nkx2.5 and GATA4 operate in combination of direct or indirect synergy to regulate cardiac gene program essential for normal cardiac development.

Csx/Nkx2.5 and Tbx5

The interaction between Csx/Nkx2.5 and *Tbx5* has attracted much attention, especially because common cardiac malformations are caused by haplo-insufficiency of each gene. Dominant mutations in human *CSX/NKX2.5* gene have been identified to be responsible for a spectrum of congenital cardiac malformations such as atrial septal defect, ventricular septal defect, tetralogy of Fallot, double-outlet right ventricle, and tricuspid valve abnormality including Ebstein's anomaly, associated with atrioventricular conduction disturbance.[19] Tbx5 is a T-box transcription factor, and heterozygous mutations of Tbx5 in humans produce Holt–Oram syndrome (HOS) characterized by upper limb malformations and a spectrum of cardiac malformations, frequently accompanied by cardiac conduction defect.[20,21] Csx/Nkx2.5 and Tbx5 interact with each other (Fig. 8.2a) via the homeodomain of Csx/Nkx2.5 and the N-terminal domain and T-box of Tbx5, and collaborate to activate the promoters of *ANP* (Fig. 8.2b) and *connexin 40,* a gap junction gene.[22,23] The region

Fig. 8.1 (*opposite*) Association of Csx/Nkx2.5 and GATA4. (A) Csx/Nkx2.5 and GATA4 are associated in mammalian cells. COS-7 cells were transiently transfected with the expression plasmids of HA-tagged Csx/Nkx2.5 and Myc-tagged GATA4. Cell lysates were immunoprecipitated with anti-HA antibody, and then subjected to immunoblotting with anti-Myc antibody. Arrow, co-immunoprecipitated GATA4 protein. (B) Csx/Nkx2.5 and GATA4 interact with each other *in vitro*. *In vitro* translated GATA4 protein labeled with ^{35}S was incubated with GST alone or GST-Csx/Nkx2.5 immobilized on glutathione-Sepharose beads, and bound proteins were analyzed by SDS-PAGE and fluorography. Arrow, GATA4 protein. (C) Csx/Nkx2.5 and GATA4 synergistic transactivate the *ANP* promoter. Expression of Csx/Nkx2.5 results in only weak transactivation, whereas overexpression of both Csx/Nkx2.5 and GATA4 strongly activate the *ANP* promoter. (D) Mutations were introduced into the two GATA sites and NKE2 either alone or in combination, and the resultant eight reporter constructs [wild type (wt) and mutants 1–7 (m1–m7)] were

cotransfected with the expression plasmids of Csx/Nkx2.5 and/or GATA4. Positive or negative results for synergism are shown on the right as (+) and (−), respectively. (E) Simultaneous overexpression of Csx/Nkx-2.5 and GATA4 but not of Csx/Nkx-2.5 or GATA4 alone induced differentiation of P19CL6noggin cells into cardiomyocytes. P19CL6noggin cells did not differentiate into beating cardiomyocytes after treatment with DMSO (c). Overexpression of BMP-2 with adenovirus induced differentiation of P19CL6noggin cells into cardiomyocytes (d). Expression plasmids containing Csx/Nkx2.5 cDNA or GATA4 cDNA were transfected into P19CL6noggin cells on day 2 by the lipofection method. Like untransfected control P19CL6noggin cells (e), the P19CL6noggin cells overexpressing Csx/Nkx-2.5 alone (f) or GATA4 alone (g) did not differentiate into beating cardiomyocytes, whereas simultaneous overexpression of both Csx/Nkx-2.5 and GATA4 in P19CL6noggin cells markedly induced their differentiation into cardiomyocytes (h). The cells were stained with MF20 or Hoechst dye (b) on day 14.

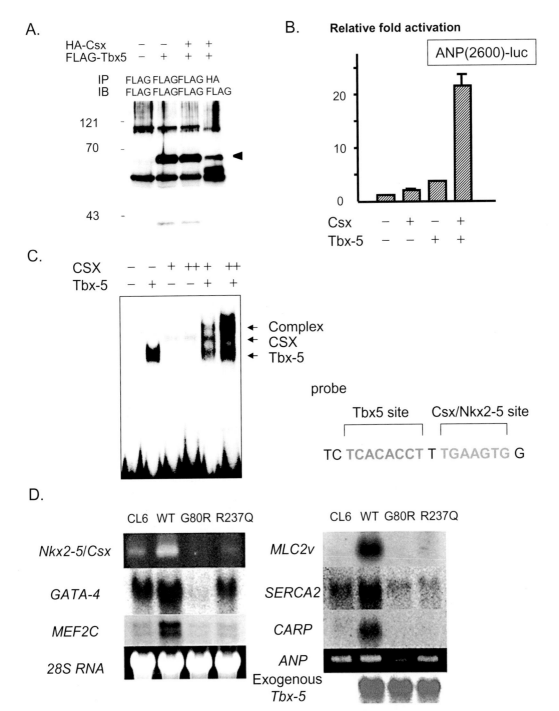

A.

HA-Csx   −   −   +   +
FLAG-Tbx5   −   +   +   +

IP   FLAG   FLAG FLAG   HA
IB   FLAG   FLAG FLAG   FLAG

121 −

70 −

43 −

B. Relative fold activation

ANP(2600)-luc

20

10

0

Csx   −   +   −   +
Tbx-5   −   −   +   +

C.

CSX   −   −   +   ++   +   ++
Tbx-5   −   +   −   −   +   +

← Complex
← CSX
← Tbx-5

probe

Tbx5 site   Csx/Nkx2-5 site

TC **TCACACCT** T **TGAAGTG** G

D.

CL6   WT   G80R   R237Q

Nkx2-5/Csx

GATA-4

MEF2C

28S RNA

CL6   WT   G80R   R237Q

MLC2v

SERCA2

CARP

ANP

Exogenous
Tbx-5

Fig. 8.2 Association of Csx/Nkx2.5 and Tbx5. (A) Csx/Nkx2.5 and Tbx5 are associated in mammalian cells. Cell lysates from COS7 cells transfected with FLAG-tagged Tbx5 and/or HA-tagged Nkx2.5 expression plasmids were incubated with anti-HA or anti-FLAG monoclonal antibody, then the immune complex precipitated with anti-mouse IgG agarose beads was subjected to immunoblotting with anti-FLAG antibody. Arrow, co-immunoprecipitated Tbx5 protein. (B) Synergistic activation of *ANP* promoter by Csx/Nkx2.5 and Tbx5. (C) Csx/Nkx2.5 bind directly to the *ANP* promoter in tandem. Competition of the binding of Tbx5 to the labeled fragment (bp −254 to −236). The Nkx2.5 binding sequence and a 'half-site' of the palindromic T (brachyury)-binding sequence (Tbx5 site) are indicated in the right. (D) Expression of cardiac genes in P19CL6 cell lines. The cell line expressing wild-type Tbx5 (WT) expresses all the cardiac genes more abundantly than parental P19CL6 cells but expression is markedly suppressed in the cell line expressing the G80R mutant. These three cell lines expressed similar amounts of exogenous Tbx5 and its mutants (exogenous Tbx5). 28S RNA demonstrates equal loading of samples.

between −270 and −240 of the *ANP* promoter is important for transactivation by Tbx5, and a half-site of a palindromic T (brachyury)-binding site flanked by a Csx/Nkx2.5-binding site is located within this region. Csx/Nkx2.5 and Tbx5 form a ternary complex together with this tandemly-arrayed cognate DNA sequence (Fig. 8.2c). Interestingly, the Tbx5 harboring G80R mutation, which causes severe cardiac defects in HOS, exhibits significantly weak synergysm on promoter activation of the *ANP* gene, compared with the wild-type Tbx5 and the Tbx5 harboring R237Q mutation, which rarely causes cardiac defects in HOS.[22] Furthermore, stable overexpression of wild-type Tbx5 promotes cardiac differentiation in P19CL6 cells with upregulation of several cardiac genes such as *Csx/Nkx2.5*, *GATA4*, *MEF2C*, *ANP*, *CARP* and *MLC2v*, whereas overexpression of the G80R mutant of Tbx5 attenuates cardiac differentiation with markedly reduced expression of these cardiac genes (Fig. 8.2d). The effects of haploinsufficiency of Tbx5 on cardiac differentiation were analyzed in a genetically engineered murine model,[23] and expression levels of *ANP* and *connexin 40* were significantly reduced in *Tbx5*-heterozygous mice, which exhibited the cardiac phenotypes of HOS. Cooperative regulation of several cardiac genes by Csx/Nkx2.5 and Tbx5 accounts for the overlapping cardiac defects produced by mutations of these transcription factors.

Other proteins that are associated with Csx/Nkx2.5

Composition of protein complexes consisting of transcription factors and cofactors is the key determinant of specificity and intensity. Recent studies have demonstrated that transcriptional activity of Csx/Nkx2.5 is modulated through physical interaction with serum response factor[24] and Tbx2,[25] besides GATA4 and Tbx5. We performed a yeast two-hybrid screening of a heart cDNA library using Csx/Nkx2.5 as a bait. Several novel proteins that associated with Csx/Nkx2.5 have been identified and functional analysis of these proteins are ongoing.

Blueprint of Csx/Nkx2.5 function in cardiogenesis has been considerably depicted, although details remain unclear. Transcriptional regulatory mechanisms have been clarified whereby protein–protein interactions involving multiple cardiac transcription factors such as Csx/Nkx2.5, GATA4 and Tbx5 allow fine-tuned gene expression. Functional analysis of the individual cardiac transcription factor and clarification of interactive roles of them will pave the way to understand the molecular basis of the gene expression program directing cardiac differentiation.

References

1 Srivastava D, Olson EN. A genetic blueprint for cardiac development. *Nature* 2000; **407**: 221–6.

2 Harvey RP. NK-2 homeobox genes and heart development. *Dev Biol* 1996; **178**: 203–16.

3 Bodmer R. The gene *tinman* is required for specification of the heart and visceral muscles in *Drosophila*. *Development* 1993; **118**: 719–29.

4 Komuro I, Izumo S. *Csx*: a murine homeobox-containing gene specifically expressed in the developing heart. *Proc Natl Acad Sci USA* 1993; **90**: 8145–9.

5 Lints TJ, Parsons LM, Hartley L, Lyons I, Harvey RP. *Nkx-2.5*: a novel murine homeobox gene expressed in early heart progenitor cells and their myogenic descendants. *Development* 1993; **119**: 419–31.

6 Lyons I, Parsons LM, Hartley L *et al.* Myogenic and morphogenetic defects in the heart tubes of murine embryos lacking the homeo box gene *Nkx2.5*. *Genes Dev* 1995; **9**: 1654–66.

7 Tanaka M, Chen Z, Bartunkova S, Yamasaki N, Izumo S. The cardiac homeobox gene *Csx/Nkx2.5* lies genetically upstream of multiple genes essential for heart development. *Development* 1999; **126**: 1269–80.

8 Biben C, Harvey RP. Homeodomain factor *Nkx2.5* controls left/right asymmetric expression of bHLH gene eHand during murine heart development. *Genes Dev* 1997; **11**: 1357–69.

9 Zou Y, Evans S, Chen J, Kuo HC, Harvey RP, Chien KR. CARP, a cardiac ankyrin repeat protein, is downstream in the *Nkx2.5* homeobox gene pathway. *Development* 1997; **124**: 793–804.

10 Bruneau BG, Bao ZZ, Tanaka M *et al.* Cardiac expression of the ventricle-specific homeobox gene *Irx4* is modulated by Nkx2.5 and dHand. *Dev Biol* 2000; **217**: 266–77.

11 Shiojima I, Komuro I, Oka T *et al.* Context-dependent transcriptional cooperation mediated by cardiac transcription factors Csx/Nkx-2.5 and GATA4. *J Biol Chem* 1999; **274**: 8231–9.

12 Kuo CT, Morrisey EE, Anandappa R *et al.* GATA4 transcription factor is required for ventral morphogenesis and heart tube formation. *Genes Dev* 1997; **11**: 1048–60.

13 Molkentin JD, Lin Q, Duncan SA, Olson EN. Requirement of the transcription factor GATA4 for heart tube formation and ventral morphogenesis. *Genes Dev* 1997; **11**, 1061–72.

14 Sepulveda JL, Belaguli N, Nigam V *et al.* GATA4 and Nkx-2.5 coactivate Nkx-2 DNA binding targets: role for regulating early cardiac gene expression. *Mol Cell Biol* 1998; **18**: 3405–15.

15 Kuo H, Chen J, Ruiz LP *et al.* Control of segmental expression of the cardiac-restricted ankyrin repeat protein gene by distinct regulatory pathways in murine cardiogenesis. *Development* 1999; **126**: 4223–34.

16 Rivkees SA, Chen M, Kulkarni J, Browne J, Zhao Z. Characterization of the murine A1 adenosine receptor promoter, potent regulation by GATA4 and Nkx2.5. *J Biol Chem* 1999; **274**: 14204–9.

17 Monzen K, Shiojima I, Hiroi Y *et al.* Bone morphogenetic proteins induce cardiomyocyte differentiation through the mitogen-activated protein kinase kinase kinase TAK1 and cardiac transcription factors Csx/Nkx-2.5 and GATA4. *Mol Cell Biol* 1999; **19**: 7096–105.

18 Monzen K, Hiroi Y, Kudoh S *et al.* Smads, TAK1, and their common target ATF-2 play a critical role in cardiomyocyte differentiation. *J Cell Biol* 2001; **153**, 687–98.

19 Schott JJ, Benson DW, Basson CT *et al.* Congenital heart disease caused by mutations in the transcription factor *NKX2-5*. *Science* 1998; **281**: 108–11.

20 Li QY, Newbury ER, Terrett JA *et al.* Holt–Oram syndrome is caused by mutations in TBX5, a member of the Brachyury (T) gene family. *Nat Genet* 1997; **15**: 21–9.

21 Basson CT, Bachinsky DR, Lin RC *et al.* Mutations in human TBX5 cause limb and cardiac malformation in Holt–Oram syndrome. *Nat Genet* 1997; **15**: 30–5.

22 Hiroi Y, Kudoh S, Monzen K *et al.* Tbx5 associates with *Nkx2.5* and synergistically promotes cardiomyocyte differentiation. *Nat Genet* 2001; **28**: 276–80.

23 Bruneau BG, Nemer G, Schmitt JP *et al.* A murine model of Holt–Oram syndrome defines roles of the T-box transcription factor Tbx5 in cardiogenesis and disease. *Cell* 2001; **106**: 709–21.

24 Chen CY, Schwartz RJ. Recruitment of the tinman homolog Nkx-2.5 by serum response factor activates cardiac alpha-actin gene transcription. *Mol Cell Biol* 1996; **16**: 6372–84.

25 Habets PE, Moorman AF, Clout DE *et al.* Cooperative action of Tbx2 and Nkx2.5 inhibits ANF expression in the atrioventricular canal: implications for cardiac chamber formation. *Genes Dev* 2002; **16**: 1234–46.

CHAPTER 9

Regulation of myocardium formation after the initial development of the linear heart tube

Maurice J. B. van den Hoff, Boudewijn P. T. Kruithof,
Andy Wessels, Roger R. Markwald, Antoon F. M. Moorman

Introduction

Well after formation of the primary linear heart tube, a second wave of myocardium formation takes place that in chicken results in the addition of: (1) the pulmonary and caval myocardium; (2) the smooth-walled atrial myocardium; (3) the myocardial atrioventricular septum; (4) the muscular tricuspid valve; (5) the muscular outlet septum and the freestanding muscular infundibulum; (6) the outflow tract. Immunohistochemical analysis showed that the formation of myocardial cells within intra- and extracardiac mesenchymal structures starts in the dorsal mesocardium at H/H19, in the atrioventricular cushion region at H/H26, and in the proximal outflow tract at H/H29, and is completed at H/H43. This myocardium is formed by recruitment of cardiomyocytes from flanking mesenchyme and/or by migration from existing myocardium (myocardialization).[1,2]

As a first attempt to approach the underlying molecular mechanisms that are responsible for the induction and regulation of this relative late process of myocardium formation, we have used an *in vitro* explant culture assay. The analysis showed that the competency to form myocardial networks *in vitro* is a characteristic of the myocardium that is flanked by intra- or extracardiac mesenchyme, i.e. the inflow tract, atrioventricular canal, and outflow tract. Early explants of these cardiac compartments do not spontaneously form myocardial networks but can

be induced to do so by conditioned medium. Addition of conditioned media derived from different late stage (H/H 26–29) cardiac compartments induces myocardial network formation early stage (H/H15–17) cardiac compartments *in vitro*. Atrial and ventricular compartments are, in general, not competent and do not produce the inducing activity, but ventricular explants do form spontaneously myocardial networks in a very limited time window (HH21–24)[1] [unpubl. obs.]. Moreover, cardiac cushion mesenchyme was found to be able to differentiate into cardiomyocytes in the *in vitro* culture assay. Taken together these observations suggest that a temporally released or secreted signal that is similar throughout the entire heart induces this late process of myocardium formation. We have previously put forward that this late formation of myocardium is the result of migration of existing cardiomyocytes into flanking mesenchyme. Recent experiments indicate that in addition to this process, mesenchymal cells also are recruited into the cardiac lineage.[1,2]

In this study we evaluated whether candidate growth factors can induce myocardial network formation in early-stage cardiac explants *in vitro*, by adding recombinant pure growth factors to the medium. The growth factors were selected based on: (1) the analysis of genetically modified mice in which congenital cardiac defects were reported;[3] (2) the analysis of early myocardium formation.[4,5]

Material and methods

The day prior to use, gels containing 1.5 mg/mL rat tail collagen type I (Collaborative Research Inc.) in Medium 199 (Life Technologies), were prepared in 24-well NUNC plates. After polymerization, the gels were equilibrated in complete medium 199 [Medium 199, penicillin/streptomycin (Life Technologies), 1% chicken serum (Life Technologies), glutamine (Life Technologies), and ITS (Collaborative Research Inc.)]. The next day, the OFT was isolated from staged chicken embryos (Drost BV, Nieuw Loosdrecht, The Netherlands), positioned on top of a drained collagen gel and allowed to attach for at least 4 h, prior to the addition of complete medium 199 or of medium that was conditioned for 1 week with the respective cardiac explants or of complete medium 199 supplemented with a recombinant purified human growth factor (Peprotech). After 5 days of culture, the gels were rinsed with PBS and fixed in ethanol at room temperature. Next, the gels were hydrated and incubated with a monoclonal directed against myosin heavy chain (MF20: Hybridoma Bank). Antibody binding was visualized using FITC-labeled rabbit anti-mouse serum (Nordic) and confocal laser scanning microscopy (Biorad MRC1024).[1,2] The extent of myocardial network formation was scored on an arbitrary scale ranging from 0 to 2: 0, is an explant from which different cell types have grown but the myocardial border is generally smooth; 1, when myocardial protrusions have formed on top of the collagen matrix; 2, when a myocardial network is formed into the matrix.

Results and discussion (Fig. 9.1)

In cultures of H/H16 OFT explants, daily inspection using Varel modulation optics revealed that endocardial cells grow out of the explants on top of the collagen matrix. Subsequently, mesenchymal cells develop in the collagen matrix below the endocardial cells. Although myocardial protrusions seem sometimes apparent, immunofluorescent identification of these cardiomyocytes is needed. When early (H/H15–17) OFTs are cultured in completed medium 199, cardiomyocytes are never observed to form myocardial networks into the collagen matrix.

Myocardial networks were formed into the collagen matrix, however, using conditioned medium derived from late OFT (H/H 26–29). These networks are generally contiguous with the original explant. These findings show that a temporally released or secreted signal induces this late process of myocardium formation.

To identify this inducing signal, we tested different growth factors, indicated to be involved in cardiovascular development,[3–5] for their ability to induce myocardial network formation in early OFT explants. Activin-a, angiotensin-II, bone morphogenetic protein (BMP)-2, BMP-4, cardiotrophin, endothelin-1, -2, -3, fibroblast growth factor (FGF)-2, insulin-like growth factor (IGF)-II, neurotrophin-3, osteopontin, platelet derived growth factor (PDGF)-BB, and transforming growth factor beta (TGFβ)-1 were each not able to induce myocardial network formation, whereas PDGF-AA and -AB, and TGFβ-2 and -3 were able to induce the formation of myocardial networks *in vitro*. TGFβ-2 and -3 induce myocardial network formation in a concentration dependent way. Maximal induction is observed at concentrations equal and higher than 10 pmol/L TGFβ-2 and 50 pmol/L TGFβ-3. TGFβ-2 and -3 have been shown to be required for endothelial cell activation and transformation in atrioventricular explant cultures.[6,7] Based on these reports and the fact that our cultures are characterized by extensive amounts of mesenchymal cells, the effect of TGFβ-2 and -3 is most probably due to stimulation of recruitment of mesenchymal cells into the cardiomyocyte lineage, which would be in line with the reported phenotype of the TGFβ2 knockout mouse.[8]

It is noteworthy that PDGF-AA stimulates myocardial network formation at low levels and inhibits at high levels, whereas PDGF-AB stimulates myocardial network formation with increasing concentrations. In general, PDGFs regulate cell proliferation, survival, morphology, and migration, as well as deposition and turnover of the extracellular matrix. In patch mice[9] and in mice in which the PDGF-receptor-α is homozygously deleted,[10] septational defects are apparent that are suggested to be the result of aberrant homing of neural crest cells. As the neural crest cells have not yet arrived in the H/H15–17 OFT, the role of PDGF signaling needs to be evaluated further.

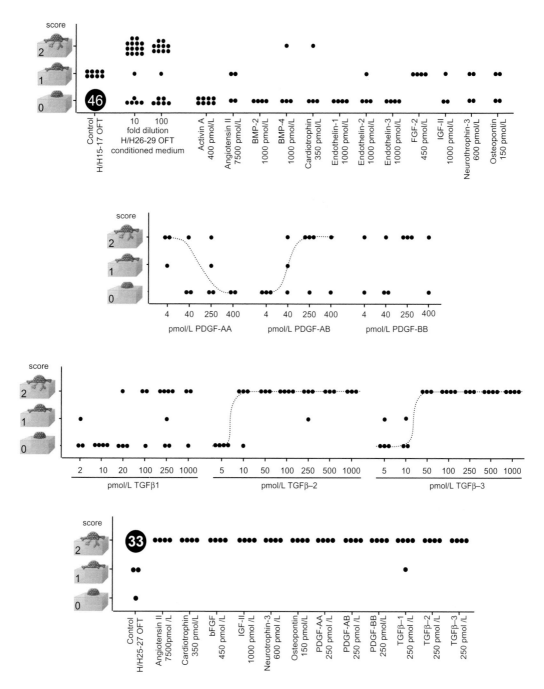

Fig. 9.1 Effects of various growth factors on myocardial network formation by outflow tracts from staged embryos explanted into a collagen matrix. The extent of myocardial network formation was scored on an arbitrary scale ranging from 0 to 2. A score 0 is assigned to an explant from which different cell types have grown but the myocardial border is generally smooth, a score 1 when myocardial protrusions have formed on top of the collagen matrix, and a score 2 when a myocardial network is formed into the matrix.

Moreover, culturing H/H25–27 OFT explants in the presence of recombinant human growth factors did not inhibit the spontaneous formation of the myocardial networks extensively. Interestingly, H/H25–27 OFT cultured in the presence of TGFβ-1, -2, or -3 resulted in an extensive turnover of the collagen gel, resulting in collapse of the gel after 5 days of culture.

References

1 van den Hoff MJB, Moorman AFM, Ruijter JM *et al.* Myocardialization of the cardiac outflow tract. *Dev Biol* 1999; **212**: 477–90.

2 van den Hoff MJB, Kruithof BPT, Moorman AFM, Markwald RR, Wessels A. Formation of myocardium after the initial development of the linear heart tube. *Dev Biol* 2001; **240**: 61–76.

3 Srivastava D, Olson EN. A genetic blueprint for cardiac development. *Nature* 2000; **407**: 221–6.

4 Lough J, Sugi Y. Endoderm and heart development. *Dev Dyn* 2000; **217**: 327–42.

5 Barron M, Gao M, Lough J. Requirement for BMP and FGF signaling during cardiogenic induction in non-precardiac mesoderm is specific, transient, and cooperative. *Dev Dyn* 2000; **218**: 383–93.

6 Ramsdell AF, Markwald RR. Induction of endocardial cushion tissue in the avian heart is regulated, in part, by TGFβ-3-mediated autocrine signaling. *Dev Biol* 1997; **188**: 64–74.

7 Boyer AS, Ayerinskas II, Vincent EB *et al.* TFGβ2 and TGFβ3 have separate and sequential activities during epithelial-mesenchymal cell transformation in the embryonic Heart. *Dev Biol* 1999; **208**: 530–45.

8 Bartram U, Molin DG, Wisse LJ *et al.* Double-outlet right ventricle and overriding tricuspid valve reflect disturbances of looping, myocardialization, endocardial cushion differentiation and apoptosis in TGFβ2-knockout mice *Circulation* 2001; **103**: 2745–52.

9 Schatteman GC, Motley ST, Effman EL, Bowen-Pope DF. Platelet-derived growth factor receptor alpha subunit deleted patch mouse exhibits severe cardiovascular dysmorphogenesis. *Teratology* 1995; **51**: 351–66.

10 Soriano P. The PDGFα receptor is required for neural crest cell development and normal patterning of the somites. *Development* 1997; **124**: 2691–700.

CHAPTER 10

The role of the extracellular matrix (ECM) in cardiac development

Robert L. Price, Thomas K. Borg, James Buggy, Wayne Carver

The regulation of heart development is a dynamic process involving both intracellular and extracellular stimuli.[1] These stimuli include mechanical, chemical, and electrical signals that are critical in regulating the form and function of the developing heart. Intimately associated with these signals are a variety of cell surface receptors that are essential in the detection of and response to these signals. Mechanical signals are generated from cell growth, muscular contraction, and non-muscle cell tension and are important in forming directional clues as well as increased growth.[2] Chemical signals are fundamental for chemotaxis, growth factor regulation, and competency signals.[3] Electrical signaling is important in both muscle and non-muscle cell populations as evidenced by changing patterns of the gap junction proteins.[4]

As the ECM changes with development of the heart so does the expression of its specific receptors. Immunocytochemical evidence indicates the temporal and spatial presence for a variety of receptors for extracellular matrix components including integrins, growth factor receptors, and extracellular proteases. The presence of the receptor as well as the ligand is critical. The absence or altered ratio of receptor to ligand can be a critical factor in morphogenesis. Angiotensin is an important hormone that interacts with specific receptors on the surface of a wide variety of cells.[5–9] In the heart, much is known concerning the expression of both the ligand and receptors in adult pathophysiology but comparatively little is known about their roles in cardiac development.[11–14] Administration of angiotensin in whole embryo culture shows abnormal looping, but knockout of angiotensin in mice is not an embryonic lethal phenotype and adult mice have only a mild cardiac phenotype.[8,11] Receptor blockade also shows an affect on cardiac development *in vitro*. Results with the knockout mice suggest that angiotensin does not play a critical role in heart development; however, another possible explanation is that angiogensin produced by the mother can cross the placenta.

To test the hypothesis that angiotensin crosses the placenta, time-pregnant rats (day 12) were injected with a mixture of various doses of nonradioactive angiotensin II and 15 Ci of ^{125}-I angiotensin II. Animals were killed after 10 min and blood, placenta, heart, and kidneys of both the mother and embryo were dissected and analyzed in a gamma counter. As expected, most of the radioactivity was found in the kidneys of the mother; however, a significant amount of radioactivity was found in the embryo (Fig. 10.1a). When the counts of the mother were subtracted from the embryonic counts, again sig-nificant counts could be observed (Fig. 10.1b).

Previous studies have shown that increased or decreased expression of angiotensin II can alter the pattern of cardiac myofibrillogenesis and development.[5,7,8] The action of angiotensin II can clearly affect a large number of cell signaling cascades, mechanical tension, and the expression of other growth factors.[6,9] Angiotensin II has been shown to alter expression of the integrin receptor family which can cause an increase in mechanical tension.[15,16] These data show that normal embryonic development requires both angiotensin and the specific receptors. Studies on the expression of the specific receptors of angiotensin II indicate that they appear to function differently in development and disease. These studies have indicated that the AT1

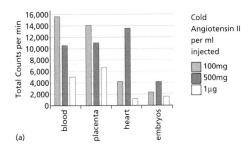

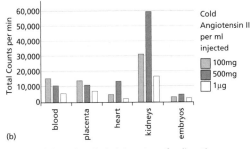

Fig. 10.1 (a) Results of administration of radioactive angiotensin II to time-pregnant rats showing the accumulation of radioactivity in various organs of the mother and fetus. (b) Accumulation of radioactivity in the fetus following subtraction of the mothers radioactivity. These data show that radioactive angiotensin II crossed the placental barrier and was incorporated into various organs of the fetus.

and AT2 receptors are present and active in development on both myocytes and fibroblasts, but it is controversial whether the AT2 receptor is active in cardiac hypertrophy. Little is known concerning the cellular localization of these receptors in the adult. Data on the expression of AT1 and AT2 are usually derived from transgenic mice where a receptor has overexpression or has been knocked out in the myocyte.[17,18] However, the fibroblast and other cell types are ignored in this approach. It is likely that there is some communication (paracrine?) between fibroblasts and myocytes and that this cellular interaction could probably involve the AT family of receptors. Future experiments manipulating both the AT1 and AT2 receptors on both fibroblasts and myocytes would be possible in 3D cultures and would provide new insight into the role of angiotensin in heart development and disease.

In the data presented here, we show that angiotensin II present in the maternal circulation is capable of crossing the placental barrier and affecting cardiac development. These data contribute to the explanation of normal development when angiotensinogen has been knocked out. This precursor molecule can obviously be replaced by the mother. What is more difficult to explain is how angiotensin converting enzyme (ACE), which is necessary for the conversion of angiotensinogen to angiotensin II, is replaced. Recent studies have shown that chymase may replace 80% of ACE at the local tissue level.[19]

The significance of these studies also lies in the fact that mothers with hypertension and/or diabetes have increased levels of angiotensin in their circulation. These increased levels of expression are likely to have an affect on the development of the heart.

Acknowledgments

These studies were supported by NIH grant HL 68038, AHA grant (RLP), HL-37669 (TKB), and NIH COBRE P20 RR1643 (TKB).

References

1 Harvey RP, Rosenthal N, eds. *Heart Development.* New York: Academic Press, 1999.

2 Sussman MA, McCulloch A, Borg TK. Dance band on the Titanic: biomechanical signaling in cardiac hypertrophy. *Circ Res* 2002; **91**: 888–98

3 Ross RS, Borg TK. Integrins and the myocardium. *Circ Res* 2001; **88**: 1112–9.

4 Kohl P, Noble D. Mechanosensitive connective tissue: potential influence on heart rhythm. *Cardiovasc Res* 1996; **32**: 62–8.

5 Yamazaki T, Komuro I, Yazaki Y. Signalling pathways for cardiac hypertrophy. *Cell Signal* 1998; **10**: 693–698

6 Schnee JM, Hsueh WA. Angiotensin II, adhesion, and cardiac fibrosis. *Cardiovasc Res* 2000; **46**: 264–8.

7 Sadoshima J, Izumo S. Mechanical stretch rapidly activates multiple signal transduction pathways in cardiac myocytes: potential involvement of an autocrine/paracrine mechanism *EMBO J* 1993; **12**: 1681–92.

8 Price RL, Potts JD, Thielen TE, Borg TK, Terracio L. Growth factor regulation of embryonic, fetal, and neonatal cardiac development. In: Tomanek RJ, Runyan R, eds. *Development of the Cardiovascular System.* New York: Springer-Verlag, 2001: 171–99.

9 Chien KR. Stress pathways and heart failure. *Cell* 1999; **98**: 555–8.

10 Masaki H, Kurihara T, Yamaki A *et al.* Cardiac-specific overexpression of angiotensin II AT2 receptor causes attenuated response to AT1 receptor-mediated pressor

and chronotropic effects. *J Clin Invest* 1998; **101**: 527–35.

11 Beinlich CJ, Morgan HE. Control of growth in neonatal pig hearts. *Mol Cell Biochem* 1993; **119**: 3–9.

12 Aoki H, Izumo S, Sadoshima J. Angiotensin II activates RhoA in cardiac myocytes: a critical role of RhoA in angiotensin II-induced premyofibril formation. *Circ Res* 1998; **82**: 666–76.

13 Price RL, Carver W, Simpson DG *et al.* The effects of angiotensin II and specific angiotensin receptor blockers on embryonic cardiac development and looping patterns. *Dev Biol* 1997; **192**(2): 572–84.

14 Ito M, Oliverio MI, Mannon PJ *et al.* Regulation of blood pressure by the type 1A angiotensin II receptor gene. *PNAS* 1995; **92**: 3521–5.

15 Burgess ML, Carver WE, Terracio L *et al.* Integrin-mediated collagen gel contraction by cardiac fibroblasts. Effects of angiotensin II. *Circ Res* 1994; **74**: 291–8.

16 Graf K, Neuss M, Stawowy P *et al.* Angiotensin II and alpha(v)beta(3) integrin expression in rat neonatal cardiac fibroblasts. *Hypertension* 2000; **35**: 978–84.

17 Unger T. The angiotensin type 2 receptor: variations on an enigmatic theme. *Journal of Hypertension* 1999; **17**(Suppl.): 1775–86.

18 Haywood GA, Gullestad L, Katsuya T *et al.* AT1 and AT2 angiotensin receptor gene expression in human heart failure. *Circulation* 1997; **95**: 1201–6.

19 Wolny A, Clozel JP, Rein J *et al.* Functional and biochemical analysis of angiotensin II-forming pathways in the human heart. *Circ Res* 1997; **80**: 219–27.

CHAPTER 11

Teratogenic effects of bis-diamine on the developing myocardium

*Nobuhiko Okamoto, Masao Nakagawa, Hidetoshi Fujino,
Setsuko Nishijima, Takashi Hanato, Tsutomu Narita,
Kyoko Yoshida-Imanaka*

Some congenital heart defects result in dispro-portional ventricular development. Conotruncal anomalies including tetralogy of Fallot (TOF) and patent truncus arteriosus (PTA) are associated with an enlarged right ventricle and hypoplastic left ven-tricle. As this ventricular disproportion is already recognized before or just after birth, it seems to be established during cardiogenesis in the embryo. However, what establishes this proportional ven-tricular development, or how the ventricular my-ocardial cells in the anomalous heart grow and proliferate, remains unclear.

N,N′-bis (dichloroacetyl) diamine-1,8-octa-methylene diamine (bis-diamine) is known to in-duce conotruncal anomaly and disproportional ventricular development in rat embryos when ad-ministered to the mother. In previous reports, this chemical was proposed to disturb the normal mi-gration of cardiac neural crest cells into the heart, leading to the induction of the conotruncal anom-alies. In order to determine the mechanisms of dis-proportional ventricular development in congenital heart defects, we morphologically analyzed the embryonic heart and investigated cardiomyocytic DNA synthesis and apoptosis.

A single dose of 200 mg of bis-diamine was ad-ministered to Wistar pregnant rats on day 9.5 of pregnancy. The embryos were removed on each em-bryonic day (ED) from 10.5 to 18.5. Morphometric analyses were performed on serial sections from each heart. Expression of cardiotrophin-1 (CT-1) and hepatocyte growth factor (HGF) was investi-gated on the sections, and CT-1 and HGF mRNAs expression was examined by RT-PCR (Fig. 11.1). Myocardial DNA synthesis was investigated using BrdU, and the labeling index (LI) was calculated for each heart. Apoptosis was also analyzed using termi-nal deoxynucleotidyl transferace-mediated dUTP nick endlabeling reaction and electrophoresis of DNA fragmentation (Fig. 11.2). Age-matched em-bryos from untreated mothers were used as controls.

The number of embryos obtained from bis-diamine treated mothers decreased as the time of pregnancy advanced, while those from control mothers were almost the same at each developmen-tal stage. The embryos treated with bis-diamine had a ventricular enlargement and an elongated outflow tract with pericardial defect in the early stages and conotruncal anomalies associated with thin left ventricular wall in the later stages. As the ventricular myocardial wall was thinner in the embryos treated with bis-diamine, bis-diamine may directly disturb early myocardial proliferation and development and subsequently induce ventricular enlargement, hydrops fetalis, and occasional fetal death.

The labeling index on ED15.5 and 16.5 was sig-nificantly lower than that in the controls. This re-duced myocardial DNA synthesis in ED15.5 and 16.5 hearts may result in the left ventricular hy-poplasia observed in neonates. The less active DNA synthesis in the embryonic hearts treated with bis-diamine does not seem to be caused by a direct effect of bis-diamine as no significant difference of LI was observed before ED15.5. A possible factor involved

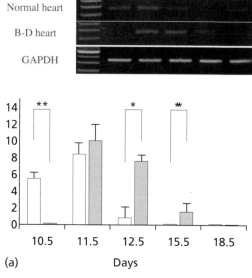

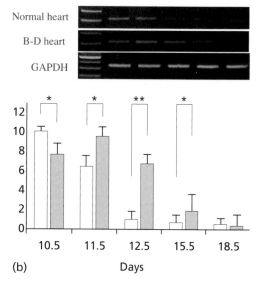

Fig. 11.1 HGF (a) and CT-1 (b) mRNAs expression. HGF mRNA expression was detected on ED10.5 in the control heart, but not detected on ED10.5 in the bis-diamine treated heart. Note the augmented expression of HGF mRNA on ED11.5 in the bis-diamine treated heart. HGF mRNA expression was still detected on ED15.5 in the bis-diamine treated heart but was absent in the control heart. The highest level of CT-1 mRNA expression was detected on ED10.5 in the control and on ED11.5 in the bis-diamine treated heart. CT-1 mRNA was highly expressed in the bis-diamine treated heart thereafter. B-D, bis-diamine; open bar, control heart; closed bar, bis-diamine treated heart.

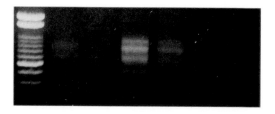

Con B-D Con B-D Con B-D
14.5 14.5 16.5 16.5 18.5 18.5

Fig. 11.2 Electrophoresis of low molecular weight cellular DNA extracted from control heart and bis-diamine treated heart. Typical DNA ladders were disclosed in the DNA fragmentation from the control heart on ED16.5. Note weak DNA ladders on ED14.5 in control and ED16.5 in treated heart.

in the decrease in the number of DNA synthesizing myocardial cells is poor development of the coronary circulation system. Recent *in vivo* and *in vitro* studies in our laboratory suggested that the pericardial defect might induce anomalous coronary arteries in rat embryos treated with bis-diamine. An acute increase of DNA synthesizing cardiomyocytes in the ventricular wall was disclosed around ED15.5 in the control, which well correlated with the establishment of the coronary vascular system in the previous report. In the bis-diamine treated embryonic hearts, normal pericardial and coronary vascular development were disturbed, and myocardial circulation and oxygenation seemed to be supplied only by endocardial blood perfusion through the trabecular of the ventricles.

HGF and HGF mRNA expression was first detected on ED10.5 in controls and on ED11.5 in hearts treated with bis-diamine. CT-1 and CT-1 mRNA expression was first detected on ED10.5 both in the bis-diamine treated and control hearts. HGF and CT-1 mRNAs expression was upregulated on ED12.5 and 15.5 in bis-diamine treated hearts. As HGF mRNA expression was detected in the early myocardial cells in primitive atria, ventricles, and outflow tract in the present study, HGF was suggested to be one the strong cardiac growth factors that promote early myocardial proliferation and differentiation. Because HGF receptors were also detected on the myocardial cells, HGF in the heart seemed to be expressed in an autocrine/paracline fashion. Therefore, an absence of HGF expression in the ED10.5 bis-diamine treated hearts may correspond to the myocardial development delay in function and differentiation caused by the immediate effect of bis-diamine. Furthermore, the upregulation of HGF mRNA expression in the bis-diamine treated hearts may be a compensatory response to the myocardial developmental delay. Recent studies have shown that CT-1 inhibits cytokine-induced apoptosis in cardiomyocytes and plays a protective role in cytokine-induced myocardial damage, including myocarditis. Therefore, although continuous expression of CT-1 mRNA in the control hearts may suggest a crucial role of myocardial proliferation, differentiation, and survival, the upregulation observed in the bis-diamine treated embryos indicates that it has a protective role from myocardial damage or loss caused by the chemical. There still remains the problem, however, of why the upregulation of HGF and CT-1 expression did not lead to

myocardial DNA synthesis and proliferation. Fewer apoptotic cells were detected in the hearts of bis-diamine treated embryos than in those of controls from ED13.5–17.5. Apoptosis detected in the endocardial or truncal cushions tissue might contribute to the abnormal truncal division or coronary artery development.

The present study shows that bis-diamine directly or indirectly disturbs normal myocardial development and that upregulation of HGF and CT-1 expression occurs in the bis-diamine treated hearts that does not lead to an augmentation of myocardial DNA synthesis but to a decrease in the number of apoptotic cells. These results indicate that the ventricular disproportion observed in the bis-diamine treated heart is probably caused by the early myocardial differentiation delay and poor proliferation and reduced apoptosis in the later stage as a result of abnormal coronary and systemic circulatory conditions.

CHAPTER 12

Proliferative responses to myocardial remodeling in the developing heart

*David Sedmera, Pavel Kucera, Frantisek Kolar,
Robert P. Thompson*

The developing myocardium of higher vertebrates grows chiefly by cell division (hyperplasia), whereas mature ventricular myocytes grow almost exclusively by increasing their size (hypertrophy). In the chick embryo, Clark et al.[1] found pure myocyte hyperplasia in response to ventricular pressure overload induced by constriction of the outflow tract (conotruncal banding). Similar effects were reported in fetal guinea pig myocardium;[2] however, the potential for hypertrophic response exists even in the fetus, as was shown in the lamb model of pulmonary artery constriction.[3] The switching from hyperplastic to hypertrophic growth occurs soon after birth in mammals,[4–6] and pressure overload created in day 5 rat pups leads already to hypertrophic response.[7] Despite these studies, the reactions of the immature myocardium to changes in loading conditions *in vivo* are underinvestigated, and even less is known about its response to experimentally decreased loading. In these proceedings we summarize our results from studies of changes in myocyte proliferative structure in four models of hemodynamic alterations with pronounced myocardial remodeling.

We analyzed proliferative responses of the myocardium by two distinct approaches. The first consists of terminal 5-bromodeoxyuridine (BrdU) labeling (up to 16 h) followed by immunohistochemical detection of S-phase cells. The labeling index (percentage of labeled myocytes) is then determined. The second approach we used is based on quantitative label dilution. The proliferating population of myocytes is pre-labeled with radioactive thymidine prior to experimental procedure. Sampling is performed at the time where desired phenotype can be clearly ascertained morphologically, and both control and experimental hearts are then processed for autoradiographic exposure yielding suitable number of grains per nucleus in the population of interest. Staining with myocyte marker (MF20 antibody detecting myosin heavy chain) and nuclear counterstaining are added. Increased proliferation of target cell population is evidenced by increased dilution of radiolabel (decreased number of grains per nucleus), while slower proliferation over that same period of time is revealed by higher retention of the initial label (higher grain counts).

In the first model system examined, we studied the effects of conotruncal banding on the proliferative structure of the chick ventricular myocardium. As was noted earlier, based on biochemistry and stereology, pure cellular hyperplasia occurs in this setting[1]; SEM study demonstrated thickening of the ventricular compact layer and trabeculae with precocious spiraling of their course,[8] suggesting accelerated morphogenesis. Pressure loading induced by conotruncal banding in chick embryonic heart led to increased cell proliferation, demonstrated more readily by the label dilution method with ^{3}H-thymidine at HH34 than by short BrdU pulses at different time points. This validated our label-dilution approach for use in embryonic systems, the main advantage being the ability to study the proliferative history in hearts with an already established phenotype of interest. We observed increased label dilution in the compact layer of both ventricles, as well as in the right ventricular trabeculae, but the cell populations destined to become the ventricular conduction system, distinguished by their permanent withdrawal from cell cycle,[9] were not affected. This shows that at such an early stage (HH21), there are already myocyte populations terminally differentiating and not responding to mechanical loading by increased cycling. Later stages were not studied, because of defective coronary development and high mortality.[10]

Next, we investigated whether myocyte hyperplasia was operative in pressure overload induced by banding of abdominal aorta in day 2 rat pups.[11] Changes in left ventricular wall thickness were already detected 24 h after the constriction, and the heart weight doubled in the most severe cases by day

10. We found increased BrdU labeling 24 h after constriction in both myocytes and nonmyocytes, and increased dilution of the radiolabel at day 21 (Fig. 12.1). After day 10, hypertrophic changes (increased cardiomyocyte width) were demonstrated, confirming the timing of transition from hyperplastic to hypertrophic growth.[6]

Our further interest was devoted to investigation of mechanisms of underloading-induced hypoplastic changes. In the chick model of the hypoplastic left heart syndrome,[8] we applied again the label-dilution technique to demonstrate decrease in the number of cell divisions over time in the hypoplastic left ventricle.[12] Interestingly, these changes were not compensated for by increased myocyte proliferation in the right ventricular wall. Decreased cell proliferation was accompanied by downregulation of PDGF-B and FGF-2, making these growth factors potential therapeutic targets for myocyte regeneration in the immature heart.

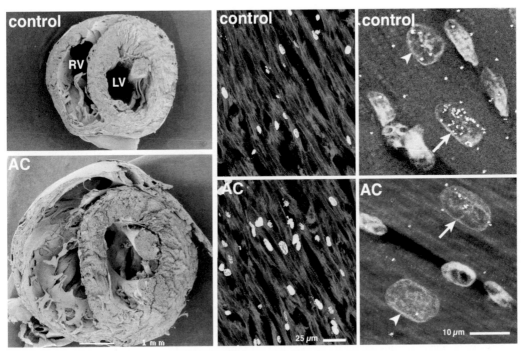

Fig. 12.1 Aortic constriction (AC) performed in neonatal rats at day 2 leads to a rapid acceleration of left ventricular growth. This is evidenced by increased heart weight and ventricular wall thickness seen on SEM micrographs of hearts sampled at day 10. The initial phase of this response is hyperplastic, as confirmed by increased BrdU labeling at day 3 (second column) and later by increased label dilution (third column). By day 10, hypertrophy starts; however, there is no evidence of myocardial fibrosis.

Ectopic electrical pacing in the adult human heart can lead, in chronic settings, to local wall thinning at the stimulation site.[13] One explanation for this observation is unequal distribution of workload, with the early-activated myocardium working less than the late-activated one.[14] This corresponds well with the fact that the apex, which is normally the first activated region of the ventricle,[15–17] is thinner than the midportion or the base.[18] We were interested to see if this situation would occur in the developing heart, which is known to react to pacing in a specific way.[19] Local decrease in wall thickness (−28%) was induced by 48 h of intermittent ventricular pacing in HH21–28 chick embryonic heart. It was mediated by localized decrease in cell proliferation, again with reduced FGF-2 levels.[18]

Interest in positional clues that may regulate proliferation during early development led to study of artificial muscular tubes *in vitro*. We hypothesized that there exists a gradient of stress–strain relationship through the wall, with higher strain found along the inner layers associated with lower rates of proliferation, and that reversal of that strain gradient would reverse the gradient of proliferation. Loops of chick ventricular muscle were dissected at HH16 and mounted on inert vascular supports (fixed vitelline veins from ED10 chick) in normal or everted position. After 2 days of concerted beating, terminal BrdU label (Fig. 12.2) demonstrated that the transmural gradient of highest proliferation along outer layers was rapidly re-established in everted muscular loops. This suggests a role of

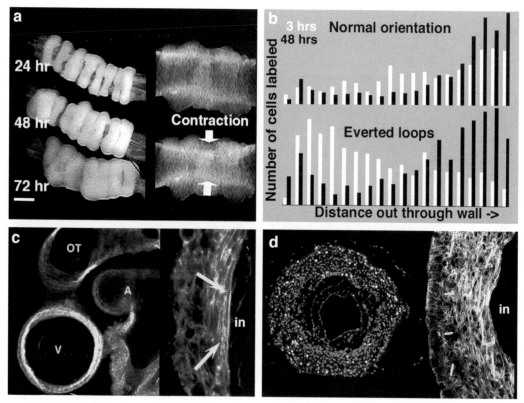

Fig. 12.2 Gradients of proliferation and differentiation in artificial myotubes. Rings cut from stage 16 chick embryonic hearts were threaded on a vitelline vein perfused via peristaltoid pump fused overnight and beat together *in vitro* (a). By 2 days in culture, original proliferative gradient, with higher proliferation in outer layers (white), was reversed in everted tubes [black (b); white dots (d)]. Phalloidin staining revealed greater circumferential alignment of sarcomeric actin along more strained inner ventricular layers in the normal heart (c). Remodeling reflecting the new geometry was observed after 48 hours in the everted loop (d). Scale bar = 200 μm.

positional information, perhaps growth factors or uneven wall strain, in regulation of cell division in the early myocardium.

The size of a cell population is not dependent only on the rate of cell proliferation. Since migration is believed to be insignificant in the working myocardium of higher vertebrates, the remaining unknown in this equation is naturally occurring cell death, or apoptosis. Apoptosis is a well-documented phenomenon in the developing heart, but seems to be very rare in ventricular myocardium[20,21] and is associated with proliferation[22] and conduction system differentiation.[23] We have therefore investigated the rates of apoptosis in all our models, since increased incidence of cell death might contribute to hypoplasia or heart failure. Apoptosis did not seem to be significantly involved in any of these settings.[12,18]

We thus conclude that experimentally induced remodeling of myocardial architecture in developing heart is based on regulation of myocyte proliferation. These studies emphasize a basic, transient property of developing myocardium and underscore the need for early corrective surgery for congenital heart disease to achieve hyperplasia-based remodeling and to prevent development of adverse myocardial structural changes.

Acknowledgments

Supported by NIH HL50582, SC COBRE in Cardiovascular Disease RR 16434–01, and March of Dimes Basil O'Connor 5-FY03–118.

References

1 Clark EB et al. Effect of increased pressure on ventricular growth in stage 21 chick embryos. *Am J Physiol* 1989; **257**: H55–61.

2 Saiki Y, Konig A, Waddell J, Rebeyka IM. Hemodynamic alteration by fetal surgery accelerates myocyte proliferation in fetal guinea pig hearts. *Surgery* 1997; **122**: 412–9.

3 Toussaint M, Bical O, Galliz P, Neveux JY. Effect of intrauterine creation of pulmonary stenosis and atresia on ventricular hypertrophy in the foetal lamb; haemodynamic, morphometric and ultrastructural study. *Eur Heart J* 1998; **19**: 654.

4 Clubb FJ Jr, Bishop SP. Formation of binucleated myocardial cells in the neonatal rat. An index for growth hypertrophy. *Lab Invest* 1984; **50**: 571–7.

5 Beinlich CJ, Rissinger CJ, Morgan HE. Mechanisms of rapid growth in the neonatal pig heart. *J Mol Cell Cardiol* 1995; **27**: 273–81.

6 Li F, Wang X, Capasso JM, Gerdes AM. Rapid transition of cardiac myocytes from hyperplasia to hypertrophy during postnatal development. *J Mol Cell Cardiol* 1996; **28**: 1737–46.

7 Campbell SE, Rakusan K, Gerdes AM. Change in cardiac myocyte size distribution in aortic-constricted neonatal rats. *Basic Res Cardiol* 1989; **84**: 247–58.

8 Sedmera D, Pexieder T, Rychterova V, Hu N, Clark EB. Remodeling of chick embryonic ventricular myoarchitecture under experimentally changed loading conditions. *Anat Rec* 1999; **254**: 238–52.

9 Cheng G et al. Development of the cardiac conduction system involves recruitment within a multipotent cardiomyogenic lineage. *Development* 1999; **126**: 5041–9.

10 Tomanek RJ, Hu N, Phan B, Clark EB. Rate of coronary vascularization during embryonic chicken development is influenced by the rate of myocardial growth. *Cardiovasc Res* 1999; **41**: 663–71.

11 Kolar F, Papousek F, Pelouch V, Ostadal B, Rakusan K. Pressure overload induced in newborn rats: effects on left ventricular growth, morphology, and function. *Pediatr Res* 1998; **43**: 521–6.

12 Sedmera D et al. Cellular changes in experimental left heart hypoplasia. *Anat Rec* 2002; **267**: 137–45.

13 Prinzen FW et al. Asymmetric thickness of the left ventricular wall resulting from asynchronous electric activation: a study in dogs with ventricular pacing and in patients with left bundle branch block. *Am Heart J* 1995; **130**: 1045–53.

14 Kappenberger L, Grobety M, Jeanrenaud X. In: Vardes PE, ed. *Cardiac Arrhythmias, Pacing & Electrophysiology.* Dordrecht: Kluwer Academic Publishers, 1998: 331–36.

15 Nygren A et al. Voltage-sensitive dye mapping of activation and conduction in adult mouse hearts. *Ann Biomed Eng* 2000; **28**: 958–67.

16 Rentschler S, Vaidya DM, Tamaddon H et al. Visualization and functional characterization of the developing murine cardiac conduction system. *Development* 2001; **128**: 1785–1792.

17 Chuck ET, Freeman DM, Watanabe M, Rosenbaum DS. Changing activation sequence in the embryonic chick heart. Implications for the development of the His-Purkinje system. *Circ Res* 1997; **81**: 470–6.

18 Sedmera D et al. Pacing-induced ventricular remodeling in the chick embryonic heart. *Pediatr Res* 1999; **45**: 845–52.

19 Grobety M, Sedmera D, Kappenberger L. The chick embryo heart as an experimental setup for the assessment of myocardial remodeling induced by pacing. *Pacing Clin Electrophysiol* 1999; **22**: 776–82.

20 Pexieder T. The tissue dynamic of heart morfogenesis. II. Quantitative investigations. A. Method and values from areas without cell death foci. *Ann Embryol Morphogen* 1973; **6**: 325–333.

21 Poelmann RE, Molin D, Wisse LJ, Gittenberger-de Groot AC. Apoptosis in cardiac development. *Cell Tissue Res* 2000; **301**: 43–52.

22 Abdelwahid E *et al.* Apoptosis in the pattern formation of the ventricular wall during mouse heart organogenesis. *Anat Rec* 1999; **256**: 208–17.

23 Cheng G, Wessels A, Gourdie RG, Thompson RP. Spatiotemporal distribution of apoptosis in embryonic chicken heart. *Dev Dyn* 2002; **223**: 119–133.

PART 3

Formation of endocardial cushions and valves

Editorial perspective

D. Woodrow Benson

The five papers in this section deal with the processes that establish the AV and semilunar valves and their spatial relationships. Cardiac valve development involves formation of early endocardial cushion swellings, endocardial–mesenchymal transformation (EMT) and invasion of neural crest-derived mesenchyme, myocardialization, proliferation, and late stages of remodeling that include apoptosis and maturation of valve leaflets. During the early stages of tubular heart development, signals released by the myocardium induce a subset of endocardial cells in the AV canal and later in the OT regions to undergo an EMT. This transformation results in formation of the endocardial cushions, which are the primordia of the cardiac valves and septa of the four-chambered heart. Although numerous genes and molecular cascades have been identified in the transformation of endocardium into cushion mesenchyme, little is known about how cushion mesenchyme subsequently differentiates into valve leaflets.

Barnett and Desgrosellier have previously reported that transforming growth factor β3 (TGFβ3) is expressed in the transforming endothelial and invading mesenchymal cells, and that bone morphogenetic protein 2 (BMP2) and 5 (BMP5) are in the AV and OT myocardium during endocardial cushion tissue formation in the chick embryo. Their *in vitro* analysis showed that at the onset of this EMT, TGFβ and BMP act synergistically with each other to induce not only the initial phenotypic changes characteristic of this phenomenon, but also mesenchymal cell invasion. The mechanism underlying this BMP–TGFβ synergy during EMT, however, remains to be clarified.

In previous studies, Baldwin and Zhou have shown that the transcription factor, nuclear factor of activated T cells (NFATc1), is required for normal valve development and that NFATc is exclusively expressed by the endocardium. To characterize the role of NFATc1 in semilunar valvulogenesis, the downstream targets of NFATc activation were identified by monitoring gene expression in an *in vitro* system using a pulmonary mesothelioma cell line (REN). Interestingly, unlike that seen in T lymphocytes, there was a prominent effect of NFATc1 activation on the suppression, rather than gene activation by both calcineurin dependent and independent mechanisms. These studies are the first to suggest a novel role for NFATc1 in regulation of the endocardial phenotype during development.

Markwald *et al.* concluded that periostin, a 90 kDa protein related to the *Drosophilia* fasciclin gene family, is expressed in cushion mesenchymal cells upon their transformation from endocardium; the cushion cells continue to express periostin as they progressively differentiate into fibrous tissue during fetal and neonatal life. Conversely, inducible repression of periostin protein correlates with differentiation of mesenchymal cells (cushion or MC3T3) into a chondrogenic or osteogenic cell type.

Suigi *et al.* localized mRNA of fibroblast growth factor (FGF) receptors (FGFR1, 2 and 3), and FGF ligands, FGF-4 and FGF-8, in developing cardiac cushion tissue implicating their role during the initial proliferative period of early valvulogenesis. Distinct patterns of FGF receptor expression were observed suggesting differing roles in regulation of the varied phases of valvulogenesis. Interestingly, they noted a pattern of FGFR3 expression restricted to the endocardium similar to that seen for NFATc (see study by Baldwin and Zhou).

Yamagishi *et al.* examined the spatiotemporal expression of Msx1 to assess the role of this homeobox gene in endocardial cushion tissue formation. Their results show that Msx1 is expressed in the transforming endothelial and invading mesenchymal cells at the onset of EMT. Further, Msx1 is required to initiate BMP/TGFβ-dependent EMT, and lies downstream of BMP signaling, but not of TGFβ. These findings suggest that Msx1 may have a key role to play in the synergistic effect of BMP and TGFβ during EMT. Further experiments will be necessary to clarify the mechanisms underlying the synergistic effect of these growth factors.

CHAPTER 13

TGFβ signaling during atrioventricular cushion transformation

Joey V. Barnett, Jay S. Desgrosellier

Congenital heart defects are the most prevalent birth defect in humans and often include valvular anomalies. Studies of the molecular regulation of cardiovascular development have identified potential mechanisms underlying these defects. We have investigated the role of transforming growth factor beta (TGFβ) receptors in the initial events of valve formation in an effort to gain insight into the molecular basis of valvular defects.

A pivotal event in valvulogenesis occurs at the tubular heart stage in the atrioventricular (AV) cushion and later in the developing outflow tract. Experiments have demonstrated a restricted localization of both the endothelial cells that can transform and myocardial cells that can signal transformation. Signals released by the myocardium induce a subset of endocardial cells to undergo an epithelial–mesenchymal transformation (EMT). These cells hypertrophy, elongate, and separate, then enter and migrate through the acellular cardiac jelly. The cushions direct one-way blood flow in the embryo and are remodeled into mature valves. Transformation has been studied extensively in avian systems where the AV cushion can be explanted onto a collagen gel[1] (Fig. 13.1). The beating myocardium compacts while endothelial cells form a monolayer on the gel surface. EMT is quantitated by measuring mesenchyme production, defined as the number of cells that enter the gel, or by determining the migration rate of individual cells.

Members of the TGFβ family play a significant role in EMT. When AV cushion endocardial cells on a collagen gel are covered with noninductive ventricular myocardium, transformation is stimulated by TGFβ2 while neutralizing antisera or antisense oligonucleotides to TGFβ[2,3] inhibit transformation. Given these data, we sought to answer the following question: If a subpopulation of AV cushion endothelial cells responds to TGFβ by undergoing transformation and adjacent ventricular cells do not, what is different about TGFβ receptor expression or coupling in AV cushion endocardial cells compared to nonresponsive cells in the ventricle?

The TGFβ family proper includes three ligands: TGFβ1, β2, and β3. Although the mRNA for these ligands have discrete and localized patterns of expression,[4] an inability to identify active ligands in the embryo has limited the assignment of ligands to specific functions. At least three cell surface receptors bind ligand. The type I TGFβ receptor (TBRI) and type II TGFβ receptor (TBRII) are serine/threonine kinases. TBRII binds TGFβ1 and β3 with high affinity, then complexes with and phosphorylates TBRI.[5] TBRII binds TGFβ2 with low affinity, although, a splice variant, TBRII-B binds TGFβ2 with high affinity.[6] Phosphorylation of TBRI results in activation of the cytoplasmic kinase domain and subsequent phosphorylation of downstream signaling molecules, including members of the Smad family of transcription factors.[7] Signaling through TBRII/TBRI mediates TGFβ effects such as growth arrest[5] and the production of plasminogen activator inhibitor 1 (PAI-1).[8] The type III TGFβ receptor (TBRIII) has a large extracellular binding

9q33-q34 and 1p32-p33, respectively. *Genomics* 1995; **28**: 356–7.

17 Sheffield VC, Pierpont ME, Nishimura D *et al.* Identification of a complex congenital heart defect susceptibility locus by using DNA pooling and shared segment analysis. *Human Mol Gen* 1997; **6**: 117–27.

18 ten dijke P, Miyazono K, Heldin CH. Signaling inputs converge on nuclear effectors in TGF-beta signaling. *Trends Biochem Sci* 2000; **25**: 64–70.

19 Ebner R, Chen R-H, Lawler S, Zioncheck T, Derynck R. Determination of type i receptor specificity by the type ii receptors for TGF-beta or activin. *Science* 1993; **262**: 900–2.

20 Macias-Silva M, Hoodless PA, Tang SJ, Buchwald M, Wrana JL. Specific activation of Smad1 signaling pathways by the BMP7 type i receptor, ALK2. *J Biol Chem* 1998; **273**: 25628–36.

21 Miettinen PJ, Ebner R, Lopez AR, Derynck R. TGF-β induced transdifferentiation of mammary epithelial cells to mesenchymal cells: involvement of type I receptors. *J Cell Biol* 1994; **127**: 2021–36.

22 Lai Y-T, Beason KB, Brames GP *et al.* Activin receptor-like kinase 2 can mediate atrioventricular cushion transformation. *Dev Biol* 2000; **222**: 1–11.

23 Hata A, Lagna G, Massague J, Hemmati-Brivanlou A. Smad6 inhibits BMP/Smad1 signaling by specifically competing with the Smad4 tumor suppressor. *Genes Dev* 1998; **12**: 186–97.

24 Barnett JV, Desgrosellier JS. TGF-beta signaling during cardiac morphogenesis. *FASEB J* 2002; **16**: A0194.

25 Galvin KM, Donovan MJ, Lynch CA *et al.* A role for smad6 in development and homeostasis of the cardiovascular system. *Nat Genet* 2000; **24**: 171–4.

CHAPTER 14

The endocardium as a unique modulator of *in utero* cardiovascular form and function

H. Scott Baldwin, Bin Zhou

Null mutations in the transcription factor, nuclear factor of activated T cells (NFATc1), have documented its requirement for normal valve development.[1,2] Our previous studies have shown that NFATc is exclusively expressed by the endocardium and that defects were preferentially detected during semilunar valve formation resulting in embryonic lethality by E14.5 in the mouse.[2] However, a detailed analysis by our collaborators has documented that defects in valvular function of the endocardial cushions can be detected as early as E11.5,[3] well before conotruncal septation is complete and prior to the onset of valve leaflet formation. Thus, physiological alterations in NFATc1 mutant embryos precede anatomical defects as detected by routine histological techniques and the role of NFATc1 in normal valvulogenesis remains obscure.

Neural crest cells are known to make a unique contribution to development of the distal outflow tract mesenchyme and the endocardium is thought to play a pivotal role as a source of proximal mesenchyme populating the endocardial cushions.[4] Therefore, we focused our attention on abnormalities in these cell populations as a potential explanation for the defects observed in the absence of NFATc1. NFATc mutant mice were bred onto the R26R reporter background where Cre-mediated excision removes a stop codon and simultaneously brings the lacZ expression cassette into a proper reading frame for immunohistological identification.[5] These mice were then crossed with transgenic animals expressing neural crest specific Cre (Wnt-1

Cre)[6] and endothelial specific Cre (Tie2-Cre)[7] to evaluate the lineage-specific contribution of each mesenchymal subpopulation to outflow tract development in NFATc1 mutant mice. Preliminary analysis of staged embryos from these matings (Plate 5a) showed a definitive, tissue-specific segregation of mesenchymal populations in wild type embryos: endothelial derived mesenchyme (EM) seemed to populate the proximal outflow tract while neural crest derived mesenchyme (NCM) was the prominent cell type in the distal outflow tract (Oft). However, in the NFATc1 null mutants (Plate 5b), this discrete tissue boundary appeared obscured suggesting that disruption of lineage-specific tissue boundaries is associated with abnormalities detected in the NFATc1 null mutants. Furthermore, no defects in the atrioventricular canal (Avc) mesenchymal cell population were detected, further supporting an enhanced sensitivity of the outflow tract to attenuated NFATc expression.

To further understand the role of NFATc1 in semilunar valvulogenesis, we have begun to analyze possible downstream targets of NFATc activation that might place NFATc1 in a clearly defined, mechanistic cascade. Because the endocardium makes up a small fraction of the total number of cells populating the cardiac outflow tract compared to myocardial and mesenchymal cells, various attempts using comparative representation display technologies of wild type and mutant embryos were unsuccessful in identifying endocardial specific candidate genes. Therefore, we have created an *in vitro* system (Fig.

14.1) to study the effects of induced NFATc activation using a pulmonary mesothelioma cell line (REN) with endothelial qualities but no detectable native expression of NFATc1 in conjunction with adenovirus infection. Two adenoviral constructs were compared (Fig. 14.1a): a control IRES-eGFP and an adenovirus containing NFATc1 in which the nuclear export signal had been deleted resulting in constitutive nuclear localization followed by an IRES-eGFP construct. The expression of eGFP by both constructs allowed cells to be FACS sorted to insure pure populations and equivalent levels of expression. When transfected into REN cells, the NFATc1 expressing virus resulted in a clear phenotypic change when compared to control virus (Fig. 14.1b). Each cell population was then cultured with or without stimulation by calcium ionophor and phorbol ester, and were also cultured in the presence or absence of cyclosporin inhibition over sequential time points to establish a dose–response curve and delineate the role of the calcineurin-calmodulin pathways. Multiple microarray analyses (Fig. 14.1c) was then used to monitor alterations in the expression of approximately 1000 different genes under control and experimental conditions. Interestingly, unlike that seen in T lymphocytes, there was a prominent effect of NFATc1 activation on the suppression, rather than activation of gene activation in

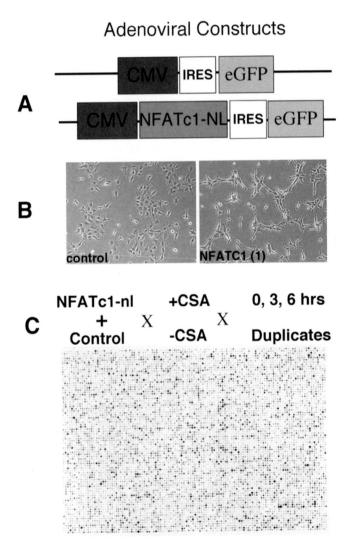

Fig. 14.1 An *in vitro* model to study the role of NFATc1. (A) Schematic of the control and treatment adenoviral constructs. These replication deficient adenoviruses used a cytomegalovirus (CMV) enhancer/promoter to drive expression of either green fluorescent protein (eGFP) alone or a mutated NFATc1 in which the nuclear export signal had been removed to induce constitutive nuclear localization and activity. A internal ribosomal entry site (IRES) was added to insure that eGFP expression was driven off the same promoter as the NFATc1 construct. (B) REN cell infected with control and NFATc1 virus documenting a morphological change associated with infectivity. (C) The schedule for cyclosporine administration and a representative microarray following mRNA extraction and hybridization.

by both calcineurin dependent and independent mechanisms. While similar mechanisms have been suggested by some previous experiments using different model systems,[8,9] these studies are the first to suggest a novel role for NFATc1 in the regulation of the endocardial phenotype during development. Further studies are underway to correlate these *in vitro* studies with those detected *in vivo* during critical periods of semilunar valvulogenesis.

References

1 de la Pompa JL, Timmerman LA, Takimoto H *et al.* Role of the NF-ATc transcription factor in morphogenesis of cardiac valves and septum. *Nature* 1998; **392**: 182–6.

2 Ranger AM, Grusby MJ, Hodge MR *et al.* The transcription factor NF-ATc is essential for cardiac valve formation [see comments]. *Nature* 1998; **392**: 186–90.

3 Phoon CKL, Ji RP, Aristizabal O *et al.* Embryonic heart failure in NFATc1-/- mice: novel mechanistic insights from *in utero* ultrasound biomicroscopy. *Circ Res* 2004; **95**: 2–9.

4 Noden DM, Poelmann RE, Gittenberger-de Groot AC. Cell origins and tissue boundaries during outflow tract development. *Trends Caridovasc Med* 1995; **5**: 69–75.

5 Soriano P. Generalized *lacZ* expression with the ROSA26 Cre reporter strain. *Nat Genet* 1999; **21**: 70–1.

6 Jiang X, Rowitch DH, Soriano P, McMahon AP, Sucov HM Fate of the mammalian cardiac neural crest. *Development* 2000; **127**: 1607–16.

7 Kisanuki YY, Hammer RE, Miyazaki J *et al.* Tie2-Cre transgenic mice: a new model for endothelial cell-lineage analysis in vivo. *Dev Biol* 2001; **230**: 230–42.

8 Feske S, Giltnane J, Dolmetsch R *et al.* Gene regulation mediated by calcium signals in T lymphocytes. *Nat Immunol* 2001; **2**: 316–24.

9 Graef IA, Chen F, Chen L, Kuo A, Crabtree GR. Signals transduced by Ca(2+)/calcineurin and NFATc3/c4 pattern the developing vasculature. *Cell* 2001; **105**: 863–75.

CHAPTER 15

Valvulogenesis: role of periostin in cushion tissue differentiation

Roger R. Markwald, Edward L. Krug, Stan Hoffman,
Ricardo Moreno-Rodriguez, Laura Villavicencio,
Corey H. Mjaatvedt, Simon J. Conway

Although 100+ genes have been identified in the transformation of endocardium into cushion mesenchyme, little genetic information is known about how cushion mesenchyme subsequently differentiates into valve leaflets. Cushion cells normally differentiate into a (myo)fibroblastic lineage but also have potential to differentiate into cardiac muscle,[1] cartilage,[2] bone and bone marrow including blood cells.[3] One candidate for regulating cushion differentiation that emerged from a gene chip (microarray) study is osteoblast specific factor 2 or periostin. Periostin is a 90 kDa protein that is related to the *Drosophila* fasciclin gene family, which is important in invertebrates in axon guidance and targeting.[4] However, in vertebrates, it seems to be more widely expressed[5,6] including the periosteum of bone and the perichondrium of cartilage. We found that the periostin mRNA is downregulated when periosteal osteoblastic ('stem') cells of bone differentiate into osteocytes. Conversely, we find that periostin is upregulated in mouse and chick cushion mesenchyme after their transformation from endocardial progenitor cells. Expression in cushion cells continues during differentiation into valve leaflets and persists, in valves, into postnatal and adult life.[6] To confirm that periostin message is also expressed as a protein, rabbit antibodies were made against synthetic peptide corresponding to amino acids 123–142 in mouse periosteum (accession no. D13664) after conjugation to keyhole limpet hemocyanin. This sequence – called peptide II – is unique to the first of four fasciclin domains in mouse periostin. On Western blots, the immunopurified antisera recognized a major band at 90 kDa in both the 14 embryonic and newborn hearts (also detected in adult hearts). Peptide II but not peptide III competitively inhibited staining of the gels (peptide III is a non-fasciclin amino acid sequence at the N-terminus) (Fig. 15.1). Using immunopurified antibodies, we confirmed that periostin protein is not expressed in the endocardium but only in the extracellular matrix surrounding its mesenchymal progeny (Plate 6). The protein was associated with cushion cell surfaces and filaments radiating into the extracellular matrix (Plate 6b). In both chick and mouse, periostin, as well as other mesenchymal markers such as JB3 and ES130, was co-expressed with a myocardial marker (MF20) in a zone of cells located at the future site where the developing leaflets will delaminate (separate) from the adjacent myocardium (Plate 6c). At such 'cleavage' sites, extracellular spaces appear, over time, which expand and coalesce resulting in partial separation of the myocardium and formation of tendinous, suspensory cords.[7] As shown in Plate 6d, some fibroblastic cells in developing tendinous cords continue to express MF20 even late into fetal life, suggesting a potential myocardial heritage. Consistent with this suggestion are cells that can be found in the 'cleavage zone' that show both mitotic nuclei and poorly organized (perhaps remnants) of striated myofibrils (Fig. 15.2). If true, this hypothesis would mean that the developing valve leaflets would *not* have to evolve a complex mechanism to hook up

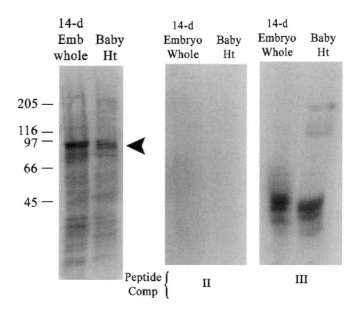

Fig. 15.1 Periostin Western blot of 14-day vs. newborn whole hearts in mice using antibody made against peptide II which completely blocked staining.

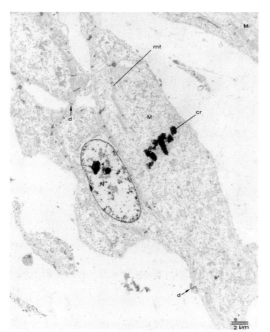

Fig. 15.2 Transmission EM of cells located in cells located at the Pn+/MF20+ interface between the cushion leaflet and myocardium. Note myofilaments (mf) are seen in a presumed myocardial cell (M) having mitotic chromosomes (cr).

with their suspensory apparatus because they would, in fact, always be in direct contact with the progenitor of the tendinous cords, i.e. the myocardial cells that co-express mesenchymal

markers (Pn, JB3 or ES130) and a striated muscle marker (MF20).[8]

Note that periostin staining is not limited to just cardiac cells but is also expressed on the surfaces of neurites extending from the neural tube (but not on cells within the tube itself) (Plate 7). This pattern of expression is consistent with its homology to fasciclins that are associated with axonal guidance in invertebrates.[9] This raises the question as to what is the potential function of periostin in valvulogenesis? Based on its expression pattern in bone and cartilage (i.e. present in osteoblasts or chondroblasts but absent in osteocytes and chondrocytes), we have proposed that periostin may promote or sustain fibrogenic differentiation and/or may inhibit mesenchymal differentiation into osteogenic or chondrogenic phenotypes.

To initially test this hypothesis, we examined periostin expression in long-term cultures of chick primary cushion mesenchymal cells. The major cushions were isolated from stage 26 chick AV canals (20+ hearts/experiment) and pooled to establish high-density cultures plated onto plastic at 50 000 cells/well. By day 14, most cultures were confluent and cells appeared homogenously mesenchymal (or fibroblastic) and expressed M38, a procollagen type I marker. There was no evidence of multilayered nodules or condensations or any marker that might have indicated chondrogenic or osteogenic differen-

BMP 2 added to "ring" cultures

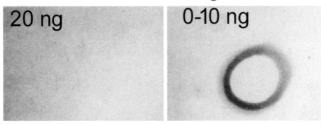

20 ng   0-10 ng

Fig. 15.3 BMP2 added to high-density cultures of cushion cells isolated from stage 26 chick hearts and cultured for 18 days. Note dense ring-like structure that forms in low levels of bone morphogenetic protein (BMP) which express Pn except at high levels.

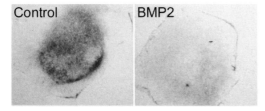

Control   BMP2

Fig. 15.4 In situ hybridization of Pn.

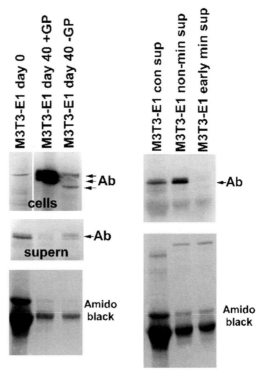

Fig. 15.5 Periostin Western blots of MC3T3 cultures +/– β-glycerophosphate.

tiation (e.g. type II collagen). On day 17, however, circular fibrous densities appeared within the cultures which grew up from the bottom of the dish into the medium (Fig. 15.3). If bone morphogenetic protein 2 (BMP2) was added to the medium (5–20 ng) at time 0 and cultures continued to day 17, the fibrous rings did not develop in the presence of 20 ng BMP2. At day 17, we examined periostin mRNA expression. While all cells expressed periostin, its expression was strongest in the developing fibrous rings (Fig. 15.4). If treated with 20 ng BMP2, message for periostin was low or absent. Thus, periostin expression correlated directly with the potential of the primary cultures to form fibrous rings. We used histological analysis to determine exactly what type of tissue was present in the fibrous rings. As shown in Plate 8, the fibrous rings were composed of dense, fibrous, collagenous tissue that expressed type I collagen (not shown), and seemed to us to be characteristic of the fibrosa layer of mature leaflets.[2] As for tissue encircled by the fibrous rings, this tissue seemed to be a mixture of poorly differentiated cells and loose fibrous tissue. However, in cultures treated with 20 ng BMP2, multiple nodules of condensed cells were present and distributed throughout the culture. Most nodules expressed type II collagen, a cartilage marker (but not periostin) (Plate 9). To fur-

ther determine if low (or suppressed) expression of periostin correlates with mesenchymal cell differentiation into chondrogenic or osteogenic lineages, we used a preosteoblastic cell line, MC3T3 (gift from Professor Amagai, Japan). These mesenchymal-like cells can be induced to form mineralized matrix if treated with β-glycerophosphate (βGP). Without such induction, they remain mesenchymal. We grew MC3T3 for 16 days with ascorbic acid (or until nodular condensations appeared) and then we added βGP and cultured for 14–24 more days. After 30 or 40 days, cultures were examined for mineralization using von Kossa staining (Plate 10) and for periostin protein expression by Western blotting (Fig. 15.5). In controls (no βGP received), periostin was expressed throughout the length of the culture. Isoforms of periostin (Pn), probably splice variants,[6] were found in both cell pellets and the supernatant (culture medium). MC3T3 cells treated with βGP formed mineralized matrix which was visualized as black precipitates stained by the von Kossa method. Such black precipitates were few or absent in controls. No or little periostin was detected in the medium. However, periostin remained detectable in the cell fraction although message was not detected (data not shown).

Thus, we tentatively conclude that periostin is expressed in cushion cells upon their transformation from endocardium and they continue to express this protein as they progressively differentiate into fibrous tissue during fetal and neonatal life. Conversely, inducible repression of periostin protein correlates with differentiation of mesenchymal cells (cushion or MC3T3) into a chondrogenic or osteogenic cell type.

Acknowledgments

Supported by NIH grants HL 19136 and 33756.

References

1 van den Hoff MJB, Kruithof BPT, Moorman FM, Markwald RR, Wessels A. Formation of the myocardium after the initial development of the linear heart tube. *Dev Biol* 2001; **240**: 61–76.

2 Icardo JM, Colvee E. Atrioventricular valves of the mouse: II. Light and transmission electron microscopy. *Anat Rec* 1995; **241**: 391–400.

3 Galvin KM, Donovan MJ, Lynch CA *et al*. A role for smad6 in development and homeostasis of the cardiovascular system. *Nat Genet* 2000; **24**: 171–4.

4 Takeshita S, Kikuno R, Tezuka K, Amann E. Osteoblastic-specific factor 2: cloning of a putative bone adhesion protein with homology with the insect protein fasiclin I. *Biochem J* 1993; **294**: 27–8.

5 Horiuchi K, Amizuka N, Takeshita S *et al*. Identification and characterization of a novel protein, *periostin*, with restricted expression to periosteum and periodontal ligament and increased expression by transforming growth factor beta. *J Bone Miner Res* 1999; **14**: 1239–49.

6 Kruzynska-Frejtag A, Machnicki M, Rogers R, Markwald RR, Conway SJ. *Periostin* (an osteoblast-specific factor) is expressed within the embryonic mouse heart during valve formation. *Mech Dev* 2001; **103**:183–8.

7 de la Cruz MV, Markwald RR. Embryological development of the ventricular inlets. Septation and atrioventricular valve apparatus. In: de la Cruz MV, Markwald RR eds. *Living Morphogenesis of the Heart*. Boston: Birkhauser (Springer-Verlag), 1998: 131–56.

8 Oosthoek PW, Wenink ACG, Vrolijk BCM *et al*. Development of the atrioventricular valve tension apparatus in the human heart. *Anat Embryol* 1998; **198**: 317–29.

9 Hortsch M, Goodman CS. *Drosophila* fasciclin 1, a neural cell adhesion molecule, has a phosphatidylinositiol lipid membrane anchor that is developmentally regulated. *J Biol Chem* 1990; **265**: 15104–09.

CHAPTER 16

Role of fibroblast growth factors in early valve leaflet formation

Yukiko Sugi, Naoki Ito, Gyorgyi Szebenyi, John F. Fallon,
Takashi Mikawa, Roger. R. Markwald

Introduction

While much has been learned about how endothelial cells transform to mesenchyme during cardiac cushion formation,[1,2] there remain fundamental questions about the developmental fate of cushions. In the atrioventricular (AV) inlets and outlet segments, cushion mesenchyme distally elongates producing bulges that project into each lumen. In the present work, we focus on the early stages of growth and development of cushion mesenchyme. Secreted growth factors are reasonable candidates for regulating these early events in valvulogenesis. Fibroblast growth factors (FGFs) belong to a structurally related heparin-binding protein family that regulate tissue differentiation and patterning[3,4] and act as potent mitogens for endothelial and mesenchymal cells.[5] In the present study, we have localized mRNA of FGF receptors (FGFR) 1, 2, and 3, and FGF ligands, FGF4 and FGF8, in developing cardiac cushion tissue during the initial proliferative period of early valvulogenesis. Based on these data, we performed the following experiments to test the hypothesis that FGF pathways play regulatory roles in cushion mesenchymal cell proliferation and elongation into prevalvular structure.

Results

Localization of FGF proteins and FGF receptor mRNA at the onset of valve formation

FGF4 protein was localized in atrial and ventricular myocardium throughout all stages (14–27) in chick embryos examined, including AV myocardium adjacent to the forming AV cardiac valves (Plate 11a). Cytoplasmic expression of FGF4 was detected in AV and OT cushion mesenchymal cells as well as AV endocardial endothelial cells. Interestingly, FGF8 protein was localized intensely on the luminal surface of the AV and OT cardiac valves (Plate 11b). Ligand distribution was also compared to FGFR expression. *In situ* hybridization data indicated that like FGF8, FGFR3 mRNA was confined to the endocardial rim of the AV cushion pads (Plate 11e,f), whereas FGFR2 was expressed exclusively in cushion mesenchymal cells (Plate 11d). FGFR1 expression like FGF4, was detected in both endocardium and cushion mesenchyme as well as in myocardium (Plate 11c).

Effect of exogenously added FGF4 on BrdU incorporation by cultured cardiac cushion mesenchymal cells

To determine if FGF4 exerted an effect on AV cushion mesenchymal cell proliferation, FGF4 was added to the medium of cultured AV cushion mesenchymal cells. AV cushion mesenchymal cells were cultured in SFM (medium 199 supplemented only with insulin, transferring, and selenium) with or without FGF4. BrdU incorporation assay provides an index of proliferation activity in cultured mesenchymal cells. As indicated in Plate 12e, as little as 10 ng/mL of FGF4 resulted in a 50% increase in the proliferative activity of mesenchymal cells.

Microinjection of FGF4 retrovirus into cushion tissue

To evaluate the effect of FGF4 on cardiac valve formation *in vivo*, FGF4 retrovirus[6] was pressure injected into cardiac cushion mesenchyme. Cushion mesenchymal cells injected *in vivo* with FGF4 virus indicated dense populations of β-gal-viral markers-positive cells and expansion of mesenchyme into the lumen (arrow, Plate 12a,b), suggesting proliferative expansion of the cushion. Control β-gal virus injected cushion mesenchyme showed normal development (not shown). None of the nine β-gal virus microinjected embryos showed any luminal expansion of cushion mesenchyme, while seven out of eight FGF4+β-gal virally injected embryos clearly demonstrated luminal expansion of β-gal positive cushion mesenchyme. Similar morphological changes were found both in outlet and inlet cushion mesenchyme.

Microinjection of FGF4 protein into cushion tissue

As shown in Plate 12d, FGF4 injected cushion mesenchyme increased the percentage of BrdU labeled mesenchymal cells (indicated by lighter color in Plate 12d) including those seen in cushions that protruded toward the lumen as compared to BSA-injected control (Plate 12c). Quantitative evaluation of the BrdU incorporation assay shows that FGF4 microinjection into the cushion tissue caused a statistically significant increase in BrdU incorporation of mesenchymal cells as compared to BSA injected controls (Plate 12f). Moreover, BSA injected control samples tended to show more BrdU positive cells near the luminal surface of the cushion, while FGF4 injected samples exhibited more BrdU positive cells in the central part of the cushion, which suggests that FGF4 injection altered (i.e. expanded) the normal distribution of BrdU positive cells.

Discussion

Our present work indicated that FGF4 was expressed in cushion mesenchymal cells in the chick (Plate 11a) and FGF8 was expressed in luminal surface of the valve in the mouse (Plate 11b), that exogenously added FGF4 induced proliferation of cushion mesenchymal cells *in vitro* (Plate 12e) and *in vivo* (*ovo*) (Plate 12c,d), and that FGF4 overexpression induced precocious extension of cushion mesenchyme into the lumen (Plate 12a,b), indicat-

ing a role of the FGF pathway in early leaflet formation. Our *in situ* hybridization data for localizing FGF receptors also support a signaling role for FGF ligands in valvulogenesis. It is presently unclear how these distinctively restricted patterns of expression for FGF receptors might interact to regulate various phases of early valvulogenesis, particularly FGFR3. It is possible that this receptor merely serves to keep the endocardium growing at a pace commensurate with cushion mesenchymal growth. However, the similarity of FGFR3 expression to that of nuclear factor activated T cells (NFATc)[7,8] may suggest another role during valvulogenesis.

It remains to be determined whether FGF signaling also interacts with other candidate regulatory molecules. In addition to simply promoting proliferation, it will be of interest to know how FGF signaling modulates or interacts with other regulatory molecules to potentially regulate further morphological changes in valve formation such as delamination from myocardium, differentiation into a myofibroblastic lineage or formation of the supporting tension apparatus.

Acknowledgement

This work was supported by NIH Grant, HL 33756 and 52813 to RRM and YS.

References

1 de la Cruz MV, Markwald RR. Embryological development of the ventricular inlets. Septation and atrioventricular valve apparatus. In: de la Cruz MV, Markwald RR, eds. *Living Morphogenesis of the Heart.* Boston, MA: Birkhauser, 1998: 131–55.

2 Eisenberg LM, Markwald RR. Molecular regulation of atrioventricular valvuloseptal morphogenesis. *Circ Res* 1995; **77:** 1–6.

3 Sugi Y, Sasse J, Lough J. Inhibition of precardiac mesoderm cell proliferation by antisense oligodeoxynucleotide complementary to fibroblast growth factor-2 (FGF2). *Dev Biol* 1993; **157:** 28–37.

4 Sugi Y, Sasse J, Barron M, Lough J. Developmental expression of fibroblast growth factor receptor-1 (*cek-1; flg*) during heart development. *Dev Dyn* 1995; **202:** 115–25.

5 Szebenyi G, Fallon JF. Fibroblast growth factors as multifunctional signaling factors. *Int Rev Cytol* 1999: **185:** 45–106.

6 Mikawa T. Retroviral targeting of FGF and FGFR in cardiomyocyte and coronary vascular cells during heart development. *Ann NY Acad Sci* 1995; **752**: 506–16.

7 de la Pompa JL Timmerman LA, Takimoto H *et al.* Role of the NF-ATc transcription factor in morphogenesis of cardiac valves and septum. *Nature* 1998; **392**: 182–6.

8 Ranger AM, Grusby MJ, Hodge MR *et al.* The transcription factor NF-ATc is essential for cardiac valve formation. *Nature* 1998; **392**: 186–90.

CHAPTER 17

Msx1 expression during chick heart development: possible role in endothelial–mesenchymal transformation during cushion tissue formation

*Toshiyuki Yamagishi, Yuji Nakajima, Katsumi Ando,
Hiroaki Nakamura*

Epithelial–mesenchymal transformation is a critical event in various developmental processes. During the early stages of heart development, endothelial cells in the atrioventricular (AV) and outflow tract (OT) regions change their phenotype to that of mesenchyme (endothelial–mesenchymal transformation, EMT), and form endocardial cushion tissue, a primordium of the valves and septa of the four-chambered heart. Maldevelopment of the endocardial cushion tissue causes various types of congenital heart defects not only in the AV canal, but also in the OT region.[1] *In vitro* assays have shown that this EMT is prompted by unknown signals produced by the subjacent AV myocardium in a spatiotemporally restricted manner.[2] Previously, we reported that transforming growth factor β3 (TGFβ3) is expressed in the transforming endothelial and invading mesenchymal cells, and that bone morphogenetic protein 2 (BMP2) and BMP5 are in the AV and OT myocardium during endocardial cushion tissue formation in the chick. Our *in vitro* analysis showed that at the onset of this EMT, TGFβ and BMP act synergistically with each other to induce not only the initial phenotypic changes characteristic of this phenomenon, but also mesenchymal cell invasion.[3–8] We are still unclear, however, of the

mechanism underlying this BMP-TGFβ synergy during EMT.

Msx is an ortholog related to the *Drosophila msh* (muscle-segment homeobox) gene and has been identified in many vertebrates, including zebrafish, frog, chick, mouse, and human.[9] During development, the *Msx1* gene is expressed in the inductive regions, in which the epithelial–mesenchymal interaction occurs extensively (such as migrating cranial neural crest cells, pharyngeal arches, tooth bud, somatopleura, limb bud, and heart).[9] Recent genetic approaches have revealed that Msx1-deficient mice are affected by cleft palate as well as abnormalities of craniofacial and tooth development.[10] Msx2 null-mutant mice display defects of skeletal organ, tooth, hair follicle, and mammary gland development. These observations suggest that *Msx* genes are essential for the regulation of cell-to-cell or cell-to-tissue communication during epithelial–mesenchymal interaction.[11]

In the present study, we investigated the spatiotemporal expression of Msx1 and its role in EMT during chick endocardial cushion tissue formation. *In situ* hybridization and immunohistochemistry revealed intense Msx1 signals in the endothelial/mesenchymal cells of the OT and AV regions at stages 14–23, during which EMT occurs extensively. Once cushion tissue formation was complete, Msx1 transcripts were seen in the cushion tissue mesenchyme until the end of the embryonic stage (stage 33). The spatiotemporal expression pattern seen for Msx1 suggests that this homeobox gene may play an important role not only in the initiation of EMT, but also in the maintenance of the cushion mesenchyme.

To try to determine whether Msx1 is required for the initiation of EMT, we cultured AV explants (preactivated endocardium + associated myocardium) from stage 14 hearts on collagen gel lattice, and treated them with antisense oligodeoxynucleotides (ODN) specific for chick Msx1 (Table 17.1). After 48 h, explants cultured with CM199 or missense ODN (2 μM) showed mesenchymal cell invasion into the gel lattice revealed to a similar extent, but in explants cultured with antisense Msx1 ODN (2 μM), this invasion was inhibited. Quantitative RT-PCR and immunocytochemistry revealed that Msx1 expression was significantly suppressed in explants treated with antisense-Msx1. These results suggest that antisense-Msx1 ODN affects the expression of the Msx1 message at the mRNA level, a perturbation that might inhibit the initiation of EMT. We next examined the expression of EMT-specific marker genes in cultured explants with or without perturbation. Quantitative RT-PCR revealed that transcripts of EMT-specific marker genes (smooth muscle α-actin, type I collagen, and fibrillin-2) were suppressed in explants treated with antisense-Msx1 ODN.

In order to test the effects of TGFβ and BMP on *Msx1* gene expression during EMT, preactivated AV endothelial monolayers from stage 14 hearts were prepared on collagen gel lattice and cultured with CM199, associated myocardium, TGFβ2 or -β3, BMP4 (a substitute for BMP2), or TGFβ + BMP4. The resulting cultures were examined to see whether they did or did not express Msx1 at the mRNA and protein levels (Table 17.2). In this experiment, endothelial cells treated with TGFβ3 (5 ng/mL) showed only the initial phenotypic changes seen in EMT (cell: cell separation, cellular hypertrophy, and migratory appendage formation on the gel surface), and they seeded few mesenchymal cells into the gel lattice. Cells treated with BMP4 displayed none of phenotypic changes of EMT.[4,6,7] In contrast, endothelial cells cultured with both TGFβ3 (5 ng/mL) and BMP4 (1 μg/mL) exhibited endothelial cell migration on the gel surface and seeded many mesenchymal cells into the gel lattice.[7]

Table 17.1 AV explant cultures treated with antisense ODN to Msx1

Culture conditions	No. of invaded mesenchymal cells (mean ± SE)
CM199	122 ± 7 (n = 73)
Missense ODN (2 μM)	85 ± 10 (n = 15)
Antisense-Msx1 ODN (2 μM)	23 ± 5 (n = 14)

AV explants prepared from stage 14 chick embryonic hearts were cultured under various conditions in a 3-D collagen gel-culture system. Antisense-Msx1 ODN (oligodeoxynucleotides), but not missense ODN, inhibited mesenchymal cell invasion into the gel lattice ($P < 0.05$, Mann–Whitney U-test). CM199, medium 199 containing 1% chick serum; n, number of explants examined.

Table 17.2 Effects of TGFβ and BMP on expression of Msx1 in preactivated AV endothelial cells

Culture conditions	Mesenchymal invasion	Msx1 expression
CM199	−	−
Myocardium	+++	+++
TGFβ2	±	−
TGFβ3	±	−
BMP4	−	+
TGFβ2 + BMP4	+	+
TGFβ3 + BMP4	+	+

Different types of AV endothelial cultures were analyzed by RT-PCR and immunocytochemistry for Msx1 expression. AV endothelial monolayers obtained from stage 14 hearts were cultured with CM199, associated myocardium, TGFβ, BMP4, or TGFβ+BMP4. When the endothelial cells were cultured with CM199 alone or with TGFβ (5 ng/mL), Msx1 expression was not observed. In contrast, when cells were cultured with myocardium or with BMP4 (1 μg/mL), Msx1 expression was observed. Combined administration of TGFβ +BMP4 also induced Msx1 expression, but the amount of Msx1 expression was no different than in cultures treated with BMP4 alone. Note that endothelial cells treated with TGFβ alone showed the initial phenotypic changes characteristic of EMT.

RT-PCR and immunocytochemistry revealed that endothelial cells cultured with associated myocardium expressed Msx1 extensively. Preactivated endothelial cells cultured with BMP4 expressed Msx1; however, the amount of Msx1 expressed in this culture condition was less than that induced by associated myocardium. Following combined administration of TGFβ + BMP4, the amount of Msx1 expression was no different than in cultures treated with BMP alone. On the other hand, cells cultured in CM199 alone or with TGFβ did not express Msx1 at all. These results indicate that BMP does not induce any of the phenotypic changes characteristic of EMT in preactivated AV endothelial cells, but that it does induce the *Msx1* gene that is required to initiate EMT. This suggests that Msx, being downstream of BMP-signaling, may play an important role in the synergistic effect that BMP and TGFβ during the formation of endocardial cushion tissue.

In the present paper, we have examined the spatiotemporal expression of Msx1 and the possible role of this homeobox gene in endocardial cushion tissue formation. Our results show that; (1) Msx1 is expressed in the transforming endothelial and invading mesenchymal cells at the onset of EMT; (2) Msx1 is required to initiate BMP/TGFβ-dependent EMT, and lies downstream of BMP signaling, but not of TGFβ. They also suggest that Msx1 may have a key role to play in the synergistic effect of BMP and TGFβ during EMT. Further experiments will be necessary to clarify the mechanisms underlying the synergistic effect of these growth factors.

References

1 Nakajima Y, Hiruma T, Nakazawa M, Morishima M. Hypoplasia of cushion ridges in the proximal outflow tract elicits formation of a right ventricle-to-aortic route in retinoic acid-induced complete transposition of the great arteries in the mouse: scanning electron microscopic observations of corrosion cast models. *Anat Rec* 1996; **245**: 76–82.

2 Mjaatvedt CH, Krug EL, Markwald RR. An antiserum (ES1) against a particulate form of extracellular matrix blocks the transition of cardiac endothelium into mesenchyme in culture. *Dev Biol* 1991; **145**: 219–30.

3 Nakajima Y, Mironov V, Yamagishi T, Nakamura H, Markwald RR. Expression of smooth muscle α-actin in mesenchymal cells during formation of avian endocardial cushion tissue: a role for transforming growth factor β3. *Dev Dyn* 1997; **209**: 296–309.

4 Nakajima Y, Yamagishi T, Nakamura H, Markwald RR, Krug EL. An autocrine function for transforming growth factor (TGF)-β3 in the transformation of atrioventricular canal endocardium into mesenchyme during chick heart development. *Dev Biol* 1998; **194**: 99–113.

5 Yamagishi T, Nakajima Y, Nakamura H. Expression of TGF β3 RNA during chick embryogenesis: a possible important role in cardiovascular development. *Cell Tissue Res* 1999; **298**: 285–93.

6 Nakajima Y, Yamagishi T, Hokari S, Nakamura H. Mechanisms involved in valvuloseptal endocardial cushion formation in early cardiogenesis: roles of transforming growth factor (TGF)-β and bone morphogenetic protein (BMP). *Anat Rec* 2000; **258**: 119–27.

7 Yamagishi T, Nakajima Y, Miyazono K, Nakamura H. Bone morphogenetic protein-2 acts synergistically with transforming growth factor-β3 during endothelial-mesenchymal transformation in the developing chick heart. *J Cell Physiol* 1999; **180**: 35–45.

8 Yamagishi T, Nakajima Y, Nishimatsu S *et al.* Expression of bone morphogenetic protein-5 gene during chick heart development: possible roles in valvuloseptal endocardial cushion formation. *Anat Rec* 2001; **264**: 313–16.

9 Davidson D. The function and evolution of Msx genes: pointers and paradoxes. *Trend Genet* 1995; **11**: 405–11.

10 Satokata I, Maas R. Msx1 deficient mice exhibit cleft palate and abnormalities of craniofacial and tooth development. *Nat Genet* 1994; **6**: 348–56.

11 Satokata I, Ma L. Ohshima H *et al.* Msx2 deficiency in mice causes pleiotropic defects in bone growth and ectodermal organ formation. *Nat Genet* 2000; **24**: 391–95.

PART 4

Segment and chamber specification

Editorial perspective

D. Woodrow Benson

The papers in this section deal with the topic of cardiac chamber specification. Better understanding of the critical steps involved in chamber specification is expected to provide improved insight into both the evolution of heart development, e.g. the number and type of cardiac chambers differs across species, and the pathogenesis of important human congenital heart defects involving cardiac chamber hypoplasia. The regulatory mechanisms governing the processes of cardiac chamber specification remain unclear. While an increasing number of examples of chamber-specific gene expression have been recognized, to date no universal mechanism has been identified.

In the study presented by Ogura, expression patterns of *Tbx5* and *Tbx20* during cardiogenesis in chick and mouse embryos were examined. *Tbx5* expression becomes restricted to the posterior part of the heart tube, and later is further restricted to the atria and the left ventricle. The ventricular septum is formed at the boundary of *Tbx5*-positive and negative domains. These observations lead to the hypothesis that *Tbx5* specifies the left ventricle and the position of ventricular septum. In search of putative right ventricle-specific *Tbx* gene(s), chick *Tbx20* is expressed in a complementary fashion, hence expressed in the *Tbx5*-negative right ventricle.

The paper by Srivastava explores the molecular and physiologic cues that initiate ventricular specification, growth, and hypertrophy. These studies reveal genetic

and epigenetic events that regulate ventricular development and provide evidence for primary defects in expansion of cardiac chambers as a potential etiology for subsets of hypoplastic right or left ventricular conditions. The conservation of the transcriptional network necessary for ventricular development across species aided these studies. In addition to transcriptional networks, there is growing evidence that epigenetic factors are critical for ventricular morphogenesis by virtue of their ability to regulate gene expression through chromatin remodeling events. Taken together these studies establish the beginnings of a roadmap to understand how some myocytes specify to become ventricular cells and then expand into a functional ventricular chamber.

The studies of Kelly *et al.* examined the extent to which cells derived from the anterior or secondary heart field (AHF) contribute to the developing heart. Evidence presented in this paper indicates that in the mouse, future right ventricular myocardium is predominantly AHF-derived. Further, the addition of future right ventricle to the linear heart tube marks the initiation of rightward looping, suggesting that the AHF contributes laterality information to the developing heart and may also contribute mechanistically to rightward looping.

Moorman *et al.* studied expression patterns of atrial natriuretic factor (Anf) in *Xenopus* embryos. The function of Anf during development is unknown, but it has been suggested to play a role in cardiomyocyte proliferation. Findings in this paper, similar to those reported in mammals and avian species, show that Anf is not expressed in the so-called primary myocardium of the linear heart tube and remains absent from those cardiac regions that do not develop into chamber my-ocardium, i.e. the inflow tract, atrioventricular canal, inner curvature, and outflow tract. Improved understanding of the regulation of chamber-specific Anf expression should improve our understanding of cardiac development.

CHAPTER 18

Tbx5 specifies the left/right ventricles and ventricular septum position during cardiogenesis

Toshihiko Ogura

T-box (*Tbx*) genes play pivotal roles during development of both vertebrate and invertebrate embryos. *Tbx* genes encode transcription factors that are characterized by a highly conserved DNA-binding domain (T-box).[1–3] The biological functions of *Tbx* genes have been investigated by *in ovo* electroporation in chick and gene targeting in mice.[4–13]

One of most well characterized is *Tbx5*, which is expressed in forelimb buds and the dorsal retina. We and another group have reported that *Tbx5* is a critical determinant of wing (forelimb).[4,5] In addition, *Tbx5* regulates pattern formation of the eye and the retinotectum projection.[6] The roles played by *Tbx5* during heart development, however, remain unclear, although mutations of human *TBX5* were found in patients with Holt–Oram syndrome (OMIM 142900).[14–16] In such patients, characteristic defects of the upper limb and heart are observed.[17]

To investigate the roles played by *Tbx5* during cardiogenesis, we examined its expression patterns in developing embryos. In both chick and mouse, *Tbx5* is expressed in the precardiac mesoderm. This expression then becomes restricted to the posterior part of the heart tube. Later, *Tbx5* expression is further restricted to the atria and the left ventricle, and a ventricular septum is formed at the boundary of *Tbx5*-positive and negative domains (Plate 13). These observations lead us to the hypothesis that *Tbx5* specifies the left ventricles and the position of ventricular septum.

Vertebrates exhibit different heart morphologies: fishes have one ventricle/one atrium. In contrast, both birds and mammals have two ventricles/two atria. Since *Tbx5* is expressed in the left ventricle, this gene could be useful for exploring evolution of vertebrate hearts, ventricle specification, and onset of congenital heart diseases. For this purpose, we performed extensive *in ovo* electroporation in chick embryos to misexpress *Tbx5* in the developing heart. In addition, we made a series of transgenic mice to explore further in mammalian hearts.

When Tbx5 was misexpressed ubiquitously, several anomalous alterations were found in the electroporated hearts (Plate 14). First, the formation of the ventricular septum was completely inhibited, resulting in a single ventricle. Second, a large dilatation of the atria was also observed. Third, the ventricular wall was thinner than that of the normal heart, and the trabecular formation was coarse and rough. Fourth, the aorta and pulmonary artery were fused and connected to the single anomalous ventricle, resulting in a double outlet left ventricle (DOLV). Although the truncal septum was formed, the conal septation and/or the conal rotation seemed to be abnormal. These morphologic changes suggest that misexpression of *Tbx5* induces aberrant differentiation of cardiac muscle cells,[18,19] suppression of ventricular septum formation, and malformation of the conotruncal septum, resulting in a complex of cardiac defects.

When misexpression was spatially partial, the left ventricle expanded, and the right ventricle shrank, with a distinct VSD (Plate 15). The relative sizes of the two ventricles suggested that the ventricular septum was shifted to the right. Conal septation and rotation defects were also observed. The atrial septum was formed, but it was membranous and thin. Trabecular formation and the thickness of the ventricular wall were not affected.

We also misexpressed the *Tbx5* gene in a restricted domain of developing hearts to make an ectopic boundary of *Tbx5*-positive and *Tbx5*-negative regions in the developing right ventricle. In such hearts, three domains were formed from the left side to the right: (1) an endogenous *Tbx5*-positive domain (the prospective left ventricle); (2) a *Tbx5*-negative area (the prospective right ventricle); (3) an ectopic *Tbx5*-positive area. Hence this restricted expression results in the extra boundary formation of *Tbx5*-positive and *Tbx5*-negative regions in the prospective right ventricle. In serial sections of these hearts, extension of trabeculae was observed. This accelerated growth of trabeculae suggests that an ectopic septum was induced at the new boundary of *Tbx5* expression. *In situ* hybridization using several septum markers, such as *BMP2, Tll-1* (*tolloid-like 1*), and *VEGF* (*vascular endothelial growth factor*),[20–24] detected clear expression of these septum markers, suggesting that restricted expression of *Tbx5* in the right ventricle induces an ectopic ventricular septum at the new border of *Tbx5* expression.

To confirm further, we made two expression constructs to target transgene expression in developing mouse hearts (Plate 16). One is a mouse *Tbx5* expression construct in which the β-MHC (myosin heavy chain) promoter was used to misexpress this gene uniformly in the ventricle.[19,20] In another construct, we used the *MLC-2v* (*myosin light chain*) promoter, which was reported to drive transgene expression in the right ventricle.[25]

When *Tbx5* was misexpressed uniformly with the β-*MHC* promoter, several morphologic changes were observed (Plate 16). First, both *eHAND* and *mANF* genes were induced almost to the right end of the developing ventricle, whereas expression of the *dHAND* gene was found to be repressed completely. Furthermore, septum formation was completely suppressed in such hearts. Instead, a tiny bulge of ventricular wall was formed in a small *eHAND/mANF*-negative region.

On the other hand, the ventricular septum formed normally in hearts of the *MLC2v-Tbx5* transgenic mice, although the right ventricle appeared to be enlarged (Plate 16). In this enlarged right ventricle, the m*ANF* gene was induced strongly. Likewise the *eHAND* gene was induced, albeit expression disappeared near the septum. In this *eHAND*-negative domain near the septum, expression of the *dHAND* gene was detected, although this gene was completely suppressed in the remaining part of the right ventricle.

Overall, these lines of evidence strongly suggest that the forced expression of *Tbx5* gene in the prospective right ventricle converts expression patterns of several right and left ventricular markers with extensive morphologic alterations.

In search of putative right ventricle-specific *Tbx* gene(s), we have found that chick *Tbx20* is expressed in a complementary fashion, hence expressed in the *Tbx5*-negative right ventricle (Plate 17). Recently, knockdown of zebrafish T-box gene *hrT* gene (*Tbx20*) resulted in upregulation of *Tbx5*. Conversely, misexpression of *hrT* induced downregulation of *Tbx5*. These data indicate that hrT regulates *Tbx5* expression in zebrafish.[26] To confirm this, we misexpressed Tbx20 in developing chick heart. As expected, expression of *Tbx5* in the left ventricle diminished, albeit weakly. In addition, the boundary of *Tbx5* expression became fuzzy and unclear. This indicates that Tbx20 regulates *Tbx5* expression also in chick heart, implying that mutually repressive actions of Tbx5 and Tbx20 are pivotal for the establishment of the right and left ventricles (Plate 18).

As mentioned previously, vertebrates exhibit different heart morphologies: fishes possess one ventricle/one atrium; amphibians, one ventricle/two atria; reptiles, two incomplete ventricles/two atria; and birds/mammals, two complete ventricles/two atria. Although we have not yet expanded our analysis to other vertebrates, the *Tbx5* and *Tbx20* genes could be good markers for exploring the evolution of heart morphology in various vertebrate animals. Our data provide important insights on cardiac development, the onset of human congenital heart diseases, and the evolution of vertebrate hearts. Although we are far from a complete understanding, precise molecular analysis of the *Tbx5* gene would provide valuable information for the comprehensive understanding of vertebrate pattern formation.

Acknowledgments

We thank Dr. Katherine E. Yutzey for providing the *β-MHC* promoter construct, Drs. Malcolm P. Logan and Cliff Tabin for the chick and mouse *HAND* genes and Dr. K.Inoue for *Zebrafish* cDNA. This work was supported by a Grant-in-Aid for Scientific Research on Priority Areas (C) from the Ministry of Education, Science Sports and Culture of Japan, Special Coordination Funds for Promoting Science and Technology from the Science and Technology Agency, Creative Basic Research from the Ministry of Education, Science Sports and Culture of Japan, the Uehara Memorial Foundation, the Inamori Foundation and the Toray Science Foundation.

References

1 Kispert A, Herrmann BG. The Brachyury gene encodes a novel DNA binding protein. *EMBO J* 1993; **12**: 3211–20.

2 Muller C, Herrmann BG. Crystallographic structure of the T domain-DNA complex of the Brachyury transcription factor. *Nature* 1997; **389**: 884–8.

3 Smith J. T-box genes: what they do and how they do it. *Trends Genet* 1999; **15**: 154–8.

4 Takeuchi JK *et al*. *Tbx5* and *Tbx4* genes determine the wing/leg identity of limb buds. *Nature* 1999: **398**: 810–14.

5 Rodriguez-Esteban C *et al*. The T-box genes Tbx4 and Tbx5 regulate limb outgrowth and identity. *Nature* 1999; **398**: 814–18.

6 Koshiba-Takeuchi K *et al*. Tbx5 and the retinotectum projection. *Science* 2000; **287**: 134–37.

7 Wilkinson DG *et al*. Expression pattern of the mouse T gene and its role in mesoderm formation. *Nature* 1990; **343**: 657–9.

8 Chapman DL, Papaioannou VE. Three neural tubes in mouse embryos with mutations in the T-box gene Tbx6. *Nature* 1998; **391**: 695–7.

9 Jerome LA, Papaioannou VE. DiGeorge syndrome phenotype in mice mutant for the T-box gene, Tbx1. *Nat. Genet* 2001; **27**: 286–91.

10 Lindsay EA *et al*. Tbx1 haploinsufficieny in the DiGeorge syndrome region causes aortic arch defects in mice. *Nature* 2001; **410**: 97–101.

11 Merscher S *et al*. TBX1 is responsible for cardiovascular defects in velo-cardio-facial/DiGeorge syndrome. *Cell* 2001; **104**: 619–29.

12 Bruneau BG *et al*. A murine model of Holt–Oram syndrome defines roles of the T-box transcription factor Tbx5 in cardiogenesis and disease. *Cell* 2001; **106**: 709–21.

13 Russ AP *et al*. Eomesodermin is required for mouse trophoblast development and mesoderm formation. *Nature* 2000; **404**: 95–9.

14 Basson CT *et al*. Mutations in human TBX5 cause limb and cardiac malformation in Holt–Oram syndrome. *Nat Genet* 1997; **15**; 30–5.

15 Li QY *et al*. Holt–Oram syndrome is caused by mutations in TBX5, a member of the Brachyury (T) gene family. *Nat Genet* 1997; **15**: 21–9.

16 Basson CT *et al*. Different TBX5 interactions in heart and limb defined by Holt–Oram syndrome mutations. *Proc Natl Acad Sci USA* 1999; **96**; 2919–24.

17 Holt M, Oram S. Familial heart disease with skeletal malformations. *Br Heart J* 1960; **22**: 236–42.

18 Hatcher CJ *et al*. TBX5 transcription factor regulates cell proliferation during cardiogenesis. *Dev Biol* 2001; **230**: 177–88.

19 Liberatore CM *et al*. Ventricular expression of tbx5 inhibits normal heart chamber development. *Dev Biol* 2000; **223**: 169–80.

20 Lyons KM *et al*. Organogenesis and pattern formation in the mouse: RNA distribution patterns suggest a role for bone morphogenetic protein-2A (BMP-2A). *Development* 1990; **109**: 833–44.

21 Lyons KM *et al*. Colocalization of BMP 7 and BMP 2 RNAs suggests that these factors cooperatively mediate tissue interactions during murine development. *Mech Dev* 1995; **50**: 71–83.

22 Clark TG *et al*. The mammalian Tolloid-like 1 gene, Tll1, is necessary for normal septation and positioning of the heart. *Development* 1999; **126**: 2631–42.

23 Tomanek RJ *et al*. Vascular endothelial growth factor expression coincides with coronary vasculogenesis and angiogenesis. *Dev Dyn* 1999; **215**: 54–61.

24 Miquerol L *et al*. Embryonic development is disrupted by modest increases in vascular endothelial growth factor gene expression. *Development* 2000; **127**: 3941–6.

25 Ross RS *et al*. An HF-1a/HF-1b/MEF-2 combinatorial element confers cardiac ventricular specificity and establishes an anterior-posterior gradient of expression. *Development* 1996; **122**: 1799–809.

26 Szeto DP, Griffin KJ, Kimelman D. HrT is required for cardiovascular development in zebrafish. *Development* 2002; **129**: 5093–5101.

CHAPTER 19

Transcriptional regulation of ventricular morphogenesis

Deepak Srivastava

Hypoplasia of either the right or left ventricle is compatible with intrauterine life but has lethal consequences in the newborn period. Although rare, the severity of hypoplastic ventricular conditions results in the single largest contribution to childhood mortality from congenital heart disease. Understanding the molecular and physiologic cues that initiate ventricular specification, growth, and enlargement is essential for future diagnostic, preventive, and therapeutic approaches. The discovery of numerous cardiac-specific transcription factors has begun to establish a network of events that regulate ventricular morphogenesis. These studies have revealed genetic and epigenetic events that regulate ventricular development and provide evidence for primary defects in expansion of cardiac chambers as a potential etiology for subsets of hypoplastic right or left ventricular conditions.

Ventricular-specific DNA-binding transcription factors

A segmental ballooning model of cardiogenesis illustrates that distinct regions of the heart are instructed to contribute to specific cardiac chambers (Plate 19).[1] The first entry into identification of chamber-specific transcription factors that might regulate this process came several years ago with the isolation of two proteins belonging to the basic helix-loop-helix (bHLH) family of transcription factors, dHAND and eHAND. While these two proteins are co-expressed throughout the linear heart tube in the chick and appear to have genetic redundancy,[2] they have chamber-specific expression pat-

terns in the mouse. Both are co-expressed in the cardiac crescent, but *dHAND* gradually becomes restricted mostly to the right ventricle and outflow tract with lower expression in the left ventricle. In contrast, *eHAND* is expressed in the outflow tract and left ventricular segments but is excluded from the right ventricular precursors as early as the straight heart tube stage.[3,4]

Hearts of mice lacking *dHAND* form normally until the straight heart tube stage, at which time *eHAND* becomes downregulated from the right ventricle. Soon thereafter, the right ventricular precursors undergo programmed cell death, presumably because this is the domain lacking any eHAND protein, resulting in a hypoplastic right ventricle.[3,5] eHAND also seems to be necessary for development of left ventricular cells,[6–8] and is absent in mice lacking the cardiac homeobox gene, *Nkx2.5*, which have only one ventricle.[4] Mice lacking *dHAND* and *Nkx2.5* are null for both *HAND* genes and fail to form any ventricular chamber,[5] consistent with the notion of genetic redundancy between *dHAND* and *eHAND*. A heart is still distinguishable, but consists only of an atrial chamber, as defined by atrial-specific markers. Interestingly, a small group of ventricular cells are specified and congregate on the ventral surface of the atrium, but fail to expand ventrally to form a chamber, supporting the 'ballooning' model of ventriculogenesis.[9] dHAND and Nkx2.5 are together necessary for expression of the ventricular-specific homeobox gene, *Irx4*, in this subdomain, consistent with the partial downregulation of *Irx4* in each single mutant.[10] In chick, Irx4 is sufficient to activate ventricular-specific gene expression and suppress atrial-specific genes,[11] suggesting that regulation of *Irx4* may in part contribute to defects in ventriculogenesis.

The transcriptional network necessary for ventricular development appears tightly conserved across species. Large-scale mutagenesis of zebrafish, which have only a single ventricular chamber and a single atrial chamber, yielded a mutant line of fish that was deficient in ventricular precursors (*hands-off*), similar to mice lacking expression of both *HAND* genes. Positional cloning of the affected locus revealed point mutations in *dHAND*,[12] the one *HAND* gene present in zebrafish,[13] consistent with the role of *HAND* genes defined in mice.

Epigenetic factors regulating ventricular development

In addition to the DNA-binding proteins described above, there is growing evidence that epigenetic factors are critical for ventricular morphogenesis by virtue of their ability to regulate gene expression through chromatin remodeling events. Covalent modification of the amino-terminal tails of histones, particularly H3 and H4, regulates higher order chromatin structure and gene expression. Modifications include acetylation of specific lysine residues (e.g. lysine-9 of histone H3) by histone acetyl transferases (HATs), deacetylation by histone deacetylases (HDACs), phosphorylation (serine-10 of histone H3) by kinases and, most recently, methylation of lysine-9 of histone H3 by histone methyl transferases (HMTs).[14–16]

mBop is expressed specifically in cardiac and skeletal muscle during development and contains two interesting domains that promote condensation of heterochromatin resulting in transcriptional silencing.[17] The mBop protein contains a MYND domain most similar to that of the ETO protein whose fusion with the AML1 protein in chronic myelogenous leukemia converts AML1, normally a transcriptional activator, into a transcriptional repressor.[18,19] The MYND domain of ETO is essential for this conversion and appears to function by recruiting the nuclear co-repressor, N-CoR, which in turn recruits the Sin3/HDAC complex to DNA sites specified by AML1 binding. mBop also recruits HDACs through the MYND domain and functions as a transcriptional repressor in part through this mechanism.[17]

It is unique that mBop also contains a SET domain that, in other proteins, contains the catalytic domain necessary for HMT activity.[20] Most of the essential residues for HMT activity are conserved in mBop, suggesting that it plays a role through regulation of the methylation state of histones. It is interesting that the lysine residues of histone tails that get methylated must first be deacetylated, raising the possibility that mBop is able to both recruit HDACS to 'prepare' specific residues, and subsequently methylate those residues.

Investigation of the *in vivo* function of mBop was undertaken by targeted disruption in mice.[17] Mouse embryos lacking mBop displayed right ventricular hypoplasia and immature ventricular cardiomyocytes; surprisingly, atrial cardiomyocytes appeared to differentiate normally. This phenotype was similar but more severe than that observed in mice lacking *dHAND*. Consistent with this, mBop was required for *dHAND* expression in the precardiac mesoderm, well before right ventricular formation, suggesting that regulation of *dHAND* may contribute to the right ventricular hypoplasia in *Bop* mutants. Consistent with mBop's effects on dHAND, *Irx4* was also downregulated in *Bop* mutants. Because mBop likely functions *in vivo* as a repressor of transcription, it is likely that there is an intermediate protein regulated by mBop that subsequently affects *dHAND* transcription and further downstream events. Identification of the molecular steps leading to mBop regulation of dHAND may yield insights into the precise targets to which mBop is recruited.

Summary

We have established the beginnings of a roadmap to understand how ventricular cells become specified, differentiate and expand into a functional cardiac chamber (Fig. 19.1). The transcriptional networks described here provide clear evidence that disruption of pathways affecting ventricular growth could be the underlying etiology in a subset of children born with malformation of the right or left ventricle. As we learn details of the precise mechanisms through which the critical factors function, the challenge will lie in devising innovative methods to augment or modify the effects of gene mutations on ventricular development. Because most congenital

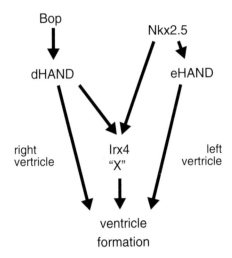

Fig. 19.1 Molecular pathway for ventriculogenesis. A model for some known genes involved in ventricular development.

heart disease likely occurs in a setting of heterozygous, predisposing mutations of one or more genes, modulation of activity of critical pathways in a preventive fashion may be useful in averting disease in genetically susceptible individuals.

Acknowledgments

This work was supported by grants from the NHLBI/NIH, March of Dimes Birth Defects Foundation and the Donald W. Reynolds Clinical Cardiovascular Center to DS.

References

1 Srivastava D, Olson EN. A genetic blueprint for cardiac development: Implications for human heart disease. *Nature* 2000; **407**:221–6.

2 Srivastava D, Cserjesi P, Olson EN. A subclass of bHLH proteins required for cardiac morphogenesis. *Science* 1995; **270**: 1995–9.

3 Srivastava D, Thomas T, Lin Q et al. Regulation of cardiac mesodermal and neural crest development by the bHLH transcription factor, dHAND. *Nat Genet* 1997; **16**: 154–60.

4 Biben C, Harvey RP. Homeodomain factor Nkx2–5 controls left/right asymetric expression of bHLH gene eHAND during murine heart development. *Genes Dev* 1997; **11**: 1357–69.

5 Yamagishi H, Yamagishi C, Nakagawa O et al. The combinatorial activities of Nkx2.5 and dHAND are essential for cardiac ventricle formation. *Dev Biol* 2001; **239**: 190–203.

6 Firulli AB, McFadden DG, Lin Q, Srivastava D, Olson EN. Heart and extra-embryonic mesodermal defects in mouse embryos lacking the bHLH transcription factor Hand1. *Nat Genet* 1998; **18**: 266–70.

7 Riley P, Anson-Cartwright L, Cross JC. The Hand1 bHLH transcription factor is essential for placentation and cardiac morphogenesis. *Nat Genet* 1998; **18**: 271–5.

8 Riley PR, Gertsenstein M, Dawson K, Cross JC. Early exclusion of hand1-deficient cells from distinct regions of the left ventricular myocardium in chimeric mouse embryos. *Dev Biol* 2000; **227**: 156–68.

9 Christoffels VM, Habets PE, Franco D et al. Chamber formation and morphogenesis in the developing mammalian heart. *Dev Biol* 2000; **223**: 266–78.

10 Bruneau BG, Bao ZZ, Tanaka M et al. Cardiac expression of the ventricle-specific homeobox gene Irx4 is modulated by Nkx2–5 and dHand. *Dev Biol* 2000; **217**: 266–277.

11 Bao ZZ, Bruneau BG, Seidman JG, Seidman CE, Cepko CL. Regulation of chamber-specific gene expression in the developing heart by Irx4. *Science* 1999; **283**: 161–4.

12 Yelon D, Ticho B, Halpern ME et al. The bHLH transcription factor hand2 plays parallel roles in zebrafish heart and pectoral fin development. *Development* 2000; **127**: 2573–82.

13 Angelo S, Lohr J, Lee KH et al. Conservation of sequence and expression of Xenopus and Zebrafish dHAND during cardiac, branchial arch and lateral mesoderm development. *Mech Dev* 2000; **95**:231–7.

14 Cheung P, Allis CD, Sassone-Corsi P. Signaling to chromatin through histone modifications. *Cell* 2000; **103**: 263–71.

15 Marmorstein R, Roth SY. Histone acetyltransferases: function, structure, and catalysis. *Curr Opin Genet Dev* 2001; **11**: 155–61.

16 Khochbin S., Verdel A, Lemercier C, Seigneurin-Berny D. Functional significance of histone deacetylase diversity. *Curr Opin Genet Dev* 2001; **11**:162–6.

17 Gottlieb PD, Pierce SA, Sims RJ et al. Bop encodes a muscle-restricted protein containing MYND and SET domains and is essential for cardiac differentiation and morphogenesis. *Nat Genet* 2002; **31**: 25–32.

18 Lutterbach B, Sun D, Schuetz J, Hiebert SW. The MYND motif is required for repression of basal transcription from the multidrug resistance 1 promoter by the t(8;21) fusion protein. *Mol Cell Biol* 1998; **18**: 3604–11.

19 Lutterbach B, Westendorf JJ, Linggi B et al. ETO, a target of t(8;21) in acute leukemia, interacts with the N-CoR and mSin3 corepressors. *Mol Cell Biol* 1998; **18**: 7176–84.

20 Rea S, Eisenhaber F, O'Carroll D et al. Regulation of chromatin structure by site-specific histone H3 methyltransferases. *Nature* 2000; **406**: 593–9.

CHAPTER 20

Fgf10 and the embryological origin of outflow tract myocardium

Robert G. Kelly, Stephane Zaffran, Margaret Buckingham, Nigel A. Brown

The vertebrate heart tube develops from cardio-myocytes of the cardiac crescent, situated in anterior lateral splanchnic mesoderm. The heart tube is initially orientated along a cranio-caudal axis with a posterior inflow (or venous) pole and an anterior outflow (or arterial) pole. Convergence of the inflow and outflow poles of the heart is brought about by rightward looping and a dorso-anterior movement of the venous pole behind the developing ventricles. Cardiac looping is initiated at embryonic day (E) 8.25 and is complete by E10.5; during this period the heart tube grows extremely rapidly in length, through addition of extra-cardiac cells to the venous and arterial poles. Cells undergoing an epithelial to myocardial transition have been described adjacent to the outflow tract of the embryonic mouse heart until E10.5 by Viragh and Challice.[1] Recently it has been demonstrated that these arterial pole precursor cells originate in the newly identified Anterior or Secondary Heart Field (AHF) situated in pharyngeal mesoderm.[2–4] Anomalies in outflow tract development and septation are among the most common features of congenital heart disease. Knowledge of the embryological origin of outflow tract myocardium, the mechanisms involved in integration of myocardial cells derived from pharyngeal mesoderm into the embryonic heart tube, and the signals coordinating growth of the myocardial wall and neural crest derived components of the outflow tract will contribute to a better understanding of normal and abnormal cardiogenesis.

We have described and analyzed the expression profile of a nuclear beta-galactosidase encoding transgene which is expressed in the right ventricle and outflow tract of the mid-gestation mouse heart.[2] At early stages of heart development the transgene is expressed in AHF cells which are contiguous with the arterial pole of the heart (Fig. 20.1). DiI labeling experiments demonstrate that these cells contribute to the myocardial wall of the embryonic outflow tract. The expression profile of this transgene results from an integration site position effect. Analysis of the flanking genomic sequence reveals that the transgene has integrated 120 kb upstream of the gene encoding fibroblast growth factor 10 (Fgf10). Comparison of the expression profile of the transgene with that of *Fgf10* transcripts supports the conclusion that *Fgf10* is the endogenous target of the regulatory elements trapped by the transgene. Genetic confirmation is provided by the fact that transgene integration has created a hypomorphic *Fgf10* allele, revealed in transgene/*Fgf10* null compound heterozygotes which display severe dysplasia of both lungs and limbs, structures which are absent in Fgf10 homozygous null embryos.[5,6]

We have examined the extent to which cells derived from the AHF contribute to the developing heart. Three lines of evidence suggest that, in the mouse, future right ventricular myocardium is predominantly AHF-derived. First, comparison of the early expression patterns of beta-galactosidase encoding transgenes, expressed in the future right and left ventricles of the mid-gestation heart, suggests that the linear heart tube contributes predominantly to the embryonic left ventricle and that only the most anterior region contains future right ventricular cells (Fig. 20.2). Second, DiI labeling of cells at the anterior end of the linear heart tube, prior to

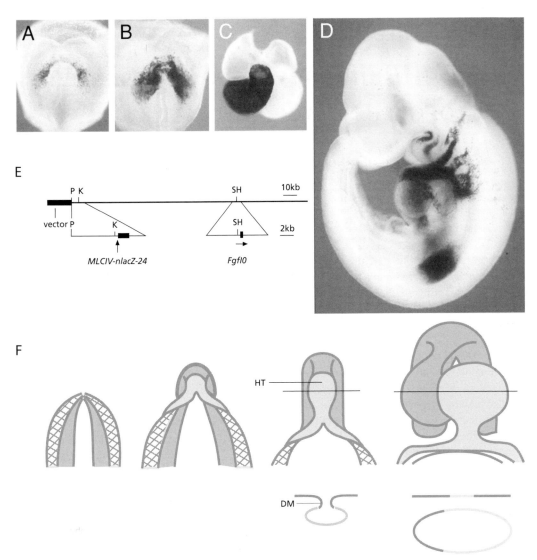

Fig. 20.1 β-galactosidase expression in *Mlc 1v-nlacZ-24* transgenic embryos. (A) At E7.5, transgene expression is observed in cells medial to the cardiac crescent. (B) At E8, expression is observed in a ring at the arterial pole of the heart tube and in bilateral wings of expression in splanchnic mesoderm dorsal to the heart tube. (C) At E 10.5, expression is observed in the embryonic right ventricle and outflow tract. (D) A left lateral view at E9.5 reveals transgene expression in pharyngeal mesoderm continuous with outflow tract myocardium. (E) Structure of mouse PAC clone RPCI21 644L10 showing the site of integration of the *Mlc 1v-nlacZ-24* transgene 120 kb upstream of *Fgf10*. (F) Cartoon showing the expression profile of the *Mlc1v-nlacZ-24* transgene (dark shading) during early heart development. HT, heart tube; DM, dorsal mesocardium. Panels reproduced with permission from Kelly *et al.*[2]

24 h of embryo culture, supports the hypothesis that the linear heart tube is fated to become the embryonic left ventricle and that the interventricular region lies close to its anterior end. Third, explant analysis confirms the future left ventricular identity of the linear heart tube and demonstrates that right ventricular and outflow tract precursors are positioned in pharyngeal mesoderm anterior to the heart tube. The addition of future right ventricular myocardium marks the initiation of rightward looping, suggesting that the AHF contributes laterality information to the developing heart, and may

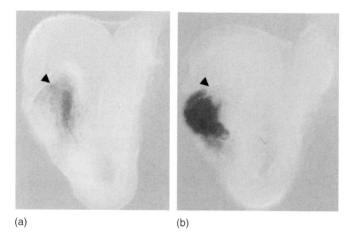

Fig. 20.2 Complementary β-galactosidase expression patterns in the heart tube of *Mlc 1v-nlacZ-24* (a) and *Mlc3f-nlacZ-2* (b) transgenic embryos at E8.25. Arrowhead, arterial pole of the heart tube in these left lateral views.

(a)   (b)

also contribute mechanistically to rightward looping. Genes encoding signaling molecules in the embryonic laterality cascade, including Nodal and Lefty2, and the transcription factor Pitx2c, are expressed in the left, but not the right, AHF.

Fgf10 has been shown to be essential for multiple steps during organogenesis.[5,6] Initial analysis of ventricular morphology of *Fgf10* null hearts reveals normal ventriculo-arterial connections and ventricular septation. Mouse embryo culture in the presence of inhibitors of all Fgf signalling, however, results in abnormal arterial pole development, including outflow tract shortening, suggesting that other Fgfs in the pharyngeal region may functionally compensate for the loss of Fgf10 in *Fgf10* null embryos. Recent data have implicated *Fgf8*, which is expressed in the pharyngeal region, in arterial pole development.[7–9] *Fgf8* is also expressed in arterial pole precursor cells, suggesting that it may functionally overlap with *Fgf10*. Identification of the AHF and the contribution of AHF-derived cardiomyocytes to the heart provides a new framework to investigate the signaling pathways involved in normal and abnormal arterial pole morphogenesis.

Acknowledgments

RK is an INSERM research fellow. NAB is supported by the British Heart Foundation (RG/98004). The laboratory of MB is supported by the Pasteur Institute, the CNRS and the ACI programme of the ministry of Research.

References

1 Viragh S, Challice CE. Origin and differentiation of cardiac muscle cells in the mouse. *J Ultrast Res* 1973; **42**: 1–24.

2 Kelly RG *et al*. The arterial pole of the mouse heart forms from Fgf10-expressing cells in pharyngeal mesoderm. *Dev Cell* 2001; **1**: 435–40.

3 Mjaatvedt CH *et al*. The outflow tract of the heart is recruited from a novel heart-forming field. *Dev Biol* 2001; **238**: 97–109.

4 Waldo KL *et al*. Conotruncal myocardium arises from a secondary heart field. *Development* 2001; **128**: 3179–88.

5 Min H *et al*. Fgf-10 is required for both limb and lung development and exhibits striking functional similarity to Drosophila branchless. *Genes Dev* 1998; **12**: 3156–61.

6 Sekine K *et al*. Fgf10 is essential for limb and lung formation. *Nat Genet* 1999; **21**: 138–41.

7 Abu-Issa R *et al*. Fgf8 is required for pharyngeal arch and cardiovascular development in the mouse. *Development* 2002; **129**: 4613–25.

8 Frank DU *et al*. An Fgf8 mouse mutant phenocopies human 22q11 deletion syndrome. *Development* 2002; **129**: 4591–603.

9 Vitelli F *et al*. A genetic link between Tbx1 and fibroblast growth factor signalling. *Development* 2002; **129**: 4605–11.

CHAPTER 21

Evolutionary conservation of atrial natriuretic factor (Anf) expression, cardiac chamber formation, and the heart-forming region

Antoon F. M. Moorman, Piet A. J. De Boer, Eric M. Small,
Paul A. Krieg, Vincent M. Christoffels

The essence of the building plan of the vertebrate chamber heart has been remarkably well conserved during vertebrate evolution (see ref. 1 for a review). The vertebrate chambered heart has evolved from a simple tubular ancestor heart. Tubular hearts are no longer present in vertebrates, but are still present in the primitive chordates, with the lancelet, *Amphioxus*, as the well-known representative. In lancelets blood is pushed ahead by waves of peristaltic contractions down to the length of the heart tube. Peristaltic hearts do not need valves. In fishes a chambered heart has developed, with an atrial chamber expanding toward the dorsal side of the heart tube and a ventricular chamber expanding toward the ventral side of the tube. The chambered heart is the more powerful heart: the fast-contracting chambers permit circulation of the blood against the higher blood pressures that were needed with the evolution of hepatic and renal filtration systems. Chambered hearts do need valves at both the inlet and the outlet of the chambers to prevent backflow of blood from an upstream compartment toward the relaxing chamber and from the contracting chamber toward an upstream compartment. It can be envisioned that as long as valves had not evolved during evolution, the parts of the original heart tube that flank the inlets and outlets of the expanding chambers, have substituted valvular function, because this type of myocardium still displays the

long-lasting peristaltic type of contraction of the original heart tube. Such a situation would be highly reminiscent of the configuration seen in avian and mammalian embryonic hearts that eventually develop into the four-chamber configuration.[2] Both in adult fish and amphibian hearts, outflow tract myocardium (conus, bulbus cordis) still surrounds the semilunar valves and has been shown to support semilunar valve function.[3,4] In human patients tachycardias originate from this region when the outflow tract myocardium apparently has not disappeared entirely.[5,6]

Cardiac chamber development in avian and mammalian species is characterized by the exclusive expression of *atrial natriuretic factor (Anf)*.[7–9] *Anf* is not expressed in the so-called primary myocardium of the linear heart tube and remains absent from those cardiac regions that do not develop into chamber myocardium, i.e. the inflow tract, atrioventricular canal, inner curvature, and outflow tract. In the formed heart, the nodal tissues that develop in these regions are devoid of Anf as well.[10] Although patterns of expression of *Anf* have not been described in the fish heart, they can be derived from electron microscopic studies reporting the presence of so-called specific myocardial granules in atrial and ventricular myocardium.[11,12] These granules have been shown to be the storage sites of Anf. From an evolutionary point of view, we judged it interesting to determine whether in an amphibian group expression of *Anf* would also identify early chamber formation. Previously we reported that Anf is expressed in the myocardium of developing *Xenopus* tadpoles.[13] However, the whole mount *in situ* hybridization experiments did not permit an unambiguous assessment of the pattern of expression in individual cardiac compartments. Therefore, we performed an *in situ* hybridization analysis on sections using a recently developed very sensitive nonradioactive *in situ* hybridization protocol.[14] Expression of *cardiac Troponin I* was used to identify the myocardium. As shown in Fig. 21.1, *Anf* is not expressed in the linear heart tube, Nieuwkoop and Faber[15] stage 30, but becomes expressed in the developing atrial and ventricular chambers as shown in a section of a stage 40 embryo in which all the cardiac compartments can be clearly recognized. The inflow tract, atrioventricular canal, and outflow tract do not express *Anf*. Later in development expression of *Anf* becomes confined to the atria.[13] This developmental pattern of expression is entirely comparable with that observed during mouse development,[9] suggesting a similar underlying regulatory mechanism that is conserved from fish to mammal. In mouse, Nkx2.5 and T-box factor Tbx5 were shown to be required for *Anf* gene expression,[16–18] whereas Tbx2 is involved in the repression of expression in the primary myocardium.[19]

The function of Anf during development is unknown, but it has been suggested to play a role in cardiomyocyte proliferation.[20,21] The temporal relationship of expression of *Anf* and chamber formation in the representatives of the different vertebrate classes might suggest causality. However, *Anf* null mutants display no developmental phenotype, although this might be owing to functional redundancy with brain natriuretic factor.[21–23] Another interesting point that deserves additional study is the presence of Anf in the hearts of primitive evertebrates such as the earthworm and the oyster,[24,25] whereas it seems no longer to be present in the primary vertebrate heart tube.

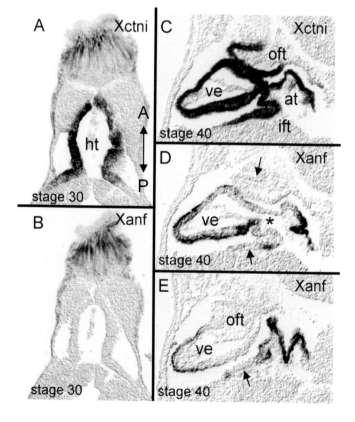

Fig. 21.1 Expression patterns of *cTnI* and *Anf* in serial sections of *Xenopus* tadpoles, visualized by non radio-active in situ hybridisation.[14] A and B show frontal sections of a stage 30 embryo; note that *cTnI* is strongly expressed in the entire heart tube, whereas *Anf* expression is not detectable. C–E show sagittal sections of a stage 40 embryo. *Anf* expression was only detectable in the forming chambers; no expression was observed inflow and outflow tracts (arrows) and in the atrioventricular canal (asterix). Ht: heart tube; ift: inflow tract; oft: outflow tract; at: atrium; ve: ventricle; A-P: antero-posterior.

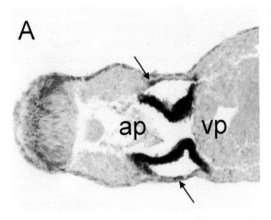

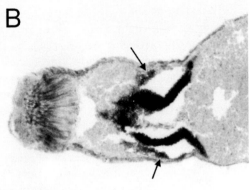

Fig. 21.2 Nonradioactive *in situ* hybridization[14] of a stage 30 *Xenopus* tadpole using a probe to *cTnI*. A and B show two different frontal sections. Long staining reaction reveals specific expression of *cTnI* in the lining of the pericardial cavity (arrows) and heavily stained myocardium of the linear heart tube. Ap, arterial pole; vp, venous pole.

A second observation worthy of note is that in early tadpoles (stage 30), cardiac Troponin I identifies not only the primary myocardium of the linear heart tube, but also the entire lining of the pericardial cavity, which is by convention called parietal pericardium (Fig. 21.2). This observation indicates that cardiogenesis is induced in the anterior mesoderm by the surrounding germ layers prior to separation of this mesoderm into a visceral and parietal layer. From studies in chicken and mouse it is known that after formation of the linear heart tube, myocardium is still added at both ends of the tube.[26–28] This myocardium originates from mesothelium and mesenchyme that is contiguous with the so-called 'primary' heart fields but went unnoticed because of technical reasons.[1] These regions have been called anterior (secondary) and posterior heart field, respectively. Taken together, the simplest description of cardiogenesis might be to consider it as a continuous recruitment of cardiac cells from the bilaterally formed 'primary' heart fields. This view does not imply that all cells within the 'primary' heart fields are similar, because they will differ owing to different positional information imposed on the fields during development.

Acknowledgments

We thank Mr J. Jansen for providing us with the *Xenopus* embryos. The Netherlands Heart Foundation (NHS) granted this work (grant no: M96.002).

References

1 Moorman AFM, Christoffels VM. Cardiac chamber formation: development, genes and evolution. *Physiol Rev* 2003; **83**: 1223–67.

2 de Jong F, Opthof T, Wilde AAM *et al.* Persisting zones of slow impulse conduction in developing chicken hearts. *Circ Res* 1992; **71**: 240–50.

3 Johansen K. Cardiovascular dynamics in fishes, amphibians and reptiles. *Ann N Y Acad Sci* 1965; **127**: 414–42

4 Satchell GH, Jones MP. The function of the conus arteriosus in the Port Jackson shark, *Heterodontus portusjacksoni.* *J Exp Biol* 1967; **46**: 373–82.

5 Kanagaratnam L, Tomassoni G, Schweikert R *et al.* Ventricular tachycardias arising from the aortic sinus of valsalva: an under-recognized variant of left outflow tract ventricular tachycardia. *J Am Coll Cardiol.* 2001; **37**: 1408–14.

6 Skromne I, Stern CD. Interactions between Wnt and Vg1 signalling pathways initiate primitive streak formation in the chick embryo. *Development* 2001; **128**: 2915–27.

7 Houweling AC, Somi S, van den Hoff MJ, Moorman AFM, Christoffels VM. The developmental pattern of ANF gene expression reveals a strict localization of cardiac chamber formation in chicken. *Anat Rec* 2002; **266**: 93–102.

8 Zeller R, Bloch KD, Williams BS, Arceci RJ, Seidman CE. Localized expression of the atrial natriuretic factor gene during cardiac embryogenesis. *Gene Dev* 1987; **1**: 693–8.

9 Christoffels VM, Habets PEMH, Franco D *et al.* Chamber formation and morphogenesis in the developing mammalian heart. *Dev Biol* 2000; **223**: 266–78.

10 Skepper JN. An immunocytochemical study of the sinuatrial node and atrioventricular conducting system of the

rat for atrial natriuretic peptide distribution. *Histochem J* 1989; **21**: 72–8.

11 Yamauchi A, Fujimaki Y, Yokota R. Fine structural studies of the sino-auricular nodal tissue in the heart of a teleost fish, misgurnus with particular reference to the caridac internuncial cell. *Am J Anat* 1973; **138**: 407–30.

12 Yamauchi A. Fine structure of the fish heart. In: Bourne GH, ed. *Heart and Heart-like Organs*. New York: Academic Press, 1980: 119–48.

13 Small EM, Krieg PA. Expression of atrial natriuretic factor (ANF) during Xenopus cardiac development. *Dev Genes Evol* 2000; **210**: 638–40.

14 Moorman AFM, Houweling AC, de Boer PAJ, Christoffels VM. Sensitive nonradioactive detection of mRNA in tissue sections: novel application of the whole-mount *in situ* hybridization protocol. *J Histochem Cytochem* 2001; **49**: 1–8.

15 Nieuwkoop PD, Faber J. *Normal Table of Xenopus laevis (Daudin)*, 1st edn. Amsterdam: North-Holland, 1956: 1–243.

16 Lyons I, Parsons LM, Hartley L *et al.* Myogenic and morphogenetic defects in the heart tubes of murine embryos lacking the homeobox gene *Nkx2–5*. *Gene Dev* 1995; **9**: 1654–66.

17 Tanaka M, Chen Z, Bartunkova S, Yamasaki N, Izumo S. The cardiac homeobox gene *Csx/Nkx2.5* lies genetically upstream of multiple genes essential for heart development. *Development* 1999; **126**: 1269–80.

18 Bruneau BG, Nemer G, Schmitt JP *et al.* A murine model of Holt-Oram syndrome defines roles of the T-box transcription factor Tbx5 in cardiogenesis and disease. *Cell* 2001; **106**: 709–21.

19 Habets PEMH, Moorman AFM, Clout DEW *et al.* Cooperative action of Tbx2 and Nkx2.5 inhibits ANF expression in the atrioventricular canal: implications for cardiac chamber formation. *Genes Dev* 2002; **16**: 1234–46.

20 Koide M, Akins RE, Harayama H, Yasui K, Yokota M, Tuan RS. Atrial natriuretic peptide accelerates proliferation of chick embryonic cardiomyocytes *in vitro*. *Differentiation* 1996; **61**: 1–11.

21 Silberbach M, Roberts CT Jr. Natriuretic peptide signalling Molecular and cellular pathways to growth regulation. *Cellular Signal* 2001; **13**: 221–31.

22 John SWM, Krege JH, Oliver PM *et al.* Genetic decreases in atrial natriuretic peptide and salt-sensitive hypertension. *Science* 1995; **267**: 279–81.

23 Vikstrom KL, Bohlmeyer T, Factor SM, Leinwand LA. Hypertrophy, pathology, and molecular markers of cardiac pathogenesis. *Circ Res* 1998; **82**: 773–8

24 Vesely DL, Giordano AT. The most primitive heart in the animal kingdom contains the atrial natriuretic peptide hormonal system. *Comp Biochem Physiol* 1992; **101**: 325–9.

25 Vesely DL, Gower WR, Giordano AT, Friedl FE. Atrial natriuretic peptides in the heart and hemolymph of the oyster, *Crassostrea virginica*: a comparison with vertebrates. *Comp Biochem Physiol* 1993; **106B**: 535–46.

26 De la Cruz MV, Sanchez-Gomez C. Straight tube heart. Primitive cardiac cavities vs. primitive cardiac segments. In: De la Cruz M, Markwald RR, eds. *Living Morphogenesis of the Heart*, 1st edn. Boston: Birkhäuser, 1998: 85–98.

27 Kelly RG, Buckingham ME. The anterior heart-forming field: voyage to the arterial pole of the heart. *Trends Genet* 2002; **18**: 210–16.

28 Kruithof BPT, van den Hoff MJB, Wessels A, Moorman AFM. Cardiac muscle cell formation after formation of the linear heart tube. *Dev Dyn* 2003; **227**: 1–13.

findings were observed in the engrailed-2 reporter mouse (conduction system like (CCS)-LacZ expressing mouse).

Wessels *et al.* provide an excellent review of approaches used to study the embryonic origins of the cardiac conduction system and introduce a new transgenic mouse model with expression of cGATA6/lacZ in the developing CCS. The cGATA6/lacZ construct is discretely expressed in the precardiac mesoderm stage suggesting that some of the molecular machinery responsible for AVCS differentiation is already in place at a very early stage of heart formation.

Nakamura and colleagues demonstrated an essential role for calreticulin, a calcium-binding protein, in cardiac development and function. Calreticulin expression was elevated in the embryonic heart and is downregulated after birth. Homozygous knockout in mice was lethal at embryonic days 14.5–16.5. Cardiac specific overexpression of calreticulin (driven by the cardiac myosin heavy chain promoter) led to severe cardiac pathology including sinus bradycardia and atrioventricular node dysfunction with progressive prolongation of the P–R interval advancing to complete heart block and sudden cardiac death. Calreticulin may be part of one pathway of events involving the endoplasmic reticulum that can cause complete heart block.

CHAPTER 22

Induction and patterning of the impulse conducting Purkinje fiber network

Takashi Mikawa, Robert G. Gourdie, Clifton P. Poma, Maxim Shulimovich, Christopher Hall, Kenneth W. Hewett, Chip Justus, Maria Reckova, David Sedmera, Kimimasa Tobita, Romulo Hurtado, David J. Pennisi, Nobuyuki Kanzawa, Kimiko Takebayashi-Suzuki

The rhythmic heartbeat is coordinated by electrical impulses initiated by, and propagated through, the cardiac excitation and conduction system.[1-3] The cardiac pacemaking impulse is rhythmically generated at the SA-node[4,5] and is conducted across the atrial chambers.[5-8] The pacemaking impulses then converge on the AV-node[1] where impulse propagation is slowed. Impulses are then rapidly propagated along the AV-bundle[9] and its branched limbs,[1] and are finally conducted into the ventricular muscle through the Purkinje fiber network.[1,10,11] Thus, the cardiac conduction system consists of several subcomponents with distinct electrophysiological characteristics. Individual conduction subcomponents are also distinguishable from each other by their expression of a unique set of proteins and genes (reviewed in refs 12–18). While little is known about how the pacemaker (SA-node) and the slow conduction component (AV-node) are established in the heart, mechanisms underlying differentiation of a fast conduction component, the Purkinje fiber network, during heart development, have begun to be uncovered in recent years. This chapter aims to review our current understanding of cellular and molecular mechanisms that induce and pattern the Purkinje fiber network (Fig. 22.1)

The first breakthrough for our dissection of the cellular and molecular components involved in Purkinje fiber differentiation and patterning came from retroviral cell lineage studies on the embryonic chick heart (reviewed in refs 12, 15, 16). It was previously thought that conduction cells differentiated from cardiac neural crest (reviewed in ref. 19). To our surprise, however, retroviral cell lineage studies in the embryonic chick heart have demonstrated that impulse-conducting Purkinje cells differentiate from myocytes, not from neural crest, exclusively along the endocardium and developing coronary arterial branches during embryogenesis[20,21] (reviewed in refs 12, 15, 16). This result provided us with a clear rationale that Purkinje fiber differentiation and patterning can be studied by addressing mechanisms which convert beating embryonic myocytes into conduction cells.

The unique site of Purkinje fiber recruitment in the embryonic heart suggested to us that paracrine signals from endocardial and arterial cells may play a role in this conversion process in the cardiomyocyte lineage. We tested this hypothesis experimentally. Using a co-culture of endocardial endothelial cells and embryonic myocytes, we have shown that induction of marker gene expression in Purkinje fibers

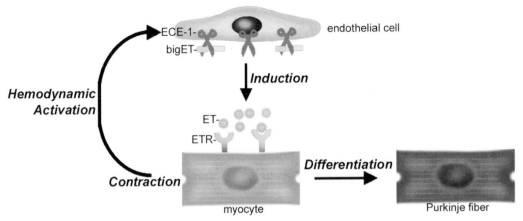

Fig. 22.1 Model for the conversion of myocytes to Purkinje fibers by endothelium-derived inductive cue(s). Recruitment of myocytes to the conduction system occurs in the embryonic chick heart only along the endocardium and coronary arterial branches. This spatially restricted conversion event seems to be triggered by hemodynamic forces created by heartbeat itself. While myocytes express endothelin receptors in the embryonic chick heart, ECE-1, one of hemodynamic-responsive factors, is expressed exclusively in coronary arterial and a subpopulation of endocardial endothelial cells. Our current working model is that hemodynamic force induces endocardial and arterial endothelial cells to upregulate the ECE-1 expression, thereby defining an activation site of this inductive signal and thus recruiting myocytes to the cardiac conduction system in a spatially restricted manner. bigET, big endothelin; ECE-1, endothelin converting enzyme-1; ET, endothelin; ETR, endothelin receptor.

does indeed depend upon signals derived from endothelial cells.[22] It has been also found that inhibition of coronary arterial branching results in loss of periarterial Purkinje fibers and that ectopic production of arterial beds in the embryonic myocardium can induce adjacent myocytes to express Purkinje fiber marker genes.[23] The data from these *in vivo* and *in vitro* experiments strongly suggested that paracrine signals derived from the endocardium and developing coronary arteries were necessary and sufficient for conversion of contractile myocytes into conduction cells in the embryonic heart. Furthermore, our survey of vessel-associated paracrine factors has identified endothelin[24] as a potent peptide for inducing myocytes to differentiate into Purkinje fibers *in vitro*[25] by switching a gene expression program from a contractile cell-type to a conduction cell-type.[26] The results have provided further evidence demonstrating that Purkinje fiber differentiation is a cell fate diversification process of the cardiomyocyte cell lineage.

The above data, however, did not explain how the inductive ET-signaling was activated specifically at the site of Purkinje fiber recruitment within the embryonic heart (i.e. exclusively along the endocardium and coronary arterial branches but not along veins or capillaries). It has been shown that active ET is produced through proteolytic processing from its precursor by ET-converting enzyme-1 (ECE-1) and triggers signaling by binding to its receptors (reviewed in refs 27, 28). Our *in situ* hybridization studies have shown that in the embryonic heart, two ET-receptors, ET_A and ET_B, are expressed by myocytes, while ET_{B2} is expressed in developing valve leaflets.[29] Importantly, however, we have found that ECE-1 is exclusively expressed in endothelial cells of the endocardium and coronary arteries, but not in veins or capillaries.[30] These expression data suggested to us that an activation site of the inductive ET-signaling may be localized in the embryonic heart by restricting ECE-1 expression. We have tested this hypothesis by ectopically co-expressing exogenous ECE-1 with ET precursor in the embryonic heart, and have found that the co-expression of these two genes is sufficient to induce myocyte conversion to conduction cells ectopically.[30] These results strongly suggest that localized expression of ECE-1 in endocardial and arterial endothelia is a key mechanism defining the site of Purkinje fiber recruitment in the embryonic myocardium.

Obvious questions to be answered next included how ECE-1 expression is restricted in a subpopulation of cardiac endothelial cells. Our preliminary studies have shown that ECE-1 expression can be upregulated and downregulated by activation and suppression, respectively, of stretch-sensitive channels. Coincident with the levels of ECE-1, Purkinje fiber differentiation, as judged by expression of conduction cell marker genes and by impulse-conduction pathways, seems to be altered. This suggests that biophysical forces acting on, and created by, the cardiovascular system during embryogenesis may play a critical role in Purkinje fiber induction and patterning (Fig. 22.1). These data from our *in vivo* and *in vitro* studies may serve as the basis for the understanding of normal and aberrant conduction system development, and may also provide rationales for future therapeutic approaches.

Acknowledgments

Supported in part by the NIH.

References

1 Tawara S. *Das Reizleitungssystem des Säugetierherzens. Eine Anatomisch-histologische Studie über das Atrioventrikularbündel und die Purkinjeschen Fäden.* Jena; Gustav Fischer, 1906.

2 Goldenberg M, Rothberger CJ. Über des Elektrogramm der spezifischen Herz-muskulatur. *Pflügers Arch* 1936; **237**: 295–306.

3 Botzler E. The initiation of impulses in cardiac muscle. *Am J Physiol* 1942; **138**: 273–82.

4 Keith A, Flack M. The form and nature of the muscular connections between the primary divisions of the vertebrate heart. *J Anat Physiol* 1907; **41**: 172–89.

5 Brooks C McC, Lu H-H. *The Sinoatrial Pacemaker of the Heart.* Springfield: Charles C. Thomas, 1972.

6 Wenckebach KF. Beiträge zur Kenntnis der menschlichen Hetztätigkeit. *Arch Anat Physiol* 1906; **1–2**: 297–354.

7 Thörel C. Vorläufige Mitteilung über eine besondere Muskelverbindung zwischen der Cava superior und dem His'schen Bündel. *Münch Med Wschr* 1909; **56**: 2159.

8 Robb JS, Petri R. Expansions of the atrio-ventricular system in the atria. In: Paes de Carvalho A *et al.*, eds. *The Specialized Tissue of the Heart.* New York: Elsevier 1961: 1–18.

9 His W. Die Tätigkeit des embryonalen Herzens und deren Bedeutung für die Lehre von der Herzbewegung beim Erwachsenen. *Arb med Klin Leipzig* 1893: 14–49.

10 Purkinje J. Mikroskopisch-neurologische Beobachtungen. *Arch Anat Physiol Wiss Med* 1845; **12**: 281–95.

11 Kölliker A. *Gewebeslehre*, 6th edn. Lpz 1902.

12 Mikawa T, Fischman DA. The polyclonal origin of myocyte lineages. *Annu Rev Physiol* 1996; **58**: 509–21.

13 Schiaffino S. Protean patterns of gene expression in the heart conduction system. *Circ Res* 1997; **80**: 749–50.

14 Moorman AFM, De Jong F, Denyn MM, Lamers WH. Development of the cardiac conduction system. *Circ Res* 1998; **82**: 629–44.

15 Mikawa T. Cardiac lineages. In: Harvey RP, Rosenthal N, eds. *Heart Development.* London: Academic Press, 1999: 19–33.

16 Mikawa T. Determination of heart cell lineages. In: Moody SA, ed. *Cell Fate Determination.* London: Academic Press, 1999: 449–60.

17 Gourdie RG, Kubalak S, Mikawa T. Conducting the embryonic heart: orchestrating development of specialized cardiac tissues. *Trends Cardiovasc Med* 1999; **9**: 18–26.

18 Welikson RE, Mikawa T. Cytoskeletal gene expression in the developing cardiac conduction system. In: Dube DK, ed. *Myofibrillogenesis.* Boston: Birkhäuser, 2002: 153–77.

19 Gorza L, Schiaffino S, Vitadello M. Heart conduction system: a neural crest derivative? *Brain Res* 1988; **457**: 360–6.

20 Gourdie RG, Mima T, Thompson RP, Mikawa T. Terminal diversification of the myocyte lineage generates Purkinje fibers of the cardiac conduction system. *Development* 1995; **121**: 1423–31.

21 Cheng G, Litchenberg WH, Cole GJ *et al.* Development of the cardiac conduction system involves recruitment within a multipotent cardiomyogenic lineage. *Development* 1999; **126**: 5041–9.

22 Pennisi DJ, Rentschler S, Gourdie RG, Fishman GI, Mikawa T. Induction and patterning of the cardiac conduction system. *Int J Dev Biol* 2002; **46**: 765–75.

23 Hyer J, Johansen M, Prasad A *et al.* Induction of Purkinje fiber differentiation by coronary arterialization. *Proc Natl Acad Sci USA* 1999; **96**: 13214–18.

24 Yanagisawa M, Kurihara H, Kimura S *et al.* A novel potent vasoconstrictor peptide produced by vascular endothelial cells. *Nature* 1988; **332**: 411–15.

25 Gourdie RG, Wei Y, Kim D, Klatt SC, Mikawa T. Endothelin-induced conversion of embryonic heart muscle cells into impulse-conducting Purkinje fibers. *Proc Natl Acad Sci USA* 1998; **95**: 6815–18.

26 Takebayashi-Suzuki K, Pauliks LB, Eltsefon Y, Mikawa T. Purkinje fibers of the avian heart express a myogenic transcription factor program distinct from cardiac and skeletal muscle. *Dev Biol* 2001; **234**: 390–401.

27 Yanagisawa H, Hammer RE, Richardson JA *et al.* Role of Endothelin-1/Endothelin-A receptor-mediated signaling pathway in the aortic arch patterning in mice. *J Clin Invest* 1998; **102**: 22–33.

28 Yanagisawa H, Yanagisawa M, Kapur RP *et al.* Dual genetic pathways of endothelin-mediated intercellular signaling

revealed by targeted disruption of endothelin converting enzyme-1 gene. *Development* 1998; **125**: 825–36.

29 Kanzawa N, Poma CP, Takebayashi-Suzuki K *et al.* Competency of embryonic cardiomyocytes to undergo Purkinje fiber differentiation is regulated by endothelin receptor expression. *Development* 2002; **129**: 3185–94.

30 Takebayashi-Suzuki K, Yanagisawa M, Gourdie RG, Kanzawa N, Mikawa T. *In vivo* induction of cardiac Purkinje fiber differentiation by coexpression of preproendothelin-1 and endothelin converting enzyme-1. *Development* 2000; **127**: 3523–32.

CHAPTER 23

Spatial correlation of conduction tissue in the ventricular trabeculae of the developing zebrafish

Norman Hu, H. Joseph Yost, Lance F. Barker, Edward B. Clark

All hearts beyond a certain critical size must contract in a more efficient manner than afforded by peristalsis alone, and excitation is coordinated by specialized conduction tissue. The terminal differentiation of cardiac myocytes during looping, septation, and trabeculation is critical to the emergence of cardiac conduction tissue and normal morphogenesis of the definite chambered heart.[1] In mammals, the neuromuscular conduction system of the ventricle transmits an electrical impulse from the atrioventricular (AV) node, through the AV bundle, the right and left bundle branches, and terminates in the fine Purkinje fibers to generate the ventricular depolarization (the initiation of ventricular contraction). In chick embryo, the central parts of the conduction tissue arise between stage 12 (2 days old) and stage 27 (5 days old), correlating with the period of trabecular formation.[2–4] The cells of the cardiac conduction system withdraw from the cell cycle earlier than the neighboring working myocardium. In fish, specialized myofibers such as the His bundle and Purkinje fibers, and the conducting tracts have not been identified. It is unclear whether trabeculated but nonseptated ventricle possesses a morphologically distinguishable conduction system. The rationale for studying the cardiac conduction system in zebrafish is that these mechanisms are phylogenetically old and conserved amongst vertebrates. Determining how the transition of the conduction system correlates with the formation of trabeculae may provide novel insight in the formation of the cardiac conduction system.

The zebrafish electrocardiogram (ECG) is similar to birds and mammals, suggesting that zebrafish have an equivalent conduction system (Fig. 23.1). Therefore, we seek to define conduction tissue using antibody techniques. In zebrafish, the first deflection of the ECG is the P wave, which represents atrial depolarization. The QRS complex proceeds almost immediately after the P wave with a relatively short P–R interval (29.1 ± 4.0 ms), and occupies only about 6% of the cardiac cycle (484.1 ± 30.6 ms). The short P–R duration in the ECG suggests that zebrafish have a less defined atrioventricular node that creates a fast transmission of the electrical impulse from the atrial depolarization to the ventricle. On the contrary, the mammalian heart retains a delay between the atrial and ventricular contractions to allow the complete contraction of the atrium before ventricular contraction starts. The duration of the QRS complex (30.5 ± 1.2 ms) is similar to the duration in P wave (28.7 ± 2.1 ms) owing to the rapid propagation of the wave of depolarization through the ventricle. The amplitude of the QRS complex is greater than the P wave since the ventricle has thicker trabeculae than those of the atrium.[5] Repolarization of the ventricle generates the T wave so that the myocardial cells can regain the negative charge and depolarize again. The duration of the T wave is considerably longer than the QRS complex since repolarization does not require spreading a rapidly propagated impulse.

The monoclonal HNK1 antibody is a sulfoglucuronyl carbohydrate originally identified on

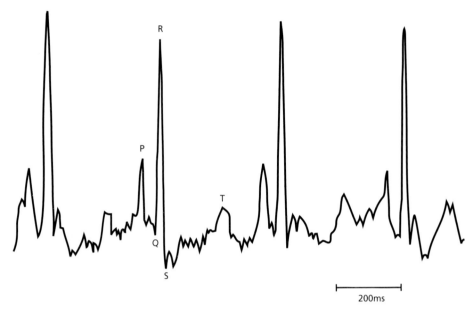

Fig. 23.1 The ECG of the zebrafish is similar to the ECG of mammalian except the zebrafish exhibits a much shorter duration in P–R interval. P wave, atrial depolarization; QRS complex, ventricular depolarization; T wave, ventricular repolarization.

human natural killer cells.[6] It reacts with the epitope expressed on the cell surface of the developing myocardium and in the migrating neural crest cells. HNK1 expression persists in 2-, 3-, and 4-day-old zebrafish, and the epitope of the conduction tissues is present in the myocardial trabeculae of both the atrium and ventricle (Plate 20). HNK1 immunoreactivity was distinctly evident in the atrioventricular and outflow tract regions, and almost the entire ventricle (Plate 21). The ventricular conduction tissue in the developing heart does not seem to be organized into segments of specialized tract (like bundle, branches, and Purkinje fibers). Instead, like the early embryonic mouse, it is being conducted by the trabeculae as a whole.[7] Fate mapping also reveals that the cardiac neural crest contributes to the formation of cardiomyocyte and pharyngeal arch development.[8] A more detailed study of neural crest-derived cells and HNK1 immunoreactivity during the critical period of looping to septated heart is necessary to elucidate the origin of the conduction system.

Materials and methods

Electrocardiogram (ECG)

ECG from the adult (6-month-old) zebrafish was acquired by placing two platinum needle electrodes on the surface of the right side of the body, one above the pectoral cartilage, and the other below the operculum close to the bulbus arteriosus. The third electrode served as the ground.

Immunohistochemistry

Whole mount immunostaining was performed on 2-, 3- and 4-day-old zebrafish. The specimens were fixed in 4% paraformaldehyde. Supernatant monoclonal HNK1 antibody (Courtesy of Dr Gary Schoenwolf's laboratory, Children's Health Research Center at the University of Utah) was used at a dilution of 1:100. Secondary antibody fluorescein-conjugated (FITC) goat anti-mouse-IgM antibodies (Roche Applied Science, Indianapolis, IN) were diluted to 1:100 to detect the primary antibody. Serial sections were digitized using a Fluoview IX70 confocal laser-scanning microscope (Olympus America Inc., Melville, NY), and images were processed with Adobe Photoshop (Adobe Systems Inc., Seattle, WA), and Scion Image (Scion Corp., Frederick, MD). 3-D volume was rendered and deconvolved with the Velocity software (Improvision, Lexington, MA).

References

1 Hu N, Sedmera D, Yost HJ, Clark EB. Structure and function of the developing zebrafish heart. *Anat Rec* 2000; **260**: 148–57.

2 Chuck ET, Freeman DM, Watanabe M, Rosenbaum DS. Changing activation sequence in the embryonic chick heart. Implications for the development of the His–Purkinje system. *Circ Res* 1997; **81**: 470–6.

3 Chuck ET, Watanabe M. Differential expression of PSA-NCAM and HNK1 epitopes in the developing cardiac conduction system of the chick. *Dev Dyn* 1997; **209**: 182–95.

4 Taber LA, Hu N, Pexieder T, Clark EB, Keller EB. Residual strain in the ventricle of the stage 16–24 chick embryo. *Circ Res* 1993; **72**: 455–62.

5 Hu N, Yost HJ, Clark EB. Cardiac morphology and blood pressure in the adult zebrafish. *Anat Rec* 2001; **264**: 1–12.

6 Abo T, Balch CM. Characterization of HNK1+ (Leu-7) human lymphocytes. II. Distinguishing phenotypic and functional properties of natural killer cells from activated NK-like cells. *J Immunol* 1982; **129**: 1758–61.

7 Viragh S, Challice CE. The development of the conduction system in the mouse embryo heart. I. The first embryonic A-V conduction pathway. *Dev Biol* 1977; **56**: 382–96.

8 Mariko Sato, Yost HJ. Cardiac neural crest contributes to cardomyogenesis in zebrafish. *Dev Biol* 2003; **257**: 127–39.

CHAPTER 24

Development of the cardiac conduction system and contribution of neural crest and epicardially derived cells

Adriana C. Gittenberger-de Groot, Nico A. Blom,
Glenn I. Fishman, Robert E. Poelmann

The cardiac conduction system (CCS) develops as a separate functional entity from the contracting embryonic myocardium. Both the working myocardium and the cardiac cells that develop into the functional conduction system differentiate from the embryonic myocardium as it is found in the straight and marginally looped early cardiac heart tube. We have been able to follow the differentiation of the conduction system initially using the HNK1 antibody in human embryos.[1-3] In later stages of cardiac development in humans, the HNK1 antibody is expressed in the myocardial areas that in subsequent development restrict the expression of HNK1 to what is generally accepted in the fully developed heart to be the definitive conduction system. On the basis of HNK1 expression, we could delineate a premature conduction system that is found in specific intersegmental or transitional zones in the developing heart. These areas are the sinoatrial transition, positioned between the sinus venosus and the developing atria, and the primary ring or fold that is found between the primitive left ventricle and the developing right ventricle. The sinoatrial transition is important for the formation of the sinoatrial conduction system whereas the primary ring or fold develops into the atrioventricular conduction system. It is interesting that both transitional zones are not lined by endocardial cushion tissue as are the other two zones of the heart, the atrioventricular canal and

the primitive outflow tract. During early development, HNK1 expression is found to be more extensive than in what eventually persists as the definitive conduction system. For the sinoatrial part we can distinguish the venous valve bases as pathways that run from the superior caval vein (later the sinus node area) to the right atrioventricular ring. There are three connections from the sinoatrial node area to the right atrial ring bundle harboring the later posterior atrioventricular node and the (transient) anterior atrioventricular node: (1) the base of the right venous valve (future right atrial terminal crest); (2) the left venous valve which is incorporated in the secondary atrial septum; (3) the septum spurium, which consists of the fused right and left venous valve that run anteriorly over the right atrial wall and connect to the anterior part of the right atrioventricular ring. This is exactly the site where in some congenital heart malformations an anterior atrioventricular node is found. The posterior fusion of the right and left venous valve in the base of the atrial septum connects to the posterior part of the right atrioventricular ring where it forms the atrial part of the atrioventricular node (Fig. 24.1a). A very interesting expression of HNK1 is seen around the pulmonary venous anlage, which in the human embryo is initially positioned slightly to the right of the developing primary septum.[2] During development, the pulmonary venous pit, which is embedded in the

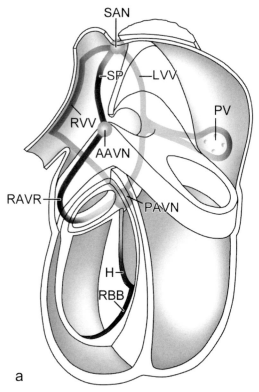

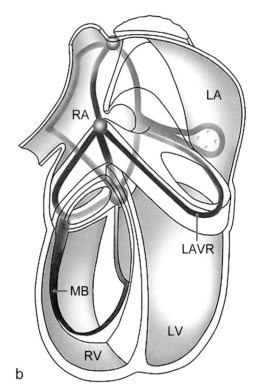

a

b

Fig. 24.1 Schematic representation of the primitive cardiac conduction system as seen with HNK1: (a) in e.g. human embryo; (b) in the mouse with the CCS/LacZ construct. AAVN, anterior atrioventricular node; H, His bundle; LA, left atrium; LAVR, left atrioventricular ring bundle; LV, left ventricle; LVV, left venous valve; MB, moderator band; PAVN, posterior atrioventricular node; PV, pulmonary veins; RAVR, right atrioventricular ring; SAN, sino atrial node; SP, septum spurium.

connection of the heart to the dorsal body wall, the so-called dorsal mesocardium, moves to the left atrium. With septation of the atrium, the pulmonary veins are disconnected from the right atrium. On the basis of these findings we are convinced that the pulmonary veins are confined within the embryonic tissue of the sinus venosus and that this tissue makes up part of the basis of the atrial septum and the dorsal wall of the left atrium.[1,2]

These data are supported by findings in the engrailed-2 reporter mouse.[4] As the insertion of the construct has proven not to be in the engrailed gene area the mouse is currently referred to as the CCS-LacZ (conduction system like) expressing mouse.[5] The marker gene is predominantly expressed in the myocardium of the embryonic heart tube but most markedly in the above-described transitional zones between the various segments of the heart. We can find it abundantly in primary fold derived structures (including the moderator band of the right ventricle), the tips of the trabeculae, and the sinoatrial transition including the three for the internodal pathways described for humans. Some parts of the expression pattern differ somewhat from the human situation as detected by HNK1 (Fig. 24.1b). There is a marked anterior band (in future the so-called Bachmanns bundle) running from the right to the left atrium just above and in connection with the anterior part of the atrioventricular ring bundle starting in a retro-aortic position at the site of the anterior atrioventricular node (not shown). The latter is with the CCS/LacZ not only encircling the right side of the atrioventricular canal but also the left side. This description was provided in the article by Rentschler *et al.*[4] No data, however, were provided on the pulmonary venous area. Recent studies of our own group using the CCS/LacZ mouse have revealed that also in this model the pulmonary veins are encircled by CCS expression during part of the development, supporting our initial hypothesis that the pulmonary veins belong to the sinus venosus area. The functional implications of the above findings might be that the areas that are prone later on in life to abnormal atrial automaticity have a common origin during embryonic life and during this period transiently express the genes that persist in the definitive conduction system.[1] It is also of importance that the CCS/LacZ expression is not only present in the future right bundle branch but continues through the moderator band all the way up to the right atrioventricular ring bundle. This finding might provide an anatomic substrate for the Mahami re-entrant tachycardia.

It is still a matter of debate which factors direct the differentiation of myocardial cells into the conduction system and working myocardium. There is circumstantial evidence that extra cardiac contributors such as neural crest cells (NCC)[6] and epicardium derived cells (EPDC)[7] might play a role in inducing the differentiation of parts of definitive CCS. NCC migrate to and into the heart. Recently we have shown that NCC differentiate not only into an autonomous nervous cell population but also provide a mesenchymal cell population that enters the heart both at the outflow and the inflow tract.[6] The latter cells could be followed in both avian and mouse (Wnt1 reporter mouse) models to flank the atrioventricular and, to a lesser extent, the sinoatrial CCS. We hypothesize that these NCC play a role in the differentiation of the central CCS by releasing growth factors during their subsequent apoptosis. It is of interest that there is a clear overlap of intracardiac NCC areas and the engrailed distribution. The

EPDC are found in the subendocardial and periarterial (avian) position and are considered to be important for differentiation of the Purkinje network of the heart. There is preliminary evidence that the close association of the NC derived autonomous nervous system and the primitive CCS areas might be instrumental in understanding some adult cardiac arrhythmias.

References

1 Blom NA, Gittenberger-de Groot AC, DeRuiter MC et al. Development of the cardiac conduction tissue in human embryos using HNK-1 antigen expression: possible relevance for understanding of abnormal atrial automaticity. *Circulation* 1999; **99**: 800–6.
2 Blom NA, Gittenberger-de Groot AC, Jongeneel TH et al. Normal development of the pulmonary veins in human embryos and formulation of a morphogenetic concept for sinus venosus defects. *Am J Cardiol* 2001; **87**: 305–9.
3 Gittenberger-de Groot AC, DeRuiter MC, Bartelings MM, Poelmann RE. In: Crawford MH, DiMarco JP, eds. *Cardiology*. London: Mosby International Limited, 2001: 2.1–2.10.
4 Rentschler S, Vaidya DM, Tamaddon H et al. Visualisation and functional characterisation of the developing murine cardiac conduction system. *Development* 2001; **128**: 1785–92.
5 Rentschler S, Zander J, Meyers K et al. Neuregulin-1 promotes formation of the murine cardiac conduction system. *Proc Natl Acad Sci USA* 2002; **99**: 10464–9.
6 Poelmann RE, Gittenberger-de Groot AC. A subpopulation of apoptosis-prone cardiac neural crest cells targets to the venous pole: multiple functions in heart development? *Dev Biol* 1999; **207**: 271–86.
7 Gittenberger-de Groot AC, Vrancken Peeters M-PFM, Mentink MMT, Gourdie RG, Poelmann RE. Epicardial derived cells, EPDCs, contribute a novel population to the myocardial wall and the atrioventricular cushions. *Circ Res* 1998; **82**; 1043–52.

CHAPTER 25

The development of the cardiac conduction system: an old story with a new perspective

Andy Wessels, Amy L. Juraszek, Angela V. Edwards, John B. E. Burch

Ever since the discovery of the cardiac conduction system (CCS), its embryonic origin has been a matter of intense debate. Before the introduction of advanced molecular tools (e.g. immunohistochemistry, *in situ* hybridization, mouse transgenics), histological criteria (such as: degree of myofibrillar development; PAS-reactivity, as indication for glycogen content)[1,2] were used to discriminate the developing CCS from its surrounding tissues. Although this histological approach has provided many insightful studies, its limitations have also resulted in inadequate interpretations of sections leading to misconceptions on the anatomy and development of the CCS. The introduction in the 1980s of immunohistochemistry (IHC) in cardiovascular developmental biology led to a significant improvement of the understanding of the issue. In the early days of IHC, the expression-domains of myosin heavy chain (MHC) isoforms were found to be informative to delineate components of the CCS. Thus, the persistence of co-expression of atrial and ventricular MHC, a characteristic feature of the primary myocardium of the early heart tube,[3] proved to be a feature of components of the developing CCS, including the proximal parts of the atrioventricular CCS (AVCS)[4,5] and the sinoatrial node (SAN).[6] It was also demonstrated that, in some species, various components of the CCS express unique MHC variants. Slow-tonic MHC (recognized by ALD58), is expressed in the distal component (Purkinje fibers) of the avian AVCS,[7] which proved to be very helpful in describing the differentiation of the Purkinje sys-

tem. In addition, it has been reported that antibodies recognizing embryonic-like MHC specifically stain discrete components of the CCS in the rat heart.[8] Subsequently, a variety of other 'markers' were found to delineate the CCS. Some of these markers were predominantly expressed in the CCS, including Cx42 in the distal AVCS of the chick heart,[9] a 55 kDa protein found in the CCS of the bovine heart,[10,11] and neurofilament in the CCS of the rabbit.[12] In contrast, in relation to the surrounding tissues, other markers were found to be expressed at extremely low levels. This included Cx43 in the proximal AVCS in several mammalian species[13] and the M-isoform of creatine kinase in the proximal AVCS in humans.[14] Although these expression profiles provided improved insight in the development and anatomy of the CCS in relatively advanced stages of development and provided tools to study the development of the CCS *in vitro* and *in vivo*, none of these markers were really useful in helping us to understand the early developmental events that underlie CCS formation. However, considerable progress in the understanding of CCS development was made when three, independently generated, antibodies (Gln2, HNK-1, and Leu7, all recognizing the same carbohydrate epitope), were found to recognize specifically the developing CCS in humans and rats.[5,15] Based on 3-dimensional reconstructions of a developmental series of serially-sectioned Gln2 stained human hearts, a model for the development of the CCS was generated that allowed us to describe development of the AVCS in re-

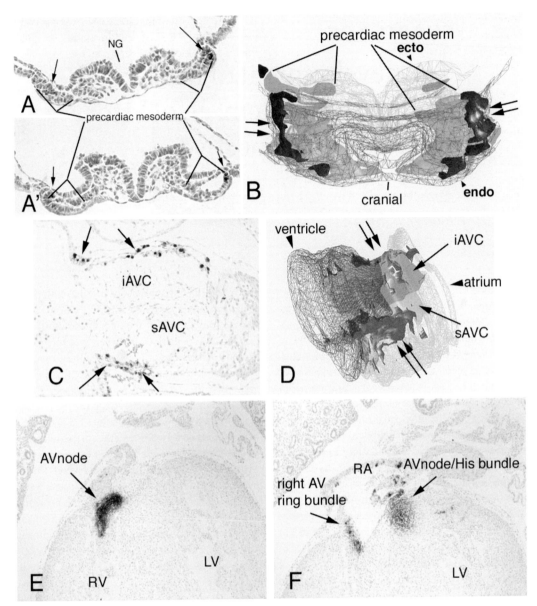

Fig. 25.1 (-1.5/+0.8)cGATA6/lacZ expression during cardiac development. Transgenic embryos at consecutive stages of development were serially sectioned and the lacZ expression pattern reconstructed using 3D-DOCTOR software (ABLE). At E7.5 [(A) and (A') are two sections from the same embryo] expression was observed in the most lateral areas of the precardiac mesoderm (black arrows/dark staining indicate transgene expression). The 3D reconstruction based on these stainings is shown in (B). At E9.5–10 (C,D) the transgene is predominantly expressed in the myocardium underneath the inferior and superior atrioventricular cushions [arrows in (C) and dark staining with double arrows in (D)]. At later stages of development [e.g. E14, (E) and (F)] the expression becomes confined to the morphologically recognizable proximal AVCS and the lateral right AV junction. As a result, at these stages the entire AV myocardium of the developing right AV junction is characterized by the expression of the cGATA6/lacZ transgene (E,F). ecto, ectoderm; endo, endoderm; iAVC, inferior atrioventricular cushion; NG, neural groove; sAVC, superior atrioventricular cushion; LV, left ventricle; RV, right ventricle.

lation to the remodeling of the embryonic AV junction.[16,17]

Despite all the CCS-related protein expression patterns discussed above, many questions related to CCS development remained unanswered. These include, but are not restricted to: (1) Does the proximal AVCS tissue derive from a common precardiac mesodermal progenitor cell population? (2) What are the molecular mechanisms that regulate the continuously changing expression profile in the developing CCS? (3) How is the 3D patterning of the CCS regulated? (4) What is the functional significance (if any) of the components of the primary ring that do not develop into morphologically recognizable components of the CCS?

The introduction of transgenic mouse technology has led to the generation of several genetically engineered mouse models that, often fortuitously, reveal new and exciting aspects of CCS development. These include the minK-lacZ mouse,[18] the cardiac-troponin I/lacZ mouse,[19] and the CCS–lacZ mouse.[20] We have recently reported on a transgenic model with expression of cGATA6-lacZ in the developing CCS.[21,22] The expression of this transgene could be traced back to the earliest stages of heart development (see Fig. 25.1). Thus, in the precardiac mesoderm stage (ED7.5) it was found in two bilateral strips of cells located in the distal-most region of the heart fields (Fig.25.1a,a',b). After the heart tube has formed and looped (e.g. ED9.5), these two areas of expression then become localized in the posterior and inferior wall of the AV canal myocardium overlying the developing major AV cushions (Fig. 25.1c,d). Eventually, in late fetal and post-natal stages, the cGATA6/lacZ transgene expression becomes largely restricted to the proximal AVCS and right AV ring bundle, expression in the distal AVCS (bundle branches and Purkinje system) or left AV junction never being observed (Fig. 25.1e,f). To the best of our knowledge, the cGATA6/lacZ construct is the only CCS-related transgene discretely expressed in the precardiac mesoderm stage. The expression profile suggests that at least some of the molecular machinery responsible for AVCS differentiation is already in place at a very early stage of heart formation. We also infer that the potential to contribute to the proximal AVCS might be restricted to a subset of myocardial cells long before the myocardial heart tube actually has been formed. This would not be surprising in light of the fact that the various components of the CCS arise within, and have distinct functional properties suited to, regions of the heart that contain functionally distinct myocardial cells that are likewise specified early in the cardiogenic program.

Acknowledgments

This work was supported by NIH Grants HL35535 (awarded to JB) and HL52813 (AW) and Core Grant CA-06927 (awarded to the FCCC). Additional support was provided from the Commonwealth of Pennsylvania.

References

1 Viragh S, Challice CE. The development of the conduction system in the mouse embryo heart. I. The first embryonic A-V conduction pathway. *Dev Biol* 1977; **56**: 382–96.

2 Viragh S, Challice CE. The development of the conduction system in the mouse embryo heart. II. Histogenesis of the atrioventricular node and bundle. *Dev Biol* 1977; **56**: 397–411.

3 de Jong F, Geerts WJ, Lamers WH, Los JA, Moorman AF. Isomyosin expression patterns in tubular stages of chicken heart development: a 3-D immunohistochemical analysis. *Anat Embryol* 1987; **177**: 81–90.

4 Wessels A, Vermeulen JLM, Virágh Sz *et al.* Spatial distribution of 'tissue specific' antigens in the developing human heart and skeletal muscle: II. An immunohistochemical analysis of myosin heavy chain isoform expression patterns in the embryonic heart. *Anat Rec* 1991; **229**: 355–68.

5 Wessels A, Vermeulen JL, Verbeek FJ *et al.* Spatial distribution of 'tissue-specific' antigens in the developing human heart and skeletal muscle. III. An immunohistochemical analysis of the distribution of the neural tissue antigen G1N2 in the embryonic heart; implications for the development of the atrioventricular conduction system. *Anat Rec* 1992; **232**: 97–111.

6 de Groot IJM, Wessels A, Virágh Sz, Lamers WH, Moorman AFM. The relation between isomyosin heavy chain expression pattern and the architecture of sinoatrial nodes in chicken, rat and human embryos. In: U. Carraro, ed. *Sarcomeric and Non-Sarcomeric Muscles: Basic and Applied Research Prospects for the 90s*. Padova: Unipress, 1988: 305–10.

7 Gonzalez-Sanchez A, Bader D. Characterization of a myosin heavy chain in the conductive system of the adult and developing chicken heart. *J Cell Biol* 1985; **100**: 270–5.

8 Gorza L, Saggin L, Sartore S, Ausoni S. An embryonic like myosin heavy chain is transiently expressed in nodal con-

duction tissue of the rat heart. *J Mol Cell Cardiol* 1988; **20**: 931–41.

9 Gourdie RG, Green CR, Severs NJ, Anderson RH, Thompson RP. Evidence for a distinct gap-junctional phenotype in ventricular conduction tissues of the developing and mature avian heart. *Circ Res* 1993; **72**: 278–89.

10 Oosthoek PW, Viragh Sz, Mayen AEM *et al.* Immunohistochemical delineation of the conduction system I: the sinoatrial node. *Circ Res* 1993; **73**: 473–81.

11 Oosthoek PW, Viragh Sz, Lamers WH, Moorman AFM. Immunohistochemical delineation of the conduction system II: the atrioventricular node and Purkinje fibers. *Circ Res* 1993; **73**: 482–91.

12 Gorza L, Vitadello M. Distribution of conduction system fibers in the developing and adult rabbit heart revealed by an antineurofilament antibody. *Circ Res* 1989; **65**: 360–9.

13 van Kempen MJA, Ten Velde I, Wessels A *et al.* Differential connexin distribution accommodates cardiac function in different species. *Microsc Res Tech* 1995; **31**: 420–36.

14 Wessels A, Vermeulen JLM, Virágh Sz *et al.* Spatial distribution of 'tissue-specific' antigens in the developing human heart and skeletal muscle. I. An immunohistochemical analysis of creatine kinase isoenzyme expression patterns. *Anat Rec* 1990; **228**: 163–76.

15 Ikeda T, Iwasaki K, Shimokawa I *et al.* Leu-7 immunoreactivity in human and rat embryonic hearts, with special reference to the development of the conduction tissue. *Anat Embryol (Berl)* 1990; **182**: 553–62.

16 Lamers WH, Wessels A, Verbeek FJ *et al.* New findings concerning ventricular septation in the human heart. Implications for maldevelopment. *Circulation* 1992; **86**: 1194–205.

17 Wessels A, Markman MW, Vermeulen JL *et al.* The development of the atrioventricular junction in the human heart. *Circ Res* 1996; **78**: 110–17.

18 Kupershmidt S, Yang T, Anderson ME *et al.* Replacement by homologous recombination of the minK gene with LacZ reveals restriction of minK expression to the mouse cardiac conduction system. *Circ Res* 1999; **84**: 146–52.

19 Di Lissi R, Sandri C, Franco D *et al.* An atrioventricular canal domain defined by cardiac troponin I transgene expression in the embryonic myocardium. *Anat Embryol* 2000; **202**: 95–101.

20 Rentschler S, Vaidya DM, Tamaddon H *et al.* Visualization and functional characterization of the developing murine cardiac conduction system. *Development* 2001; **128**: 1785–92.

21 Davis DL, Edwards AV, Juraszek AL *et al.* A GATA-6 gene heart-region-specific enhancer provides a novel means to mark and probe a discrete component of the mouse cardiac conduction system. *Mech Dev* 2001; **108**: 105–19.

22 Wessels A, Phelps A, Trusk, TC *et al.* Mouse models for cardiac conduction system development. In: *Development of the Cardiac Conduction System. Novartis Foundation Symposium.* Chichester: Wiley, 2003; **250**: 44–59; discussion 59–67, 276–9.

26 CHAPTER 26

The role of calreticulin in cardiac development and function

Kimitoshi Nakamura, Fumio Endo, Marek Michalak

Animal models for defects of cardiac development and function have been generated and related knowledge has accumulated. The models reveal that defects in cardiac function are closely linked to abnormalities during embryonic development, and understanding of heart development helps us to clarify the mechanisms of heart disease.

Development of the embryonic heart is regulated by diverse components including transcription factors, intracellular signaling, and cell to cell contact. Calreticulin, one of the proteins regulating intracellular signaling, is a ubiquitous Ca^{2+}-binding protein, located to the endoplasmic reticulum lumen. The protein has been implicated in many functions, including regulation of intracellular Ca^{2+} homeostasis, chaperone activity, gene regulation, and cell adhesion. The expression of calreticulin is elevated in the embryonic heart and is downregulated after birth. To understand the physiological function of calreticulin, we used gene targeting to generate a knockout mouse. Homozygous mice were lethal at embryonic days 14.5–16.5, probably owing to a marked decrease in ventricular wall thickness. Calreticulin deficient cells exhibited impaired nuclear import of nuclear factor of activated T cell (NF-AT) transcription factor indicating that calreticulin plays a role in cardiac development as a component of the transcription pathway.

The molecular details underlying calreticulin deficient mice are not yet understood. Impaired nuclear import of NF-AT, however, suggests that Ca^{2+}-dependent pathways may underlie the embryonic lethality. To test this hypothesis we reconstitut-ed the hearts of calreticulin-deficient mice with a truncated, Ca^{2+}-independent, constitutively active form of calcineurin to re-establish the Ca^{2+}-dependent cascade downstream of calreticulin (Plate 22). Overexpression of activated calcineurin reverses the defect in cardiac development observed in calreticulin-deficient mice and rescues them from embryonic lethality. Reversal of embryonic lethality owing to calreticulin-deficiency by activated calcineurin underscores the impact of calreticulin–calcineurin functions on the Ca^{2+}-dependent signaling cascade during early cardiac development. These findings show that calreticulin and calcineurin play fundamental roles in Ca^{2+}-dependent pathways essential for normal cardiac development and explain the molecular basis for the rescue of calreticulin deficient phenotype.

Next, we generated transgenic mice that overexpress calreticulin in the heart and we investigated physiological consequences of continued high expression of the protein in the postnatal heart. Cardiac specific overexpression of calreticulin was driven by the cardiac myosin heavy chain promoter. The transgenic mice showed that postnatally elevated expression of calreticulin leads to severe cardiac pathology including sinus bradycardia and atrio-ventricular node dysfunction with progressive prolongation of the P–R interval followed by complete heart block and sudden cardiac death. Cardiomyocytes overexpressing calreticulin have a decreased density of L-type Ca^{2+} channels. The transgenic mice seemed to be a model of postnatal arrhythmia and cardiac-related sudden death. Calreticulin may be part of one pathway of events involving the endoplasmic reticulum that can cause complete heart block.

Our results demonstrate an essential role for cal-reticulin during embryogenesis and cardiac function. Transgenic models with cardiac defect facilitate elucidation of mechanisms involved in heart disease, and contribute to the development of new approach to the disease.

References

1 Masaeli N, Nakamura K, Zvaritch E *et al*. Calreticulin is essential for cardiac development. *J Cell Biol* 1999; **144**: 857–68.

2 Nakamura K, Bossy-Wetzel E, Burns K *et al*. Changes in endoplasmic reticulum luminal environment affect cell sensitivity to apoptosis. *J Cell Biol* 2000; **150**: 731–40.

3 Guo L, Lynch J, Nakamura K *et al*. COUP-TF1 Antagonizes Nkx2.5-mediated activation of the calreticulin gene during cardiac development. *J Biol Chem* 2001; **276**: 2797–801.

4 Nakamura K, Robertson M, Liu G *et al*. Complete heart block and sudden death in mice overexpressing calreticulin. *J Clin Invest* 2001; **107**: 1245–53.

5 Nakamura K, Zuppinni A, Lynch J *et al*. Functional specialization of calreticulin domains. *J Cell Biol* 2001; **154**: 961–72.

6 Gao B, Adhikari R, Howarth M *et al*. Assembly and antigen-presenting function of MHC class I molecules in cells lacking the ER chaperone calreticulin. *Immunity* 2002; **16**: 99–109.

7 Arnaudeau S, Frieden M, Nakamura K, Castelbou C, Michalak M, Demaurex N. Calreticulin differentially modulates calcium uptake and release in the endoplasmic reticulum and mitochondria. *J Biol Chem* 2002; **277**: 46696–705.

8 Guo L, Nakamura K, Lynch J *et al*. Cardiac specific expression of calcineurin reverses embryonic lethality in calreticulin-deficient mouse. *J Biol Chem* 2002; **277**: 50776–9.

PART 6

Coronary artery development

Editorial perspective

Michael Artman

Mechanisms governing the formation of the coronary arteries and their proper connection to the aortic sinuses remain incompletely defined. Although much has been learned regarding coronary artery morphogenesis, relatively little is known about the molecular mechanisms and signaling processes that drive coronary artery formation in normal and abnormal cardiovascular development.

It has been shown previously that the proximal coronary arteries form by inward endothelial growth toward the aorta. Ando *et al.* further refined this concept by demonstrating that multiple endothelial strands penetrate the aortic wall at several sites followed by fusion of endothelial strands at the facing sinuses. Interestingly, at the same time there is regression of the endothelial strands that have penetrated the noncoronary sinus. Lastly, the tunica media develops in the proximal coronary arteries. The signals that promote regression of the endothelial strands at the noncoronary sinus and coalescence and ongoing development of the definitive coronary arteries remain to be determined.

Tenascins are a family of extracellular matrix proteins that might play a role in vasculogenesis in the developing heart. It has been shown that cells derived from the proepicardial organ adhere to the surface of the heart and spread over it to become epicardial cells which are vascular cell precursors. Imanaka-Yoshida *et al.* studied the potential role of tenascin-C (TNC) and tenascin-X (TNX) in this process, since tenascins have been implicated in morphogenesis, cell motility, and epithelial–mesenchymal and/or mesenchymal–epithelial transformation. TNC was highly expressed in the mesenchymal cells of the proepicardial organ, but once cells migrated to the surface of the heart, TNC expression decreased. In contrast, TNX was highly expressed after the epicardial covering was completed, but in contrast to TNC, TNX was not expressed in the cells of the proepicardial organ or during migration of the proepicardial cells. It may be that TNC allows the initial migration of cells from the proepicardial organ and then TNX serves to sustain this process. However, much remains to be determined regarding the role of tenascins and other extracellular matrix proteins in these processes. As demonstrated by Hanato *et al.*, the bis-diamine model of abnormal cardiovascular development includes significant coronary artery abnormalities. Thus, application of this technique might be a useful model for future studies of normal and abnormal coronary artery development.

CHAPTER 27

Development of proximal coronary artery in quail embryonic heart

Katsumi Ando, Yuji Nakajima, Toshiyuki Yamagishi, Sadamu Yamamoto, Hiroaki Nakamura

Several investigators have shown that the proximal segment of the coronary arteries develops by endothelial ingrowth from the peritruncal ring (PR) of the coronary vasculature, rather than by endothelial outgrowth from the aorta.[1–3] In chick embryo, Aikawa and Kawano were the first to describe that at the onset of the formation of the proximal coronary arteries, multiple 'primitive' coronary arteries originate from the right and left coronary sinuses, and then decrease in number to form definitive coronary arteries on each side.[4] Later, Poelmann et al. reported that multiple endothelial strands grow into the aorta from the PR at several sites, and that the capillary network persists at only two of these sites to form definitive coronary arteries.[5] At this stage, the first vascular smooth muscle cells come to surround the right and left coronary arteries (HH 32; 7.5 days incubation).[6] Not withstanding the above observations, the exact process involved in the formation of the proximal coronary arteries remains unclear. In the present paper, we made detailed observations of the formation of the main coronary trunks in quail embryos using double immunostaining for an endothelial marker (QH1, IgG1) and anti-smooth muscle α-actin (1A4, IgG2a) in serial sections cut parallel to the aortic orifice.[7,8] In addition, using the confocal microscope, we observed the initial development of the endothelial strands (anlagen of the proximal coronary arteries) that penetrate the aortic wall.

The development of the proximal coronary arteries in staged embryos is summarized in Table 27.1. At 5 days of incubation, QH1-positive subepicardial sinusoidal structures were observed surrounding both the aortic and pulmonary trunks (PR of the coronary vasculature); however, there was no visible connection between the PR and the aortic lumen. At 6 days of incubation, QH1-positive endothelial strands that seemed to begin to connect the PR with the aortic lumen were found in the aortic wall facing the future left or right coronary sinus (much as described by Aikawa and Kawano[4]). No QH1-positive endothelial strands were detectable in the wall of the pulmonary trunk in any of the serial sections we examined. At 7 days of incubation, multiple QH1-positive endothelial strands were penetrating the aortic wall of the right and left coronary regions (the facing sinuses). In three out of five embryos, QH1-positive endothelial strands were penetrating the aortic wall facing the noncoronary cusp; indeed, endothelial strands with an apparent lumen were observed penetrating the aortic wall of the noncoronary sinus. At 8 days of incubation, all embryos possessed a single right coronary trunk and four out of five a single left coronary trunk (one embryo exhibited two left proximal coronary arteries). At this stage, QH1-positive endothelial strands penetrating the noncoronary sinus were seen in three out of five embryos. By 9 days of incubation, the right and left proximal coronary trunks were completed in all five embryos examined. At this stage, there were no QH1-positive endothelial strands in the aortic wall facing the noncoronary sinus, and the right and left coronary orifices were manifest as a large concavity surrounded by a thick smooth muscle cell layer (tunica media of the coronary artery).

Table 27.1 Summary of development of proximal coronary vessels in staged embryos

Days of incubation	No. of penetrating vessels (average)		
	RCS	LCS	NCS
5 (n = 3)	0	0	0
6 (n = 5)	1.4	0.8	0
7 (n = 5)	3.6	3.4	1.6
8 (n = 5)	1.0	1.2	0.6
9 (n = 5)	1.0	1.0	0

At 5 days of incubation, there was no QH1-positive endothelial connection between the peritruncal ring and the aortic lumen. At 6 days of incubation, QH1-positive endothelial strands began to penetrate into RCS and LCS. At 7 days of incubation, more than 3 endothelial strands were penetrating into RCS and LCS, and in 3 out of 5 hearts, endothelial strands were penetrating NCS. By 9 days of incubation, the right and left proximal coronary trunks were completed, and no QH1-positive endothelial strands were observed penetrating NCS. RCS, right coronary sinus; LCS, left coronary sinus; NCS, noncoronary sinus; N, number of hearts examined.

Several investigators have noted that while multiple endothelial strands of the coronary arterial analagen from PR connect to the aorta, only one channel survives in each of the two sinuses to become the definitive right and left proximal coronary arteries and their orifices.[3–5] In our observations, multiple endothelial strands penetrating the aortic wall facing the right and left coronary sinuses seemed to become fused to each other. Thus, a reticular structure consisting of endothelial strands with decidual tissues could be clearly seen in the aortic wall. We suggest that the fusion of the endothelial strands penetrating the wall facing each sinus may contribute to the generation of a single proximal coronary trunk. On the other hand, we could not find such a reticular structure with a decidual-tissue involvement in the noncoronary sinus region. This may be because the sparse penetration of fewer endothelial strands in this region perturbes the fusion of the endothelial strands within the wall of the

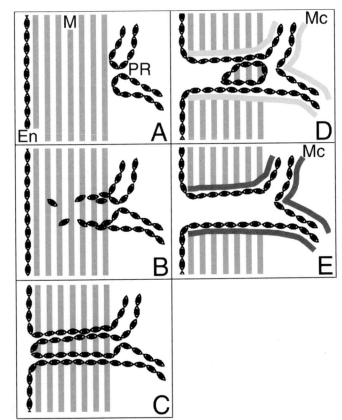

Fig. 27.1 Schematic representation of developing proximal coronary artery. (A) Peritruncal ring (PR) of coronary vasculature surrounds the aorta; (B) Endothelial strands are established by vasculogenesis in the outside-to-inside direction; (C) Multiple endothelial strands with lumens penetrate the aortic wall at several sites.; (D) Fusion of the multiple endothelial strands occurs, and the tunica media of the coronary artery develops; (E) A single coronary trunk surrounded by a well-developed tunica media is completed. En, aortic endothelium; M, tunica media; Mc, tunica media of coronary artery; PR, peritruncal ring.

noncoronary sinus. In addition, a thick tunica media was observed surrounding the right and left proximal coronary arteries penetrating the aortic wall, while only weak anti-smooth muscle actin immunoreactivity was seen in cells surrounding the endothelial strands penetrating the noncoronary sinus. It seems likely that the definitive proximal coronary segments are demarcated from the aortic media (a derivative of the pharyngeal mesenchyme and ectomesenchyme) by the newly formed coronary artery tunica media (a derivative of the proepicardial organ).

Next, using the confocal microscope we examined the details of the process by which endothelial strands develop from PR. Thick (50 μm) sections across the cardiac base of day-6 embryos ($n = 5$) were prepared and stained with QH1 antibody. The resulting sections were scanned using a laser confocal microscope, and the images reconstructed. Confocal microscopic observation showed that QH1-positive discontinuous endothelial progenitors, which did not make contact either with the PR of the coronary vasculature or with the aortic endothelium, were situated within the aortic wall. Some QH1-positive cells were seen connecting either with PR or with both PR and the aortic lumen. We found no endothelial progenitors connecting with the aortic lumen alone. In addition, we found no case in which the coronary orifice did not connect with PR. These observations strongly suggest that the formation of endothelial strands occurs by vasculogenesis in an outside-to-inside (PR-to-aortic) direction.

In the present paper, we have analyzed the development of the proximal coronary arteries, and we propose a new morphologic mechanism to explain the development of the proximal coronary arteries and their orifices (Fig. 27.1): (1) multiple endothelial strands penetrate the aortic wall at several sites; (2) fusion of the multiple endothelial strands occurs at the facing sinuses, while at the same time the endothelial strands penetrating the noncoronary sinus disappear; (3) a coronary artery tunica media develops, and demarcates the definitive proximal coronary arteries from the aortic media. Further investigations will be needed to reveal the molecular mechanisms underlying the development of the coronary arteries.

References

1 Bogers AJJC, Gittenberger-de Groot AC, Dubbeldam JA, Huysmans HA. The inadequacy of existing theories on development of the proximal coronary arteries and their connexions with the arterial trunks. *Int J Cardiol* 1988; **20**: 117–23.

2 Bogers AJJC, Gittenberger-de Groot AC, Poelmann RE, Peault BM, Huysmans HA. Development of the origin of the coronary arteries, a matter of ingrowth or outgrowth? *Anat Embryol* 1989; **180**: 437–41.

3 Waldo KL, Willner W, Kirby ML. Origin of the proximal coronary artery stems and a review of ventricular vascularization in the chick embryo. *Am J Anat* 1990; **188**: 109–20.

4 Aikawa E, Kawano J. Formation of coronary arteries sprouting from the primitive aortic sinus wall of the chick embryo. *Experientia* 1982; **38**: 816–18.

5 Poelmann RE, Gittenberger-de Groot AC, Mentink MM, Bokenkamp R, Hogers B. Development of the cardiac coronary vascular endothelium, studied with antiendothelial antibodies, in chicken-quail chimeras. *Circ Res* 1993; **73**: 559–68.

6 Vrancken Peeters M-PFM, Gittenberger-de Groot AC, Mentink MM *et al.* The development of the coronary vessels and their differentiation into arteries and veins in the embryonic quail heart. *Dev Dyn* 1997; **208**: 338–48.

7 Coffin JD, Poole TJ. Endothelial cell origin and migration in embryonic heart and cranial blood vessel development. *Anat Rec* 1991; **231**: 383–95.

8 Skalli O, Ropraz P, Trzeciak A *et al.* A monoclonal antibody against alpha-smooth muscle actin: a new probe for smooth muscle differentiation. *J Cell Biol* 1986; **103**: 2787–96.

CHAPTER 28

Possible roles of the extracellular matrix in coronary vasculogenesis of mouse

Kyoko Imanaka-Yoshida, Mari Hara, Miyuki Namikata, Keiichi Miyamoto, Takashi Hanato, Noriko Watanabe, Masao Nakagawa, Toshimichi Yoshida

During development, blood vessels arise through two mechanism: angiogenesis and vasculogenesis.[1] While angiogenesis refers to the formation of capillaries from preexisting vessels, the formation of new capillaries by angioblasts which differentiate *in situ* is termed vasculogenesis. The heart is vascularized by vasculogenesis by cells that originate from the outside the primitive heart tube.[2] Angiogenesis and vasculogenesis sometimes overlap and require common mechanisms such as endothelial cell proliferation, migration, formation, and reorganization of 3-D structures, which are mediated by cell–extracellular matrix interaction.

The tenascins are a family of extracellular matrix proteins.[3] Tenascin-C (TNC) is transiently expressed in restricted sites during morphogenesis and tissue remodeling often associated with cell motility such as migration or epithelial–mesenchymal/mesenchymal–epithelial transformation.[4] Several lines of evidence suggest that TNC is involved in neovascularization in cancer invasion and wound healing in adult tissues.[5] Another member of the family, Tenascin-X (TNX), is more ubiquitously expressed but is predominantly expressed in the heart and blood vessels, and is often complimentary to TNC. Mutation of the TNX gene is reported to cause vascular disease.[6] These findings suggest that TNC and TNX may regulate the embryonic development of coronary vessels.

To study the roles of TNC and TNX in coronary vasculo/angiogenesis, we first analyzed the expression of TNC and TNX in mouse embryos by immunohistochemistry, *in situ* hybridization and RT-PCR. Initially, the primitive heart tube consists of only a two-cell population; myocardial cells and endocardial cells both originating from the lateral plate mesoderm.[7] At E9–9.5, mesenchymal cells at the base of the sinus venosus form a cauliflower-like structure and extend villous projections toward the heart. This transitory structure is called the proepicardial organ (PEO). At E 9.5, cell aggregates detach from PEO, adhere to the surface of the heart and spread over the heart to become epicardial cells,[8] which are precursors of vascular cells and interstitial fibroblasts.[9–12] Strong expression of TNC expression was observed in the mesenchymal cells of the PEO (Fig. 28.1). However, once the cells were transferred onto the surface of the heart, the expression of TNC was diminished. This expression pattern suggests that TNC can be involved in the initial step of cell migration from PEO. Proepicardial strands also extend over the inner surface of the pericardial cavity.[13,14] Interestingly, the cell inner surfaces of the pericardium continue to express TNC. Cardiomyocytes at this stage may send some signal to inhibit the expression of TNC of proepicardial cells.

After the total surface of the heart is ensheathed by a single layer of epicardium by E10.5, some epicardial cells undergo epithelial–mesenchymal transformation, delaminate, and invade the myocardium, which gives rise to the vascular endothelium, smooth muscle, and interstitial fibroblasts.[10,12,14–19]

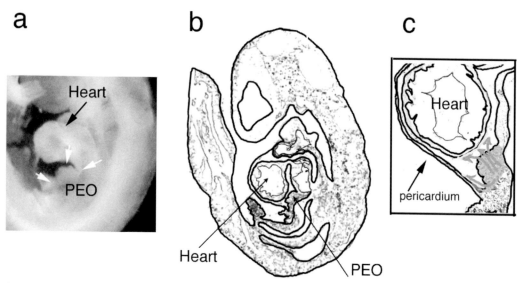

Fig. 28.1 *In situ* hybridization for TNC of E9.5 mouse embryo (a). Diagram of the embryo showing proepicardial organ (PEO) (b). Cells from PEO transfer onto the surface of the heart and spread over the heart to become epicardial cells. Cells also migrate along the inner surface of the pericardial cavity.

Generally, TNC expression is closely associated with cell motility; however, during epicardial cell migration and epithelial–mesenchymal transformation, TNC is not detected in the epicardium or myocardium.

In contrast, TNX is dramatically upregulated around E11 after the epicardial covering is completed, although it is not expressed in PEO nor during the migration of proepicardial cells. Whole-mount immunohistochemistry showed that TNX initially appeared along the interventricular groove and AV groove and eventually covered the entire surface of the heart by E12. Histological sections of the immunostained heart demonstrated that TNX was detected around the subepicardial cells that form vascular channels. In the E12.5 embryo, TNX was also detected associated with cells invading the ventricular myocardium as well as with channel-like structures in the myocardium. TNX seems to play an important role in vascular channel formation, while TNC is not involved in coronary vasculogenesis. However, around E13, preceding the connection of primitive coronary arteries to the aorta, TNC became detectable associated with the capillary plexus at a peritruncal ring around the aorta. TNC might be related with development of the proximal coronary arteries and their orifice formation.

To examine the process of coronary vessel formation *in vitro*, we tried to explant a culture of PEO. When the explants were plated on coverslips coated with rat tail collagen I, fibronectin, or laminin, the cells quickly spread and formed an epithelial sheet. When PEO was cultured on the collagen gel or in the gel, small outgrowths of cells were seen around the explants 3–4 days after plating. Around day 5, cord-like structures began to grow from the explants, gradually elongated, increased in number, and formed a branching network of structures (Fig. 28.2). A histological section demonstrated that the cells migrated into the gel and formed tube-like structures with lumens which were similar to the primitive vascular channels in the embryonic heart. The cells forming channels were TNX-positive, similar to the observation *in vivo*. This result indicates that PEO contains angioblasts or their precursors that have the ability to differentiate to vascular cells and form vascular channels without signals from other tissues such as cardiomyocytes or the liver, and that PEO apparently needs a particular extracellular environment to form vascular channel structures.

Vasculo/angiogenesis is a multistep process requiring various cell activities. TNC and TNX can take part in its regulation as significant extracellular factors. PEO explant culture in a 3-D collagen gel

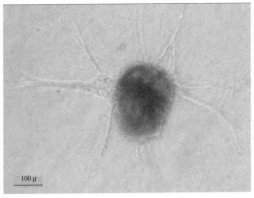
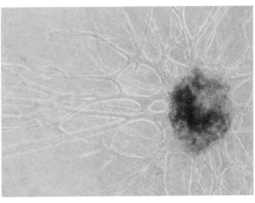

(a)

100 µ

(b)

Fig. 28.2 Proepicardial organ explant culture on collagen gel. (a) Day 5, (b) Day 10.

system could provide a useful approach to understand the complex nature of coronary vasculo/angiogenesis.

Methods

Antibodies

A mouse monoclonal antibody against TNC, clone 4F10TT, was raised by immunization of a TNC-null mouse with purified human glioma TNC.[20] Polyclonal anti-TNX antibodies were raised in rabbits against a fusion protein of the EGF-like repeats of murine TNX.[21]

Immunohistochemistry

Immunostaining of tissue sections was performed as previously described.[20,22]

In situ hybridization

Whole mount *in situ* hybridization of mouse embryos was carried out as described.[23] *In situ* hybridization of the tissue sections was performed as previously described.[20,22]

RT-PCR

RT-PCR of TNC and β-actin was performed as previously described.[24] The forward and reverse primers for TNX were 5'-GCCTCTTCCCCTC CACCTTCTCTACA-3' and 5'-GTCTCGATCAC GGGCAGAAAAGACA-3', respectively, and the expected size of the PCR fragment was 553 bp.

PEO culture

Only the tip region of PEO was dissected from E9.5 mouse embryos with tungsten needles and placed

on a collagen gel or coverslips coated with various substrates.

Collagen gel

Type I collagen was purified from rat tail tendon and collagen gel was prepared as previously described.[25] Briefly, 5 volumes of collagen solution (2.2 mg/mL), 5 volumes of 2× concentrated DMEM and 1 volume of FCS were mixed and warmed to 37 °C to allow gels to form.

References

1 Risaw W. Mechanisms of angiogenesis. *Nature* 1997; **386**: 671–4.

2 Bernanke DH, Velkey JM. Development of the coronary blood supply: changing concepts and current ideas. *Anat Rec* 2002; **269**; 198–208.

3 Erickson HP. Tenascin-C, tenascin-R and tenascin-X: a family of talented proteins in search of functions. *Curr Opin Cell Biol* 1993; **5**; 869–76.

4 Jones FS, Jones PL. The tenascin family of ECM glycoproteins: structure, function, and regulation during embryonic development and tissue remodeling. *Dev Dyn* 2000; **218**: 235–59.

5 Zagzag D, Capo V. Angiogenesis in the central nervous system: a role for vascular endothelial growth factor/vascular permeability factor and tenascin-C. Common molecular effectors in cerebral neoplastic and non-neoplastic 'angiogenic diseases'. *Histol Histopathol* 2002; **17**: 301–21.

6 Burch GH *et al.* Tenascin-X deficiency is associated with Ehlers-Danlos syndrome. *Nat Gen* 1997; **17**: 104–8.

7 Linask KK, Lash JW. Early heart development: dynamics of endocardial cell sorting suggests a common origin with cardiomyocytes. *Dev Dyn* 1993; **196**: 62–9.

8 Komiyama M, Ito K, Shimada Y. Origin and development of the epicardium in the mouse embryo. *Anat Embryol* 1987; **176**: 183–9.

9 Mikawa T, Cohen-Gould L, Fischman DA. Clonal analysis of cardiac morphogenesis in the chicken embryo using a replication-defective retrovirus. III: Polyclonal origin of adjacent ventricular myocytes. *Dev Dyn* 1992; **195**: 133–41.

10 Mikawa T, Gourdie RG. Pericardial mesoderm generates a population of coronary smooth muscle cells migrating into the heart along with ingrowth of the epicardial organ. *Dev Biol* 1996; **174**: 221–32.

11 Poelmann R, Gittenberger-de Groot A, Mentink M, Bokenkamp R, Hogers B. Development of the cardiac coronary vascular endothelium, studied with antiendothelial antibodies, in chicken-quail chimeras. *Circ Res* 1993; **73**: 559–68.

12 Dettman RW, Denetclaw W Jr, Ordahl CP, Bristow J. Common epicardial origin of coronary vascular smooth muscle, perivascular fibroblasts, and intermyocardial fibroblasts in the avian heart. *Dev Biol* 1998; **193**: 169–81.

13 Manner J. Experimental study on the formation of the epicardium in chick embryos. *Anat Embryol* 1993; **187**: 281–9.

14 Perez-Pomares JM, Macias D, Garcia-Garrido L, Munoz-Chapuli R. The origin of the subepicardial mesenchyme in the avian embryo: an immunohistochemical and quail-chick chimera study. *Dev Biol* 1998; **200**: 57–68.

15 Mikawa T, Fischman DA. Retroviral analysis of cardiac morphogenesis: discontinuous formation of coronary vessels. *Proc Nat Acad Sci U S A* 1992; **89**; 9504–8.

16 Gittenberger-de Groot AC, Vrancken Peeters, MP, Mentink MM, Gourdie RG, Poelmann RE. Epicardium-derived cells contribute a novel population to the myocardial wall and the atrioventricular cushions. *Circ Res* 1998; **82**: 1043–52.

17 Manner J. Does the subepicardial mesenchyme contribute myocardioblasts to the myocardium of the chick embryo heart? A quail-chick chimera study tracing the fate of the epicardial primordium. *Anat Rec* 1999; **255**; 212–26.

18 Vrancken Peeters MP, Gittenberger-de Groot AC, Mentink MM, Poelmann RE. Smooth muscle cells and fibroblasts of the coronary arteries derive from epithelial–mesenchymal transformation of the epicardium. *Anat Embryol* 1999; **199**: 367–78.

19 Vrancken Peeters MP *et al.* The development of the coronary vessels and their differentiation into arteries and veins in the embryonic quail heart. *Dev Dyn* 1997; **208**: 338–48.

20 Imanaka-Yoshida K *et al.* Tenascin-C is a useful marker for disease activity in myocarditis. *J Pathol* 2002; **197**: 387–94.

21 Hasegawa K. *et al.* Differential expression of tenascin-C and tenascin-X in human astrocytomas. *Acta Neuropathol* 1997; **93**: 431–7.

22 Imanaka-Yoshida K *et al.* Tenascin-C modulates adhesion of cardiomyocytes to extracellular matrix during tissue remodeling after myocardial infarction. *Lab Invest* 2001; **81**: 1015–24.

23 Wei L *et al.* Rho kinases play an obligatory role in vertebrate embryonic organogenesis. *Development* 2001; **128**: 2953–62.

24 Noda N *et al.* Expression of tenascin-C in stromal cells of the murine uterus during early pregnancy: induction by interleukin-1 alpha, prostaglandin E2 and prostaglandin F2 alpha. *Biol Reprod* 2000; **63**: 1723–30.

25 Fujita Y, Yoshida T, Sakakura Y, Sakakura T. Reconstruction of pleomorphic adenoma of the salivary glands in three-dimensional collagen gel matrix culture. *Virchows Arch.* 1999; **434**: 137–43.

CHAPTER 29

Abnormal coronary development in bis-diamine treated embryo

*Takashi Hanato, Masao Nakagawa, Nobuhiko Okamoto,
Setsuko Nishijima, Hidetoshi Fujino, Yoshihiro Takeuchi*

Conotruncal anomalies, including tetralogy of Fallot, truncus arteriosus communis, and aortic arch anomalies, are often associated with anomalous coronary arteries.[1,2] However, the pathological mechanisms of anomalous coronary arteries associated with the conotruncal defects[3–5] as well as the developmental anatomy of coronary vasculatures have not been fully demonstrated. N,N′-bis(dichloroacetyl)diamine-1,8-octa-methylene diamine (bis-diamine) induces conotruncal anomaly in rat embryos when administered to the mother.[6–8] To determine whether anomalous coronary arteries are associated with the cardiac defects caused by bis-diamine, we morphologically studied rat embryos treated with bis-diamine.

Materials and methods

A single dose of 200-mg bis-diamine conjugated with 1 mL of 1% gum was administered to pregnant rats at 10.5 embryonic days (ED) of gestation. ED were dated from midnight prior to the presence of a vaginal plug. Controls received 1 mL of 1% gum at ED10.5. Embryos removed from the mothers at ED20.5 were used for morphological analysis of coronary arteries. The distributional patterns of coronary arteries were examined by injecting India ink into the aorta. To have the aorta accessible for ink injection, a midsternal thoracotomy was performed with iridectomy scissors. The beating of the heart was stopped in diastole by dripping a 20% KCl solution (4°C) over its surface. A solution of India ink and 1% arabia gum diluted in phosphate buffered saline (PBS) was then slowly injected into the ascending aorta. Injections were given through a micropipette. Following ink injections, the hearts were removed and fixed in Carnoy's solution (ethanol: chloroform: glacial acetic acid = 6: 3: 1) for 3 h. The coronary vasculature of each heart was studied under a stereoscope. Histological sections from each heart were examined under microscope.

Results

The incidence of congenital heart anomalies, anomalous coronary arteries, and defects of the left diaphragm in bis-diamine-treated embryos at ED20.5 (*n* = 52) are presented in Table 29.1. Thirty-six (69%) of 52 embryos had truncus arteriosus communis and 12 (23%) had tetralogy of Fallot. Aortic arch anomalies were detected in 6 (11.5%). No cardiovascular anomaly was observed in the controls. A single right coronary artery or hypoplastic left

Table 29.1 Incidence of conotruncal anomalies, abnormal coronary arteries, and defects of the left diaphragm in control and bis-diamine-treated embryos

	Control (n = 20)	Bis-diamine treated (n = 52)
Heart anomalies	None	48 (92%) TA 36; TF 12[a]
Coronary anomalies	None	48 (92%)
LDD[b]	None	52 (100%)

[a] TA, truncus arteriosus communis; TF, tetralogy of Fallot.
[b] LDD, defect of left diaphragm.

Table 29.2 Coronary vascularization in the embryonic rat heart

	Control			Treated		
Site	ED15	ED16	ED17	ED15	ED16	ED17
CA proximal	+/–	+	++	+/–	+	++
CA distal	+/–	++	++	–	–	–
Distance of extra–myocardial layer (μm)	18.75	11.25	2.5	34.5	31.25	18.75

–, Nothing; +/–, endothelial lined channel (only blood island); +, vascular channel; ++, complete coronary artery.

coronary artery was detected in all the embryos and was associated with truncus arteriosus communis or tetralogy of Fallot. Abnormal distributions of coronary arteries were also detected in all embryos. There was no relationship between the type of coronary artery anomalies and cardiac defects. Histological sections revealed incomplete hatching and abnormal connection of the aorta to the coronary vasculature. Serial sections from younger embryos treated with bis-diamine disclosed poor epicardial development and disturbed vascular channel formation (Table 29.2; Plate 23). No abnormal coronary arteries were detected in the embryos that did not have a cardiac anomaly. All the embryos treated with bis-diamine had a defect in the left diaphragm. Controls had neither abnormal coronary arteries nor a defect in the diaphragm.

Discussion

In this study, we demonstrated that bis-diamine induced anomalous coronary arteries, including a single right coronary artery and a hypoplastic left coronary artery, in association with conotruncal defects. As the conotruncal anomalies were experimentally produced by ablation of the cardiac neural crest in chick embryos,[9,10] bis-diamine is supposed to disrupt the migration of neural crest cells into the heart in early rat embryos. Hood and Rosenquist,[11] and Poelman et al.[12] suggested the possible contribution of the neural crest cells to the development of coronary vasculature. Although we found no evidence to support their speculation, this study revealed poor development of the coronary vasculature near the truncus arteriosus and incomplete hatching and abnormal connection of the aorta to the coronary vasculature. These findings suggested that bis-diamine disturbed the formation

of vascular channels and subsequently induced abnormal development of the coronary vasculature. As the anomalous coronary arteries, including an aplastic or hypoplastic left coronary artery, were always associated with a conotruncal anomaly in this study, it may be possible that abnormal truncal division secondarily disrupted the spatial relationship between the coronary ostium and vasculature.

References

1 Fellows KE, Freed MD, Keane JF et al. Results of routine preoperative coronary angiography in tetralogy of Fallot. *Circulation* 1975; **51**: 561–6.
2 Dabizzi RP, Caprioli G, Aiazzi L et al. Distribution and anomalies of coronary arteries in tetralogy of Fallot. *Circulation* 1980; **61**: 95–102.
3 Bogers AJJC, Bartelings MM, Bokenkamp R et al. Common arterial trunk, uncommon coronary arterial anatomy. *J Thorac Cardiovasc Surg* 1993; **106**: 1133–7.
4 Conte G, Pellegrini A. On the development of the coronary arteries in human embryos, stage 14–19. *Anat Embryol* 1984; **169**: 209–18.
5 Bogers AJJC, Gittenberger-de Groot AC, Dubbeldam JA, Huysmans HA. The inadequacy of existing theories on development of the proximal coronary arteries and their connections with the arterial trunks. *Int J Cardiol* 1988; **20**: 117–23.
6 Taleporos P, Salgo P, Oster G. Teratogenic action of a bis(dichloroacetyl) diamine on rats. Patterns of malformations produced in high incidence at time-limited periods of development. *Teratology* 1978; **18**: 5–16.
7 Jackson M, Connel MG, Smith A, Drury J, Anderson RH. Common arterial trunk and pulmonary atresia: close developmental cousins? Results from a teratogen induced animal model. *Cardiovasc Res* 1995; **30**: 992–1000.
8 Okamoto N, Satow Y, Lee JY et al. Morphology and pathogenesis of the cardiovascular anomalies induced by bis-(dichloroacetyl) diamine in rats. In: Takao A, Nora JJ eds.

Congenital Heart Disease: Causes and Processes. New York: Futura, 1984: 199–221.

9 Kirby ML, Turnage KL, Hays BM. Characterization of conotruncal anomalies following ablation of 'cardiac' neural crest. *Anat Rec* 1985; **213**: 84–93.

10 Nishibatake M, Kirby ML, Van Mierop LHS. Pathogenesis of persistent truncus arteriosus and dextroposed aorta in the chick embryo after neural crest ablation. *Circulation* 1987; **75**: 255–64.

11 Hood LC, Rosenquist TH. Coronary artery development in the chick: Origin and deployment of smooth muscle cells, and the effects of neural crest ablation. *Anat Rec* 1992; **234**: 291–300.

12 Poelmann RE, Gittenberger-de Groot Ac, Mentink MMT, Bokenkamp R, Hogers B. Development of the cardiac vascular endothelium, studied with anti-endothelial antibodies in chicken-quail chimeras. *Circ Res* 1993; **73**: 559–68.

PART 7

Models of congenital cardiovascular malformations

Editorial perspective

D. Woodrow Benson

A large number of genetically engineered mice have a cardiac phenotype, but such models have rarely predicted the genetic basis of viable, human congenital heart malformations. As illustrated by the chapters in this part, the identification of single gene mutations resulting in human cardiac malformations has provided new tools to study the pathogenesis of congenital heart disease in animal models.

The paper by Bruneau describes mice with haploinsufficiency of $Tbx5$ ($Tbx5^{del/+}$). $Tbx5^{del/+}$ mice have all the major hallmarks of Holt–Oram syndrome, confirming that haploinsufficiency of Tbx5 causes Holt–Oram syndrome. Affected mice demonstrate atrial septal defects, ventricular septal defects and AV conduction abnormalities. Variations in severity of phenotype between strains and within an outbred strain of almost genetically identical animals, as is seen in humans with heterozygous $TBX5$ mutations populations, supports a role for genetic modifiers as modulators of penetrance and expressivity.

FOG-2 is a multi-zinc finger protein and a member of the Friend of GATA family of transcriptional modulators. To elucidate FOG-2's role in cardiac development, Svensson *et al.* generated a mouse deficient in FOG-2 using standard gene targeting techniques. Homozygous mice died *in utero*; cardiac examination revealed cardiac malformations that included pulmonic stenosis, double outlet right ventricle, atrial and ventricular septal defects, absent coronary arteries, and tricuspid atresia. During a functional analysis of the FOG-2, they determined that zinc fingers 1 and 6 of FOG-2 were capable of binding GATA4 and identified a binding site for the transcriptional co-repressor C-terminal binding protein-2 (CtBP-2) in the C-terminal portion of the FOG-2 protein. Taken together, these results demonstrate the importance of FOG-2 for cardiac formation and indicate that transcriptional repressors are required for the regulation of heart development.

The chromosomal abnormality, del22q11, is frequent cause of congenital cardiac defects in humans. The deletion spans about 3 Mbp of DNA and includes approximately 30 genes. *TBX1* is contained in the deleted region; haploinsufficiency of *Tbx1* results in a mouse phenotype reminiscent of del22q11 in humans. In order to define Tbx1-related regulatory cascades, Yamagishi and Sirvastava searched for the *cis*-regulatory elements that control *Tbx1* expression during development. Their studies show that *Tbx1* is directly regulated by Foxc1 and Foxc2 in the head mesenchyme, and Foxa2 in the pharyngeal endoderm, through a common Fox binding element upstream of *Tbx1*. Shh signaling functions to maintain the expression of *Foxa2*

the decreased cx40 expression in $Tbx5^{del/+}$ mice. The first is that the decrease in *cx40* mRNA levels (>90% decrease) is not proportional to the 50% loss of Tbx5, which shows that the regulation of *cx40* by Tbx5 is not linear, and perhaps involves cooperative interactions between multiple Tbx5 binding sites. The second is that the decrease in *cx40* expression may be in itself sufficient to explain the conduction defects in $Tbx5^{del/+}$ mice (and in Holt–Oram syndrome) independent of the ASDs. One might argue that the conduction defects are secondary to the structural defects, but several points argue against this. One is that the decrease in *cx40* expression occurs at stage in mouse embryogenesis prior to that at which formation of the atrial septum occurs. The other is that within a family with a *TBX5* mutation, one can find individuals with ASDs but no AV block, or AV block without an ASD, thus suggesting that the two are unrelated except for the *TBX5* mutation.[11] Another intriguing observation from cx40-deficient mice is that a proportion of these have ASDs and VSDs.[8] However, these may occur as a result of impaired neural crest cell function/migration, and are perhaps distinct from those caused by Tbx5 deficiency. We are currently generating transgenic mice

that express cx40 in the heart independent from Tbx5 in order to rescue the defective cx40 levels in $Tbx5^{del/+}$ mice; this may conclusively show what portion of the $Tbx5^{del/+}$ phenotype can be attributed to cx40 deficiency.

The decrease in *cx40* expression may explain the conduction system defects caused by Tbx5 haploinsufficiency, but it might not explain the ASDs and VSDs. The underlying basis for these defects is still unknown. Preliminary analysis has not uncovered dramatic changes in cell proliferation or apoptosis in the hearts of $Tbx5^{del/+}$ mice [unpubl. data]. It is however possible that a small population of cells are slightly impaired in their proliferative capacity, and that these changes, although sufficient to cause these structural defects, have to date escaped detection. $Tbx5^{del/+}$ mice have much thinner atrial walls than their wild-type littermates (Fig. 30.1), lending support for the notion of decreased proliferation. Similarly, ventricular septa of $Tbx5^{del/+}$ mice are disorganized and hypocellular (Fig. 30.1). Perhaps also, as suggested by *in vitro* data, Tbx5 is involved in cell migration and motility,[8] and that this is the process that is impaired in the formation of the septa. On the other hand, it appears that fundamen-

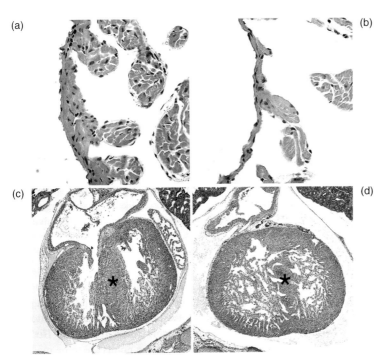

(a)

(b)

(c)

(d)

Fig. 30.1 Histology of wild-type (a,c) and $Tbx5^{del/+}$ (b,d) mouse hearts from 8-week-old adult animals (a,b) and E16.5 fetuses (c,d). (a), (b) Close-ups (magnification × 40) of the atrial wall. Note the considerably thinner wall in the $Tbx5^{del/+}$ animal (b). (c), (d) Sections (magnification × 10) through the ventricles. Note the acellular and disorganized ventricular septum in the $Tbx5^{del/+}$ animal (d). *, ventricular septum.

tal changes in gene expression and patterning occur in $Tbx5^{del/+}$ mice, as can be seen at E9.5–10.5 by increased right ventricular expression of *ANF*, as well as ectopic expression of this gene in the interventricular groove where the interventricular septum will arise (ref. 7 and Plate 24) Microarray analysis will hopefully assist in uncovering genes other than *cx40* that are misregulated in $Tbx5^{del/+}$ mice, and lead us in the right direction to uncover the mechanisms underlying the structural defects in Holt–Oram syndrome. For example, we have shown that Tbx5 controls limb formation by activating, in concert with Wnt signals, a fibroblast growth factor signaling cascade;[1] perhaps similar pathways downstream of Tbx5 exist in the developing heart.

The observation that a 50% decrease in the levels of a transcription factor such as Tbx5 would cause such dramatic heart defects and profound changes in the expression of downstream target genes points to very accurate responses to Tbx5 levels. We have recently made use of a hypomorphic allele of *Tbx5* (A. Mori and B.G.B, unpublished data) to uncover a much finer degree of gene regulation. The *Tbx5* hypomorphic allele expresses some *Tbx5* mRNA, but less than wild-type levels. Thus in the heterozygous state, it expresses less than wild-type but more than $Tbx5^{del/+}$ mice, and in the homozygous state it expresses less than $Tbx5^{del/+}$ mice but more than $Tbx5^{del/del}$ mice. Thus using all these lines of mice we have several graded intermediate levels of *Tbx5* expression ranging between 0 and 100%. In mice heterozygous for the hypomorphic allele, ASDs are found, but conduction defects are less severe, showing a marked and precise sensitivity to decreased Tbx5 dosage. Furthermore, mice homozygous for the hypomorphic allele have defects in morphogenesis that are not quite as severe as in embryos lacking all Tbx5 protein. In these embryos, many genes that are downregulated in $Tbx5^{del/del}$ embryos are also affected, but some escape downregulation, again showing that the dosage of Tbx5 is crucial for regulation of downstream target genes at all dosage levels. This extraordinary rheostat-like control by Tbx5 may be as a result of numbers of Tbx5 binding sites in the promoters of downstream genes. Preliminary analyses, however, have not revealed any strong correlation between sensitivity to Tbx5 dosage and numbers of T-box binding sites. Tbx5 can synergis-

tically activate some promoters in combination with Nkx2–5;[6,13] it may be that it is a combination of numbers of Tbx5 binding sites with Nkx2–5 or other types of binding sites that dictates the degree of sensitivity to Tbx5 levels. These precise differential Tbx5 dosage sensitivities from one gene to the next provide a useful mechanism to generate diversity of transcriptional responses in different cell types at various times in development.

We have gained much information from the generation of a mouse model of Holt–Oram syndrome. However, more questions have been raised than answered, which points to the complexities underlying the development of CHDs. The transcriptional integration of multiple cellular processes in different cell types at various stages of heart development is all potentially disrupted to varying degrees by mutations in genes such as Tbx5. Identifying these components and their complex interplay during heart development will be the key to understanding CHDs.

Acknowledgments

The author's research is supported by the Canadian Institutes of Health Research, the Heart and Stroke Foundation of Ontario, and the March of Dimes Birth Defects Foundation. The author holds of a Canada Research Chair in Developmental Cardiology.

References

1 Agarwal P, Wylie JN, Galceran J et al. Tbx5 is essential for forelimb bud initiation following patterning of the limb field in the mouse embryo. *Development* 2003; **130**: 623–33.

2 Basson CT, Bachinsky DR, Lin RC et al. Mutations in human TBX5 cause limb and cardiac malformation in Holt–Oram syndrome. *Nat Genet* 1997; **15**: 30–5.

3 Basson CT, Cowley GS, Solomon SD et al. The clinical and genetic spectrum of the Holt–Oram syndrome (heart-hand syndrome). *N Engl J Med* 1994; **330**: 885–91.

4 Benson DW, Silberbach GM, Kavanaugh-McHugh A et al. Mutations in the cardiac transcription factor NKX2.5 affect diverse cardiac developmental pathways. *J Clin Invest* 1999; **104**: 1567–73.

5 Bevilacqua LM, Simon AM, Maguire CT et al. A targeted disruption in connexin40 leads to distinct atrioventricular conduction defects. *J Interv Card Electrophysiol* 2000; **4**: 459–67.

6 Bruneau BG. Mouse models of cardiac chamber formation and congenital heart disease. *Trends Genet* 2002; **18**: S15–S20.

7 Bruneau BG, Nemer G, Schmitt JP *et al*. A murine model of Holt–Oram syndrome defines roles of the T-box transcription factor Tbx5 in cardiogenesis and disease. *Cell* 2001; **106**: 709–21.

8 Hatcher CJ, Kim MS, Mah CS *et al*. TBX5 transcription factor regulates cell proliferation during cardiogenesis. *Dev Biol* 2001; **230**: 177–88.

9 Hiroi Y, Kudoh S, Monzen K *et al*. Tbx5 associates with Nkx2–5 and synergistically promotes cardiomyocyte differentiation. *Nat Genet* 2001; **28**: 276–80.

10 Kirchhoff S, Kim JS, Hagendorff A *et al*. Abnormal cardiac conduction and morphogenesis in connexin40 and connexin43 double-deficient mice. *Circ Res* 2000; **87**: 399–405.

11 Kirchhoff S, Nelles E, Hagendorff A *et al*. Reduced cardiac conduction velocity and predisposition to arrythmias in connexin40-deficient mice. *Curr Biol* 1998; **8**: 299–302.

12 Li QY, Newbury-Ecob RA, Terrett JA *et al*. Holt–Oram syndrome is caused by mutations in *TBX5*, a member of the Brachyury (T) gene family. *Nat Genet* 1997; **15**: 21–9.

13 Schott J-J, Benson DW, Basson CT *et al*. Congenital heart disease caused by mutations in the transcription factor *NKX2–5*. *Science* 1998; **281**: 108–11.

14 Simon AM, Goodenough DA, Paul DL. Mice lacking connexin40 have cardiac conduction abnormalities characteristic of atrioventricular block and bundle branch block. *Curr Biol* 1998; **8**: 295–8.

CHAPTER 31

The role of the transcriptional co-repressor FOG-2 in cardiac development

Eric C. Svensson, Jeannine Wilk, Rodney Dale, Melinda Modrell

Cardiac development is a complex process regulated by a number of transcription factors, only some of which are currently known.[1–5] To date, most of these factors are strong transcriptional activators such as GATA4, MEF2C, and Nkx2.5.[6–9] Recently, the importance of transcriptional repressors to heart development is becoming apparent. We and others have previously identified FOG-2, a multi-zinc finger protein and a member of the FOG family of transcriptional modulators.[10–13] FOG-2 is first expressed in the developing heart and septum transversum at mouse embryonic day 8.5, and is subsequently expressed in the developing brain and gonads as well as at low levels in the liver and lung. FOG-2 physically interacts with the N-terminal zinc finger of GATA4 and represses GATA4's ability to activate transcription of a number of GATA-dependent cardiac promoters *in vitro*.[12]

To elucidate FOG-2's role in cardiac development, we generated a mouse deficient in FOG-2 using standard gene targeting techniques.[14,15] Disruption of the FOG-2 gene resulted in embryonic lethality at mid-gestation, with homozygous deficient mice displaying signs of embryonic heart failure. A histologic examination of these embryos revealed cardiac malformations that included pulmonic stenosis, double outlet right ventricle, atrial and ventricular septal defects, the failure to form coronary arteries, and tricuspid atresia. Taken together, these results demonstrate the importance of FOG-2 for cardiac formation and indicate that transcriptional repressors are required for the regulation of heart development.

To obtain a better understanding of function of FOG-2 in cardiac morphogenesis, we undertook a functional analysis of the FOG-2 protein to determine the critical regions of FOG-2 mediating GATA4 binding and repression.[16] Our analysis indicated that zinc fingers 1 and 6 of FOG-2 were capable of binding GATA4. We also identified a binding site for the transcriptional co-repressor C-terminal binding protein-2 (CtBP-2) in the C-terminal portion of the FOG-2 protein. However, this site was not required for repression of GATA-mediated transcription *in vitro*. Instead, we found that the N-terminal 226 amino acids of FOG-2 were necessary for this repression and sufficient to mediate repression when fused to a heterologous DNA binding domain.

During our isolation of FOG-2 cDNA clones from a mouse embryonic day 13 cDNA library, we isolated an alternative FOG-2 transcript containing 240 bp of unique 5' sequence which we designated FOG-2B. To determine the origin of this sequence, we assembled a genomic map of the FOG-2 gene from the human sequences present in Genbank. We found that the FOG-2 gene was composed of eight exons and spanned over 500 kb of genomic DNA (Fig. 31.1). Further, the unique sequence of the FOG-2B transcript was encoded by an alternative exon located between exon 1A and 2. To determine the pattern of expression of this transcript, we isolated total RNA from embryonic day 13.5 mouse hearts as well as adult heart, brain, and liver. RT-PCR analysis using primers specific for the FOG-2A or FOG-2B transcripts is shown in Fig. 31.2. As we have shown previously, FOG-2A is present in embryonic

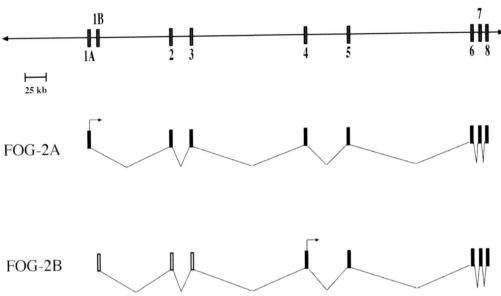

Fig. 31.1 Genomic organization of the human FOG-2 gene. Schematic illustration of the FOG-2 gene (above) and transcripts (below). Genomic data derived from Genbank. For each FOG-2 transcript, the translation initiation site is indicated with an arrow. Exons containing coding sequences are indicated by black shading.

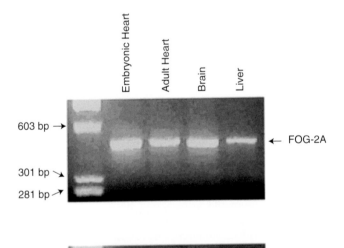

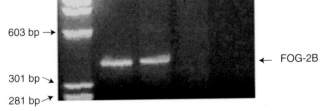

Fig. 31.2 FOG-2A and FOG-2B are differentially expressed. RT-PCR analysis of mRNA from embryonic day 13.5 heart, adult heart, brain, and liver using primers specific for the FOG-2A (top panel) or FOG-2B (bottom panel) transcript.

and adult heart, brain, and liver. In contrast, the FOG-2B transcript is only expressed in embryonic and adult heart. These results demonstrate that FOG-2B is an alternative transcript of the FOG-2 gene expressed in a distinct pattern from FOG-2A.

Owing to the lack of an initiator methionine in exon 1B, translation of the FOG-2B transcript is predicted to be initiated from a methionine in exon 4. The resulting protein is an N-terminal truncation of FOG-2A, lacking the N-terminal 132 amino acids but still containing all eight zinc finger motifs. To determine if this protein was capable of binding to GATA4, *in vitro* binding assays were performed as previously.[16] The results indicate that FOG-2B is able to bind to GATA4 as expected based on our previous functional analysis of FOG-2A (data not shown).

To test the function of FOG-2B, we transfected NIH 3T3 fibroblasts with expression vectors encoding GATA4 and either FOG-2A or FOG-2B, along with a reporter construct containing the atrial naturetic factor (ANF) promoter driving expression of human growth hormone. As we have shown previously, FOG-2A efficiently represses transcriptional activation of the ANF promoter by GATA4.[16] In marked contrast, FOG-2B is unable to repress GATA4 transactivation under these conditions (data not shown).

In summary, we have described an alternative transcript of the FOG-2 gene that is expressed in a distinct tissue-restricted pattern. Further, this transcript encodes an N-terminal truncation of FOG-2A that is capable of binding GATA4 but unable to repress GATA-mediated transactivation of cardiac promoters. The importance of this transcript for cardiac development is currently under investigation.

References

1 Srivastava D, Olson EN. A genetic blueprint for cardiac development. *Nature* 2000; **407**: 221–6.

2 Fishman, MC, Olson EN. Parsing the heart: genetic modules for organ assembly. *Cell* 1997; **91**: 153–6.

3 Harvey RP. Cardiac looping – an uneasy deal with laterality. *Sem Cell Dev Biol* 1998; **9**: 101–8.

4 Olson EN, Srivastava D. Molecular pathways controlling heart development. *Science* 1996; **272**: 671–6.

5 Sucov HM. Molecular insights into cardiac development. *Annu Rev Physiol* 1998; **60**: 287–308.

6 Molkentin JD, Lin Q, Duncan SA, Olson EN. Requirement of the transcription factor GATA4 for heart tube formation and ventral morphogenesis. *Genes Dev* 1997; **11**: 1061–72.

7 Kuo CT *et al.* GATA4 transcription factor is required for ventral morphogenesis and heart tube formation. *Genes Dev* 1997; **11**: 1048–60.

8 Lyons I *et al.* Myogenic and morphogenetic defects in the heart tubes of murine embryos lacking the homeobox gene Nkx2–5. *Genes Dev* 1995; **9**: 1654–66.

9 Lin Q, Schwarz J, Bucana C, Olson EN. Control of mouse cardiac morphogenesis and myogenesis by transcription factor MEF2C. *Science* 1997; **276**: 1404–7.

10 Lu JR *et al.* FOG-2, a heart- and brain-enriched cofactor for GATA transcription factors. *Mol Cell Biol* 1999; **19**: 4495–502.

11 Holmes M *et al.* hFOG-2, a novel zinc finger protein, binds the co-repressor mCtBP2 and modulates GATA-mediated activation. *J Biol Chem* 1999; **274**: 23491–8.

12 Svensson EC, Tufts RL, Polk CE. Leiden JM. Molecular cloning of FOG-2: a modulator of transcription factor GATA-4 in cardiomyocytes. *Proc Natl Acad Sci USA* 1999; **96**: 956–61.

13 Tevosian SG *et al.* FOG-2: a novel GATA-family cofactor related to multitype zinc-finger proteins Friend of GATA-1 and U-shaped. *Proc Natl Acad Sci USA* 1999; **96**: 950–5.

14 Svensson EC *et al.* A syndrome of tricuspid atresia in mice with a targeted mutation of the gene encoding Fog-2. *Nat Genet* 2000; **25**: 353–6.

15 Tevosian SG *et al.* FOG-2, a cofactor for GATA transcription factors, is essential for heart morphogenesis and development of coronary vessels from epicardium. *Cell* 2000; **101**: 729–39.

16 Svensson EC, Huggins GS, Dardik FB, Polk CE, Leiden JM. A functionally conserved N-terminal domain of the friend of GATA-2 (FOG-2) protein represses GATA4-dependent transcription. *J Biol Chem* 2000; **275**: 20762–9.

CHAPTER 32

Molecular mechanisms regulating tissue-specific expression of *Tbx1*

Hiroyuki Yamagishi, Deepak Srivastava

22q11.2 deletion syndrome (22q11DS) is the most frequent chromosomal microdeletion syndrome in humans and is characterized by congenital cardiac and craniofacial defects.[1–3] Haplo-insufficiency of *Tbx1* in mice results in aortic arch malformations, whereas a homozygous mutation causes pharyngeal arch defects and most features of 22q11DS.[4–6] Consistent with the mutant phenotype, *Tbx1* is expressed in the head mesenchyme, pharyngeal mesoderm, and pharyngeal endoderm,[4–8] but the developmental program in which it functions is unknown.

In order to define Tbx1-related regulatory cascades, we searched for the *cis*-regulatory elements that control *Tbx1* expression during development.[9] Transgenic expression of the *lacZ* marker under control of the 5' genomic region (12.8 kb long) of *Tbx1* recapitulated the endogenous expression of *Tbx1* (Plate 25a–c). To localize the regulatory elements responsible for embryonic expression of *Tbx1*, we constructed a series of deletions of the 12.8 kb genomic fragment and analyzed their ability to direct *lacZ* expression from a heterologous promoter in F_0 transgenic mice at embryonic day (E) 9.5. As shown in Plate 25, these analyses identified the critical *cis*-element(s) necessary for *Tbx1* expression in the pharyngeal endoderm and head mesenchyme within a 1.1 kb region (Plate 25a–f).

The temporospatial expression pattern of *Tbx1* during early embryogenesis was determined using stable transgenic mouse lines bearing *lacZ* under control of the 12.8 kb upstream fragments described above. At E7.5, the 12.8 kb transgene directed *lacZ* expression in the paraxial mesodermal cells that give rise to cranial mesenchyme, but not in the lateral plate mesoderm or cardiac crescent that forms the heart tube (Plate 25g,l). Slightly later (E8.5), *lacZ* expression was observed in a segment of the cranial mesoderm including the first pharyngeal arch mesoderm (Plate 25h,m). At E9.5, the transgene directed high levels of *lacZ* expression in the mesoderm-derived head mesenchyme and the mesodermal core of the pharyngeal arches (Plate 25i,k,n–p). *LacZ* expression in pharyngeal endoderm became detectable at this stage and was pronounced in the pharyngeal pouches. Expression was not detectable in pharyngeal arch mesenchyme derived from neural crest cells, consistent with the endogenous *Tbx1* expression previously shown by RNA *in situ* hybridization. At E10.5, *lacZ* expression was maintained in the head mesenchyme, pharyngeal mesoderm and endoderm, and began to extend to the precursors of the vertebral column (Plate 25j).

Although expression of *Tbx1* in the developing heart had not been detectable by mRNA expression analyses, a recent study using mice harboring the *lacZ* gene targeted into the *Tbx1* locus demonstrated *Tbx1* expression in the cardiac outflow tract between E9.5 and E12.5.[10] *LacZ* expression under control of the 12.8 kb fragment was detectable in the myocardial and endocardial layer of the outflow tract between E8.5 and E10.5 (Plate 25k,p), but not in the conotruncal cushion, indicating that *Tbx1* may be expressed in the recently identified cells of the anterior heart tube that are derived from anterior or secondary heart field.[11,12]

We have previously reported regulation of *Tbx1* by a secreted molecule, Sonic hedgehog (Shh), in mouse and chick embryos.[8] *Shh*-null mice die soon after birth and have numerous craniofacial and car-

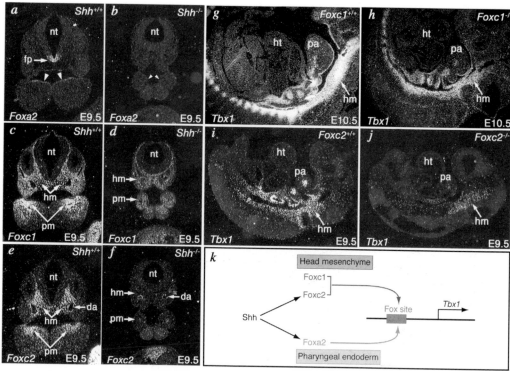

Fig. 32.1 Shh regulation of *Tbx1* is directly mediated by Fox proteins. (a),(b) Radioactive *in situ* hybridization on transverse sections of E9.5 mouse embryos showed that *Foxa2* is downregulated in floor plate (fp) of neural tube (nt) and pharyngeal endoderm (arrowheads) of *Shh*[-/-] embryos compared with wild type (*Shh*[+/+]) embryos. (c),(d) *Foxc1* was expressed normally in the head mesenchyme (hm) and pharyngeal arch mesenchyme (pm) of *Shh* mutant embryos compared with wild type embryos. (e),(f) *Foxc2* was downregulated in the head mesenchyme and pharyngeal arch mesenchyme of *Shh* mutant embryos compared with wild type embryos. *Foxc2* expression in dorsal aortae (da) was normal in *Shh* mutant embryos. (a), (c) and (e) are serial sections from a wild type embryo, and (b), (d) and (f) are serial sections from a *Shh* mutant embryo. (g)-(l) Radioactive *in situ* hybridization on sagittal sections of E9.5–10.5 mouse embryos showed that *Tbx1* was expressed, but partially downregulated in the head mesenchyme of *Foxc1* or *Foxc2* mutant (*Foxc1*[-/-] or *Foxc2*[-/-]) embryos compared with wild type (*Foxc1*[+/+] or *Foxc2*[+/+]) embryos. (k) A proposed model for molecular regulation of *Tbx1*. ht, heart; pa, pharyngeal arch.

diac defects[13] that are distinct, but overlapping, with defects in *Tbx1* mutants. We, therefore, crossed *Tbx1-lacZ* transgenic mice into the *Shh*-null background to examine whether this enhancer is dependent on Shh signaling.[9] At E9.25, *lacZ* expression was relatively normal compared with wild type. At E9.5, however, *lacZ* expression was downregulated in pharyngeal arches and the head mesenchyme of *Shh* mutant embryos. These results suggest that the *Tbx1* enhancer responds to Shh signaling and promotes maintenance, rather than induction, of *Tbx1* expression.

We inspected the 1.1 kb enhancer, which is required for pharyngeal endoderm and head mes-enchyme expression, for binding sites of transcription factors using the MatInspector V.2.2 based on TRANSFAC 4.0.[14] Alignment of the 1.1 kb enhancer with the corresponding human *TBX1* upstream sequence revealed a consensus-binding site (GCCT GTTTGTTTT) for the winged helix/forkhead, or Fox, family of transcription factors that was completely conserved across species.[9] To determine if the Fox binding site was required for *Tbx1* expression *in vivo*, we mutated this site in the context of the 1.1 kb enhancer and generated transgenic embryos. *LacZ* expression in pharyngeal endoderm and head mes-enchyme was abolished in 6/6 embryos harboring the mutant transgene. This result identified *Tbx1* as a direct transcriptional target of Fox transcription factors during development *in vivo*.

Of the numerous Fox factors, Foxc1 and Foxc2 (formerly Mf1 and Mfh1, respectively), are closely related Fox proteins with virtually identical DNA-binding domains that are expressed in the mesoderm-derived head mesenchyme and play redundant roles in cardiovascular development.[15–19] Embryos lacking either *Foxc1* or *Foxc2*, and most compound heterozygotes, die perinatally from aortic arch defects including interruption of the aortic arch (IAA), reminiscent of mice heterozygous for a *Tbx1* mutation.[4–6] In contrast, Foxa proteins, also known as hepatocyte nuclear factors (HNF)-3, are expressed in the pharyngeal endoderm and one member, Foxa2 (HNF-3β), is essential for endoderm development.[20,21]

To determine if the conserved Fox binding site was capable of binding Foxa2, we performed electrophoretic mobility shift assays (EMSA) with ^{32}P-labeled oligonucleotides containing the *cis*-element.[9] Foxa2 protein specifically shifted this element and DNA-binding was effectively competed by an excess of unlabeled cognate competitor but not by a mutated oligonucleotide, suggesting that Foxa2 specifically interacts with the Fox consensus site in the *Tbx1* enhancer. Similar studies using Foxc1 or Foxc2 protein also demonstrated interaction with varying affinities for this site.

We transiently transfected HeLa cells with a luciferase reporter cloned downstream of the Fox binding element (FBE) in the 1.1 kb *Tbx1* enhancer.[9] Transfection with expression vectors of Foxa2, Foxc1, or Foxc2 activated this reporter by approximately 5-, 20-, or 25-fold, respectively. Similar results were obtained in COS-7 cells. These results suggest that Foxa2, Foxc1, and Foxc2 can bind and directly activate transcription through the consensus Fox *cis*-element upstream of *Tbx1*.

To test whether Fox proteins might serve as a transcriptional link between Shh signaling and *Tbx1* expression, we examined expression of these Fox factors in *Shh*-null mice by section *in situ* hybridization.[9] Previous studies demonstrated that the expression of *Foxa2* was downregulated in the neural tube floor plate of *Shh*-null mice from E8.5. Transverse section of E9.5 embryos showed Foxa2 expression in pharyngeal endoderm in wild type, and that *Foxa2* expression in pharyngeal endoderm was dependent on Shh signaling. Serial transverse sections demonstrate that Foxc2 expression was undetectable, while Foxc1 expression was detectable in *Shh* mutants. These results suggest a requirement of Shh signaling for Foxa2 and Foxc2 expression that in turn activates Tbx1.

Foxc1 or *Foxc2* mutant embryos have aortic arch defects similar to *Tbx1* heterozygotes and survive until E18.5,[16–18] allowing us to test whether these factors are involved in regulation of *Tbx1* regulation *in vivo*. The expression of *Tbx1* was partially downregulated in either *Foxc1* or *Foxc2*-null embryos, suggesting that Foxc1 and Foxc2 may regulate *Tbx1* in a dose-dependent and redundant fashion.

Taken together, we propose a model for tissue-specific regulation of *Tbx1*[9] (Fig. 32.1k). *Tbx1* is directly regulated by Foxc1 and Foxc2 in the head mesenchyme, and Foxa2 in the pharyngeal endoderm, through a common Fox binding element upstream of *Tbx1*. Shh signaling functions to maintain the expression of *Foxa2* and *Foxc2*, which subsequently activate *Tbx1* expression. This model provides insight into novel molecular mechanisms underlying the pathogenesis of 22q11DS and cardiovascular development. Elucidating such molecular pathways may reveal genetic modifiers for the highly variable phenotype of 22q11DS and may eventually lead to novel methods of prevention of this disease.

Acknowledgments

We thank Drs J. Maeda, T. Hu, J. McAnally, C. Yamagishi, S. J. Conway, T. Kume, N. Miura, J. A. Richardson and E. N. Olson; S. Johnson for preparation of figures. This work was supported by a grant from the American Heart Association, Texas Affiliate to HY, and from the NHLBI/NIH, March of Dimes Birth Defects Foundation and Smile Train Inc. to DS.

References

1 Scambler PJ. The 22q11 deletion syndromes. *Hum Mol Genet* 2000; **9**: 2421–6.

2 Lindsay EA. Chromosomal microdeletions: dissecting del22q11 syndrome. *Nat Rev Genet* 2001; **2**: 858–68.

3 Yamagishi H. The 22q11.2 deletion syndrome. *Keio J Med* 2002; **51**: 77–88.

4 Lindsay EA, Vitelli F, Su H *et al.* Tbx1 haploinsufficiency in the DiGeorge syndrome region causes aortic arch defects in mice. *Nature* 2001; **410**: 97–101.

5 Merscher S, Funke B, Epstein JA *et al*. TBX1 is responsible for cardiovascular defects in velo-cardio-facial/DiGeorge syndrome. *Cell* 2001; **104**: 619–29.

6 Jerome LA, Papaioannou VE. DiGeorge syndrome phenotype in mice mutant for the T-box gene, Tbx1. *Nat Genet* 2001; **27**: 286–91.

7 Chapman DL, Garvey N, Hancock S *et al*. Expression of the T-box family genes, *Tbx1–Tbx5*, during early mouse development. *Dev Dyn* 1996; **206**: 379–90.

8 Garg V, Yamagishi C, Hu T *et al*. Tbx1, a DiGeorge syndrome candidate gene, is regulated by sonic hedgehog during pharyngeal arch development. *Dev Biol* 2001; **235**: 62–73.

9 Yamagishi H, Maeda J, Hu T *et al*. Tbx1 is regulated by tissue-specific forkhead proteins through a common Sonic hedgehog-responsive enhancer. *Genes Dev* 2003; **17**: 269–81.

10 Vitelli F, Morishima M, Taddei I, Lindsay EA, Baldini A. Tbx1 mutation causes multiple cardiovascular defects and disrupts neural crest and cranial nerve migratory pathways. *Hum Mol Genet* 2002; **11**: 915–22.

11 Waldo KL, Kumiski DH, Wallis KT *et al*. Conotruncal myocardium arises from a secondary heart field. *Development* 2001; **128**: 3179–88.

12 Kelly RG, Brown NA, Buckingham ME. The arterial pole of the mouse heart forms from Fgf10-expressing cells in pharyngeal mesoderm. *Dev Cell* 2001; **1**: 435–40.

13 Chiang C, Litingtung Y, Lee E *et al*. Cyclopia and defective axial patterning in mice lacking Sonic hedgehog gene function. *Nature* 1996; **383**: 407–13.

14 Quandt K, Frech K, Karas H, Wingender E, Werner T. MatInd and MatInspector: new fast and versatile tools for detection of consensus matches in nucleotide sequence data. *Nucleic Acids Res* 1995; **23**: 4878–84.

15 Winnier GE, Hargett L, Hogan BL. The winged helix transcription factor MFH1 is required for proliferation and patterning of paraxial mesoderm in the mouse embryo. *Genes Dev* 1997; **11**: 926–40.

16 Iida K, Koseki H, Kakinuma H *et al*. Essential roles of the winged helix transcription factor MFH-1 in aortic arch patterning and skeletogenesis. *Development* 1997; **124**: 4627–38.

17 Kume T, Deng KY, Winfrey V *et al*. The forkhead/winged helix gene Mf1 is disrupted in the pleiotropic mouse mutation congenital hydrocephalus. *Cell* 1998; **93**: 985–96.

18 Winnier GE, Kume T, Deng K *et al*. Roles for the winged helix transcription factors MF1 and MFH1 in cardiovascular development revealed by nonallelic noncomplementation of null alleles. *Dev Biol* 1999; **213**: 418–31.

19 Kume T, Jiang H, Topczewska JM, Hogan BL. The murine winged helix transcription factors, Foxc1 and Foxc2, are both required for cardiovascular development and somitogenesis. *Genes Dev* 2001; **15**: 2470–82.

20 Weinstein DC, Ruiz I, Altaba A *et al*. The winged-helix transcription factor HNF-3 beta is required for notochord development in the mouse embryo. *Cell* 1994; **78**: 575–88.

21 Ang SL, Rossant J. HNF-3 beta is essential for node and notochord formation in mouse development. *Cell* 1994; **78**: 561–74.

CHAPTER 33

Tbx1 and DiGeorge syndrome: a genetic link between cardiovascular and pharyngeal development

Huansheng Xu, Masae Morishima, Antonio Baldini

The pharyngeal apparatus is a transient, vertebrate-specific, modular structure made of pharyngeal arches and pouches. Arches and pouches develop progressively, in a cranial-caudal direction. Proper development of these is critical for separation of the pulmonary and systemic circulation, thymic, parathyroid and thyroid development, and for development of the mandible, maxilla, external and middle ear.[1] Developmental defects of the pharyngeal apparatus underlie many birth defects including cardiovascular anomalies, mainly affecting outflow tract and aortic arch, craniofacial defects, velo-pharyngeal insufficiency, and developmental defects of the ear. DiGeorge syndrome (DGS) is a typical disorder of the pharyngeal apparatus. The phenotype includes, but is not limited to, craniofacial abnormalities, congenital heart disease, thymic and parathyroid aplasia or hypoplasia. The great majority of DGS cases is caused by a heterozygous deletion of chromosome 22q11.2 (*del22q11*). *Del22q11* is the most common chromosomal deletion associated with birth defects in humans (reviews in refs 2–4). The common deletion spans about 3 Mbp of DNA and includes approximately 30 genes. We generated the first animal model of this syndrome by engineering a multi-gene chromosomal deletion of the murine region homologous to *del22q11*. Heterozygously deleted mice, referred to as *Df1/+* mice, have cardiovascular defects similar to those observed in *del22q11* patients.[5] They also show thymic and parathyroid abnormalities.[6] Later, we and others have identified *Tbx1* as the gene haplo-

insufficient in *Df1/+* mice.[7–9] *Tbx1+/−* mice have the same cardiovascular phenotype as *Df1/+* mice while *Tbx1−/−* animals have severe abnormalities affecting all the segments of the pharyngeal apparatus, and have severe aortic arch and outflow tract defects.[7,8,10] In particular, the outflow tract defects are complex as they affect septation and alignment. The latter is a malalignment between the inter ventricular foramen and the infundibulum. We have proposed that the outflow tract septation failure is the result of defective neural crest cell migration into the truncal cushions, while the alignment defect may be owing to loss of function of *Tbx1* in the secondary heart field.[10,11] If this hypothesis is correct, the two types of outflow tract defects (affecting septation and alignment) should be separable. The currently available mutants of *Tbx1*, however, do not allow us to dissect this phenotype. Therefore, we have generated a new allelic series of the *Tbx1* gene to initiate detailed genetic dissection of its function and improve the disease model. One of these alleles carries a PGK-neo cassette inserted into intron 5 (Fig. 33.1). This allele expresses a low amount of mature *Tbx1* RNA message (as tested by RT-PCR) and, therefore, functions as an hypomorphic allele. We have performed initial experiments with mice carrying this allele, which we named *Tbx1^neo^*. Phenotypic analyses have revealed differences between *Tbx1−/−* and *Tbx1^neo/neo^* that underscore the high sensitivity of some morphogenetic processes to *Tbx1* RNA dosage. For example, proper closure of the secondary palate was almost never observed in our

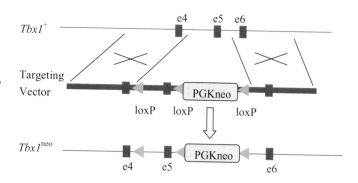

Fig. 33.1 Schematic representation of the hypomorphic allele *Tbx1^neo^*. This allele has been obtained by inserting a PGK-neo cassette into exon 5 of the *Tbx1* gene by homologous recombination in mouse embryonic stem cells. The amount of *Tbx1* RNA message produced by this allele is much lower than that produced by the wild type allele (not shown).

Tbx1–/– animals, while in *Tbx1^neo/neo^* the palate is always closed, hence a minimal amount of *Tbx1* message is sufficient to correct this abnormality. The external ear defects were also less severe in *Tbx1^neo/neo^* animals. However, our data indicate that normal development of the cardiovascular system, requires higher dosage of *Tbx1* RNA message. *Tbx1^neo/+^* animals have the same arch defects as *Tbx1*+/– animals, and *Tbx1^neo/neo^* animals have cardiovascular abnormalities very similar but not identical to those seen in *Tbx1*–/– animals. In particular, aortic arch and outflow septation defects were not distinguishable between the two sets of mutants. However, the alignment defect typical of the 5 *Tbx1*–/– mutants was substantially less severe in about half of the *Tbx1^neo/neo^* animals. In *Tbx1*–/– fetuses (E18.5), the truncus originates entirely from the right ventricle while the left ventricle communicates with the outflow indirectly, through a large ventricular septal defect (VSD) (Plate 26, central panel). In these animals, there is no continuity between the truncal valve and the mitral valve (not shown). In contrast, in three out of five *Tbx1^neo/neo^* fetuses so far examined, the truncus overrides a subvalvular VSD and communicates directly with both the left and right ventricles (Plate 26, right panel). In addition, there is continuity between the truncal valve and the mitral valve (not shown). Hence, there is a nearly complete correction of the alignment defect. These initial data indicate that the outflow septation defect and the malalignment defect can occur independently and suggest that the two types of defects may derive from different pathogenetic mechanisms. Interestingly, the type of outflow-ventricular alignment found in the *Tbx1^neo/neo^* fetuses resembles more closely the congenital heart defects found in *del22q11* patients.[12,13] Therefore, manipulation of the *Tbx1* RNA dosage should lead to improved mouse models of the *del22q11* syndrome.

However, *Tbx1* RNA dosage is not the only parameter that affects penetrance and expressivity of the mutant phenotype. Interactors and target loci are likely to contribute substantially to phenotypic variability. Potential targets of the Tbx1 transcription factor are members of the fibroblast growth factor (*Fgf*) family of genes. It has been shown that dosage reduction of *Fgf8* RNA dosage in mouse cause phenotypic abnormalities reminiscent of those seen in *del22q11* patients and *Tbx1* mouse mutants.[14,15] We have shown that *Fgf8* interacts genetically with *Tbx1* because *Fgf8* mutation enhances the aortic arch and thymic phenotype of *Tbx1*+/– mice.[11] In addition, *Fgf8* and *Fgf10* have Tbx1-dependent expression domains.[11,16] We propose that downregulation of some *Fgf* genes may play a pathogenetic role in the *Tbx1* mutant phenotype and possibly in the human *del22q11* phenotype.

Future research will further dissect the *Tbx1* mutant phenotype by genetic manipulation of the gene, establish the pathogenetic significance of genetic interactions with *Fgf* genes, and identify direct targets of Tbx1.

Acknowledgments

This research is supported by grants from the National Institutes of Health, USA.

References

1 Graham A. The development and evolution of the pharyngeal arches. *J Anat* 2001; **199**: 133–41.

2 Scambler PJ. The 22q11 deletion syndromes. *Hum Mol Genet* 2000; **9**: 2421–6.

3 Lindsay EA. Chromosomal microdeletions: dissecting del22q11 syndrome. *Nat Rev Genet* 2001; **2**: 858–68.

4 McDermid HE, Morrow BE. Genomic disorders on 22q11. *Am J Hum Genet* 2002; **70**: 1077–88.

5 Lindsay EA *et al.* Congenital heart disease in mice deficient for the DiGeorge syndrome region. *Nature* 1999; **401**: 379–83.

6 Taddei I, Morishima M, Huynh T, Lindsay EA. Genetic factors are major determinants of phenotypic variability in a mouse model of the DiGeorge/del22q11 syndromes. *Proc Natl Acad Sci U S A* 2001; **98**: 11428–31.

7 Lindsay EA *et al.* Tbx1 haploinsufficieny in the DiGeorge syndrome region causes aortic arch defects in mice. *Nature* 2001; **410**: 97–101.

8 Jerome LA, Papaioannou VE. DiGeorge syndrome phenotype in mice mutant for the T-box gene, *Tbx1. Nat Genet* 2001; **27**: 286–91.

9 Merscher S *et al.* TBX1 is responsible for cardiovascular defects in velo-cardio-facial/DiGeorge syndrome. *Cell* 2001; **104**: 619–29.

10 Vitelli F, Morishima M, Taddei I, Lindsay EA, Baldini A. Tbx1 mutation causes multiple cardiovascular defects and

11 Vitelli F *et al.* A genetic link between Tbx1 and fibroblast growth factor signaling. *Development* 2002; **129**: 4605–11.

12 Momma K, Kondo C, Matsuoka R, Takao A. Cardiac anomalies associated with a chromosome 22q11 deletion in patients with conotruncal anomaly face syndrome. *Am J Cardiol* 1996; **78**: 591–4.

13 Marino B, Digilio MC, Toscano A, Giannott, A, Dallapiccola B. Congenital heart defects in patients with DiGeorge/velocardiofacial syndrome and del22q11. *Genet Couns* 1999; **10**: 25–33.

14 Abu-Issa R, Smyth G, Smoak I, Yamamura K-I, Meyers EN. Fgf8 is required for pharyngeal arch development and cardiovascular patterning in the mouse. *Development* 2002; **129**: 4613–25.

15 Frank DU *et al.* An Fgf8 mouse mutant phenocopies human 22q11 deletion syndrome. *Development* 2002; **129**: 4591–603.

16 Kochilas L *et al.* The role of neural crest during cardiac development in a mouse model of DiGeorge syndrome. *Dev Biol* 2002; **251**: 157–66.

disrupts neural crest and cranial nerve migratory pathways. *Hum Mol Genet* 2002; **11**: 915–22.

CHAPTER 34

New insights into the role of *Tbx1* in the DiGeorge mouse model

Lazaros Kochilas, Jun Liao, Sandra Merscher-Gomez,
Raju Kucherlapati, Bernice Morrow, Jonathan A. Epstein

The velo-cardio-facial syndrome (VCFS)/DiGeorge syndrome (DGS) is a common human genetic disorder characterized by numerous phenotypic abnormalities including cardiovascular defects.[1] Most patients are hemizygous for a 1.5–3.0 Mb region of 22q11 (DGCR). Mice hemizygous for the 1.5 Mb orthologous area on mouse chromosome 16 (Lgdel/+) exhibit similar defects reminiscent of human DGS. A series of complementation experiments using mouse transgenic lines (BAC transgenics) that contained extra human copies of some of the deleted genes implicated a small group of genes within the deleted area as possible candidates for the cardiovascular abnormalities.[2–4] Subsequent analysis identified *Tbx1* as the critical gene with a dose dependent function.[5] BAC transgenic mice overexpressing *Tbx1* and three other genes in a wildtype background, also show DGS phenotypes, including reduced viability, cardiovascular defects, ear disorders, thymus hypoplasia, and cleft palate.[4] To further study the *Tbx1* dosage effect, the BAC transgenic mice were crossed with *Tbx1* mutant mice. After obtaining *Tbx1* heterozygotes that also carry BAC transgenes, the offspring were crossed again with *Tbx1* heterozygotes to generate BAC transgenic mice in *Tbx1* null background (Plate 27). Transgenic mice in wild type background show reduced viability, while transgenic mice in *Tbx1* null background have normal mendelian ratio. The reason for the decreased viability of the *Tbx1* overexpressing mice is their increased incidence of cardiovascular anomalies: 28% in transgenics in *Tbx1* null background, compared with 53% in transgenics in *Tbx1* heter-

ozygous background and 64% in transgenics in wild type background [unpubl. data]. These results suggest that *Tbx1* null mutation can rescue cardiovascular defects in BAC transgenic mice and that overexpression of *Tbx1* is responsible for cardiovascular defects in BAC transgenic mice.

These studies demonstrate that both increased and decreased *Tbx1* level can cause cardiovascular defects similar to those observed in DGS and indicate that Tbx1 might have a paradoxical dosage effect on mouse embryonic development. Many of the affected organs have neural crest contributions, suggesting that *Tbx1* and the other genes within the DGCR could be related to abnormal neural crest development. Interestingly, though, *Tbx1* is not expressed by neural crest cells but by the pharyngeal endoderm and core mesenchyme through which neural crest migrates.[6] We therefore examined whether haplo-insufficiency of the mouse orthologous DGCR, that includes *Tbx1*, affects neural crest migration. For this purpose, we utilized a binary Cre-lox system to activate β-galactosidase expression in Pax3-expressing cells and their descendants to fate map neural crest precursors in Lgdel/+ embryos (Plate 28). Pax3-expressing neural crest precursors are fated to invade the cardiac outflow tract and to populate the aorticopulmonary septum and the aortic arch of both wild type and Lgdel/+ embryos, although in the latter a more scattered and less dense pattern of neural crest derivatives is observed in the endocardial cushions, which is consistent with the findings of other investigators in a similar mouse model.[7,8] Several neural crest markers were tested by *in situ* hybridization and there was no detectable difference of expression in affected embryos. We also crossed mice containing loxP sites surrounding the Lgdel area with Pax3pro-Cre transgenic mice to create a hemizygous deletion of the entire interval in neural crest cells. We examined cardiovascular anatomy by corrosion casting and gross dissection and we were unable to find any cardiovascular abnormalities in the mice with the hemizygous neural crest-specific inactivation of the Lgdel genes.[7]

Together these results suggest that the cardiovascular defects seen in this mouse model of DGS are not caused by absence of neural crest cells in the pharyngeal region. Hence, Lgdel genes including *Tbx1* are not required for cardiac neural crest migration but could affect neural crest development in a non cell-autonomous fashion. For instance, they could affect the neural crest differentiation into smooth muscle cells in the aortic arch arteries. Neural crest cells encasing the arch arteries differentiate into smooth muscle and invest the medial layer of these vessels. To answer this question we used a mouse in which *lacZ* had been inserted into the SM22α locus as a sensitive assay for smooth muscle differentiation.[9] This early marker of smooth muscle differentiation is reduced or absent in specific segments of the 4th and 6th aortic arches of Lgdel/+ embryos.[7]

Since *Tbx1* is expressed by adjacent mesenchyme, these results suggest a model in which *Tbx1* induces the secretion of a critical growth factor that is required for proper differentiation or survival of nearby neural crest derivatives. Fibroblast growth factors (*Fgfs*), such as *Fgf8*, that are downregulated in other models of abnormal arch formation,[10] could mediate interactions between endoderm or ectoderm and migrating neural crest cells. At E11.5, we noted a specific loss of pharyngeal expression of *Fgf8* in the endoderm of the third pharyngeal pouch of *Tbx1*$^{-/-}$, while the expression in the pharyngeal ectoderm and mesenchyme was preserved. *Fgf10*, a related member of the *Fgf* family, is likewise downregulated in the mesenchymal tissue adjacent to pharyngeal endoderm in the region of the developing 4th aortic arch of *Tbx1*$^{-/-}$ embryos.[7] Since *Tbx1* is also expressed by pharyngeal endoderm, these results suggest that *Tbx1* may function upstream of *Fgf* signaling in this tissue and in adjacent structures. Fibroblast growth factors (*Fgfs*), such as *Fgf8* and *Fgf10*, could mediate interactions between sur-

rounding tissues and migrating neural crest cells and recent data suggest a genetic link between *Tbx1* and *Fgf* signaling.[11]

In conclusion our studies demonstrate that mice with abnormal *Tbx1* dosage display cardiovascular defects similar to those observed in DGS. Hemizygosity of the mouse DGCR does not eliminate cardiac neural crest migration. However, neural crest cells in these embryos are defective in their ability to differentiate into smooth muscle. This defect involves both 4th and 6th aortic arches and is associated with inappropriate regression of aortic arch segments, thus accounting for the anomalies observed in Lgdel/+ mice and perhaps in humans with DGS.

References

1 Goldmuntz E, Emanuel BS. Genetic disorders of cardiac morphogenesis. The DiGeorge and velocardiofacial syndromes. *Circ Res* 1997; **80**: 437–43.

2 Lindsay EA *et al.* Congenital heart disease in mice deficient for the DiGeorge syndrome region. *Nature* 1999; **401**: 379–83.

3 Lindsay EA *et al.* Tbx1 haploinsufficieny in the DiGeorge syndrome region causes aortic arch defects in mice. *Nature* 2001; **410**: 97–101.

4 Merscher S *et al.* TBX1 is responsible for cardiovascular defects in velo-cardio-facial/DiGeorge syndrome. *Cell* 2001; **104**: 619–29.

5 Jerome LA, Papaioannou VE. DiGeorge syndrome phenotype in mice mutant for the T-box gene, Tbx1. *Nat Genet* 2001; **27**: 286–91.

6 Garg V *et al.* Tbx1, a DiGeorge syndrome candidate gene, is regulated by sonic hedgehog during pharyngeal arch development. *Dev Biol* 2001; **235**: 62–73.

7 Kochilas LK *et al.* The role of neural crest during cardiac development in a mouse model of DiGeorge syndrome. *Dev Biol* 2002; **251**: 157–66.

8 Vitelli F *et al.* Tbx1 mutation causes multiple cardiovascular defects and disrupts neural crest and cranial nerve migratory pathways. *Hum Mol Genet* 2002; **11**: 915–22.

9 Zhang, JC *et al.* Analysis of SM22alpha-deficient mice reveals unanticipated insights into smooth muscle cell differentiation and function. *Mol Cell Biol* 2001; **21**: 1336–44.

10 Wendling O *et al.* Retinoid signaling is essential for patterning the endoderm of the third and fourth pharyngeal arches. *Development* 2000; **127**: 1553–62.

11 Vitelli F. A genetic link between Tbx1 and fibroblast growth signaling. *Dev Biol* 2002; **129**: 4605–11.

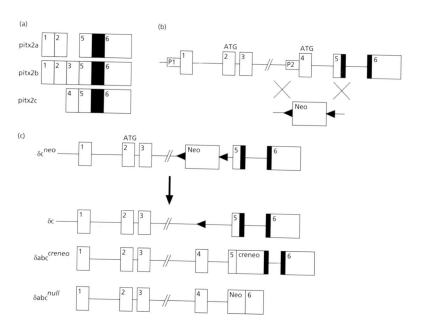

Plate 1 (a)–(c) Gene targeting strategy to generate the *Pitx2* δc and *cre* knock-in, δ*abc^creneo*, alleles. (a) Summary of exon use by *Pitx2* isoforms. (b) *Pitx2* genomic structure and *Pitx2c* specific targeting strategy. Boxes, exons; straight lines, introns. P1 and P2, two promoters that regulate expression of different isoforms. (c) *Pitx2* δc targeted allele before and after *PGKneomycin* removal.

E18.5

+/+   dc/dc

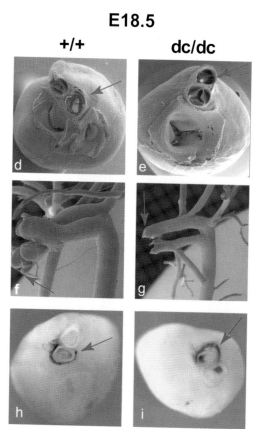

E11.5

+/+   dc/dc

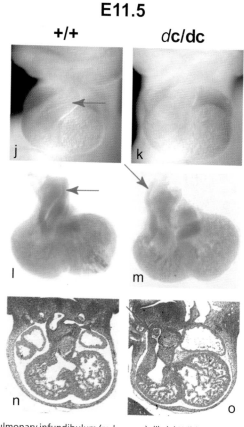

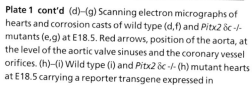

Plate 1 cont'd (d)–(g) Scanning electron micrographs of hearts and corrosion casts of wild type (d,f) and *Pitx2* δc -/- mutants (e,g) at E18.5. Red arrows, position of the aorta, at the level of the aortic valve sinuses and the coronary vessel orifices. (h)–(i) Wild type (i) and *Pitx2* δc -/- (h) mutant hearts at E18.5 carrying a reporter transgene expressed in pulmonary infundibulum (red arrows). (j)–(o) Wild type (j,l,n) and *Pitx2* δc -/- mutant (k,m,o) hearts at E11.5 showing OFT cushions (red arrows mark apposition lines). Frontal views of fresh (j,k) and alcian blue stained (l,m) hearts, and coronal sections (n,o).

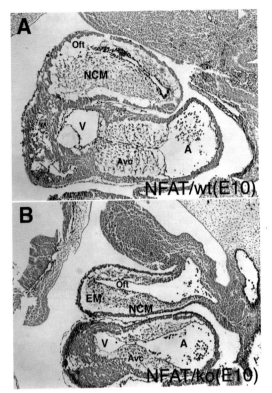

Plate 5 Sagittal section through the heart of an embryonic day 10 (E10) mouse embryo that was either (A) heterozygous (NFATc-/WT) or (B) homozygous (NFATc-/ko) for a null mutation in the NFATc1 gene. To perform a lineage analysis of endocardial cushion derived mesenchyme, these mice were bred into the R26R reporter line and crossed into the Tie2-Cre transgenic line to specifically identify all endothelial cells and their progeny (blue-X-gal staining). In the heterozygous (A) embryo all of the mesenchyme in the distal outflow tract (Oft) is derived from the neural crest (NCM) with little or no contribution from endothelial derived mesenchyme. In the atrioventricular canal (AVC), most, if not all of the mesenchyme in the endocardial cushion is derived from endocardium as evidenced by X-gal staining. However, in the null mutant heart (B) there is now an increase in the component of endothelial derived mesenchyme (EM) in the Oft suggesting either an increase in endothelial proliferations and / or an increase in epithelial to mesenchymal transformation of Oft endocardium.

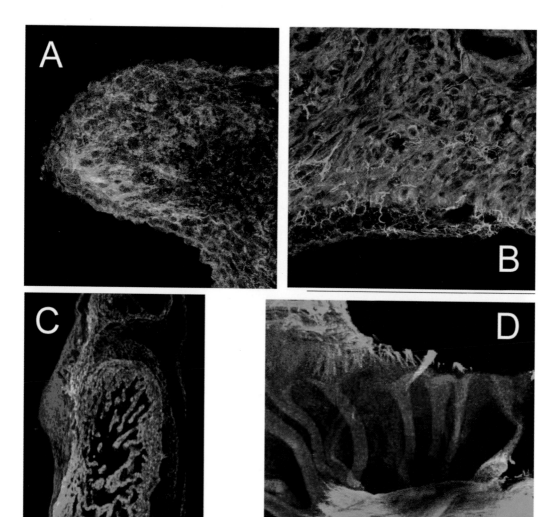

Plate 6 (A) A 9-day mouse AV cushion showing that Pn staining is upregulated in transformed mesenchyme. (B) A 12.5-day mural leaflet demonstrating extracellular Pn+ filaments. (C) Stage 29 chick AV cushion co-stained with a myocardial marker MF20 and ES130, a mesenchymal marker to show co-localization occurs in cells located at the interface where the cushion delaminates from the myocardium. (D) Stage 42 chick AV leaflets co-stained with ES130 (red) and MF20 (green) to demonstrate that some cells within the developing tendinous cords express MF20.

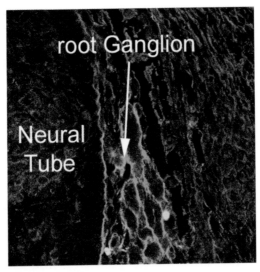

Plate 7 Periostin staining of the anterior neural tube region of a day 10.5 mouse.

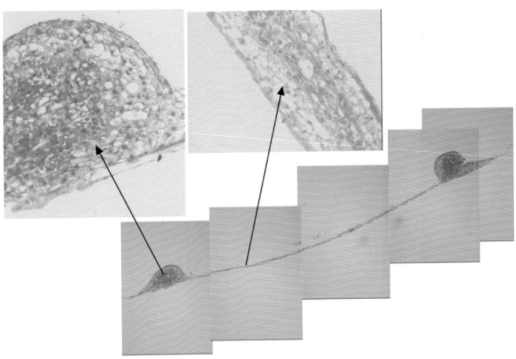

Plate 8 Histology showing that rings are dense fibrous tissue (type I collagen+) compared to circumscribed undifferentiated, loose mesenchymal tissue (magnification × 20).

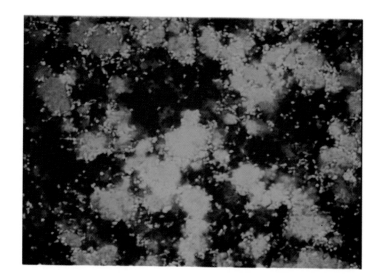

Plate 9 Staining of type II collagen in day-17 cushion cultures treated with 20 ng bone morphogenetic protein (BMP).

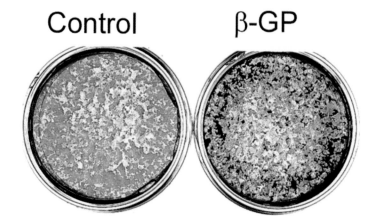

Plate 10 MC3T3 cultures at 40 days with β-glycerophosphate or without and stained with von Kossa stain (magnification × 10).

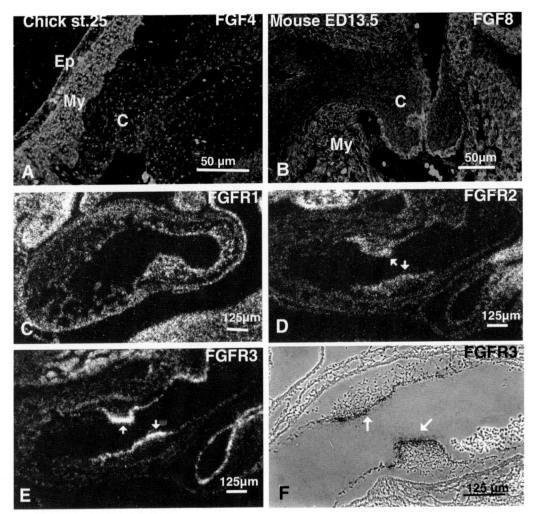

Plate 11 (A) Immunohistochemical localization of FGF4 in the stage 25 chick heart. FGF4 was detected in the cushion mesenchymal cells (C) as well as in the myocardial cells (My). Punctate cytoplasmic staining of FGF4 was seen in both myocardial (My) and cushion mesenchymal (C) cells. (B) Immunohistochemical localization of FGF8 in the embryonic day (ED) 13.5 mouse heart. FGF8 was expressed primarily in the luminal endocardial rim of the cushion (C) as well as in the myocardial cells (My). (C) FGFR1 mRNA expression was detected throughout the heart including myocardium and cushion mesenchyme. (D) FGFR2 mRNA, however, was expressed intensely in the cushion mesenchymal cells (arrows) but little signal was detectable in the myocardium. (E) Most strikingly, FGFR3 mRNA expression was confined to the endocardium of the cardiac cushion (arrows). (F) High power view of FGFR3 mRNA expression in the cardiac cushion tissue (bright field view). This bright field picture indicates a restricted pattern of FGFR3 mRNA expression to cushion endocardial endothelial cells (arrows). Note cushion mesenchymal cells have few silver grains.

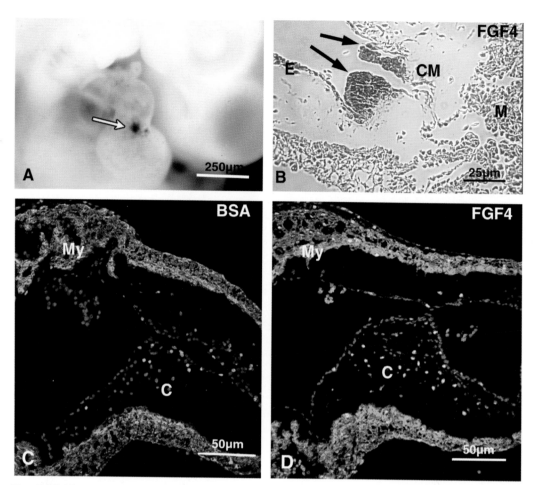

Plate 12 (A), (B) FGF4 overexpression induces expansion of cardiac cushion mesenchyme *in ovo*. Replication-defective retrovirus encoding FGF4 and bacterial ß-galactosidase (FGF4 + ß-gal) or ß-galactosidase (ß-gal) was microinjected into the sinistro-ventral conal cushion (SVCC) of the heart of stage 17 chick embryos. Whole embryos were incubated to stage 24 then processed with X-gal histochemistry to detect viral reporter ß-galactosidase expression. A total of 17 chick embryos was successfully microinjected with virus specifically into cardiac cushions. Eight out of 17 embryos were microinjected with FGF4+ß-gal virus and nine were microinjected with ß-gal control virus. microinjected. None of nine ß-gal microinjected embryos showed expansion of cushion mesenchyme. Seven out of eight FGF4 + ß-gal embryos injected with virus clearly demonstrated luminal expansion of ß-gal positive cushion mesenchyme. Arrow, intense viral ß-galactosidase staining in the heart (A). A paraffin section of the same embryo shows the outgrowth of a bud-like expansion of cushion tissue stained with X-gal (arrows) (B). (C), (D) FGF4 protein injection stimulates BrdU incorporation by cardiac cushion mesenchymal cells *in ovo*. Recombinant human FGF4 was microinjected into cushion mesenchyme of the inner curvature at stages 17–18. Embryos were incubated another 18 h to evaluate the proliferative effect of FGF4. BrdU was applied topically to the embryo for 3 h before the termination of the incubation *in ovo*. After the fixation and paraffin embedding, sections were immunostained with an anti-BrdU monoclonal antibody (green). Myocardium was immunostained with MF20 (blue) and all nuclei were stained with propidium iodide (red). Note that the increased incidence of BrdU-positive nuclei (yellow, after overlay of triple labeled immunofluorescent microphotographs) nuclei in the FGF4 injected cushion mesenchyme (D) as compared to the BSA injected control (C). BSA injected control samples tend to show more BrdU positive cells near the luminal surface of the cushion (C), while FGF4 injected samples show more BrdU positive cells in the central part of the cushion (D).

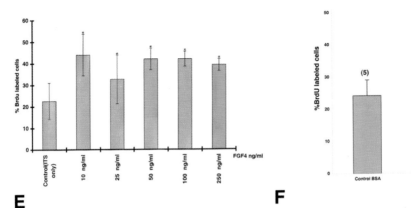

E   **F**

Plate 12 cont'd (E) Quantitative analysis of exogenous FGF4 mediated proliferation in culture. BrdU positive and negative nuclei in the cultured AV cushion mesenchymal cells from stage 25 chick embryos were cultured for 2 days in the serum-free medium 199 with FGF4 at final concentrations of 0–250 ng/mL. BrdU was added to the medium 2 h before the termination of the culture. BrdU-incorporated nuculei were counted to determine the percentage of cells which were in cell-cycle transit as a index of proliferation. A total of 500 nuclei in each culture well was evaluated in random fields. Vertical bars indicate ± 1 SD of the mean. Six wells of mesenchymal cells were evaluated for each dosage of the culture. FGF4 (as low as 10 ng/mL in SFM) promoted proliferation of mesenchymal cells. Asterisk, significant difference at the 1% level of confidence using Student's *t*-test. (F) Quantitative analysis of FGF4 protein-mediated cardiac cushion mesenchyme proliferation *in ovo*. Six μm serial paraffin sections at every 24 μm were subjected to quantitative evaluation of BrdU incorporation into nuclei as an index of proliferation. BrdU positive and negative nuclei in cushion mesenchymal cells were counted to determine the percentage of cells that were in cell-cycle transit. Vertical bars indicate ± 1 SD of the mean. BrdU incorporation in FGF4 microinjected samples is statistically higher than that in the control BSA injected cushion mesenchyme. Asterisk, significant difference at the 1% level of confidence using Student's *t*-test. Numbers of chick embryos used for quantitative evaluation indicated in parenthesis.

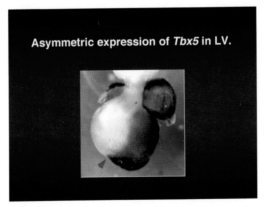

Plate 13 Asymmetric expression of *Tbx5*. Expression of *Tbx5* is restricted to the left ventricle, making a clear boundary at the position of ventricular septum (red arrow head).

RCAS-Tbx5

TYPE1

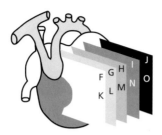

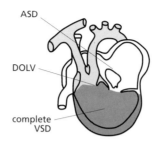

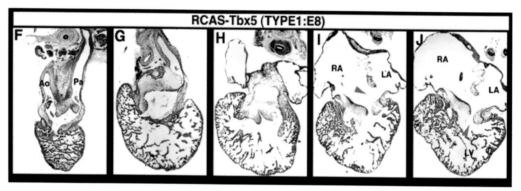

Plate 14 Misexpression of Tbx5 in the entire heart ventricle. Ventricular septum formation was severely disturbed, resulting in a single ventricle. The ventricular wall was thin, and the trabeculae were coarse and rough. Both right and left atria were dilated with an atrial septum defect (ASD). The aorta and pulmonary artery were fused at their base and connected to the single ventricle, resulting in a double outlet left ventricle (DOLV).

RCAS-Tbx5

TYPE2

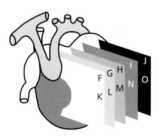

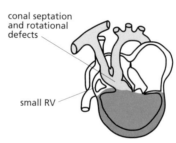

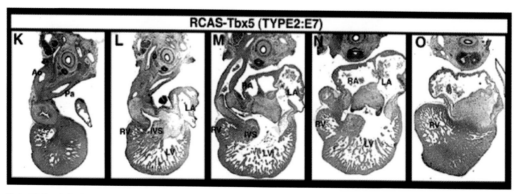

Plate 15 Partial misexpression of Tbx5 in the heart ventricle. The left ventricle expanded and the right ventricle shrank. The relative sizes of these two ventricles indicate a shift of the ventricular septum formation to the right, although the trabecular formation and the thickness of ventricles were not affected. Conal septation/rotation defects were also observed. The atrial septum formed, but it was thin and membranous.

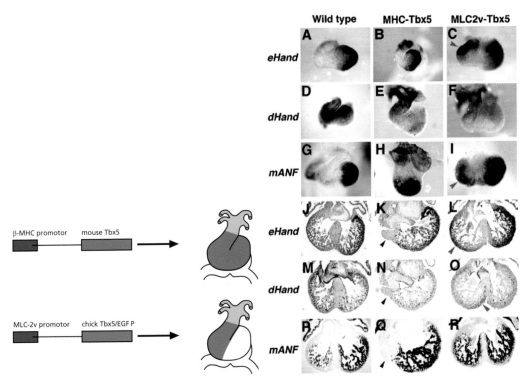

Plate 16 Misexpression of Tbx5 in mouse heart. (B), (H), (H) and (Q) In the *MHC-Tbx5* transgenic mice, both *eHAND* and *mANF* were induced in the entire ventricle, whereas *dHAND* was repressed. (K) Ventricular septum formation was disrupted with a tiny bulge at the right-most end (black arrowhead). (C), (F), and (I) In the *MLC-2v-Tbx5* transgenic mice, the right ventricle expanded, as indicated by a red arrowhead. In this portion, both the *eHAND* and *mANF* genes were induced, and the *dHAND* gene was repressed. (L), (O), and (R) Histologic analysis revealed the swelling of the right ventricle, as indicated by a red arrowhead in (L). In this swelling, *eHAND* was induced in a gradient manner, as indicated by a red arrowhead in (L), leaving an *eHAND*-negative part near the septum. (O) In this small part, *dHAND* is expressed, as indicated by a red arrowhead, whereas this gene is repressed in the rest of right ventricle. (R) *mANF* was induced in the right ventricle of this transgenic mouse.

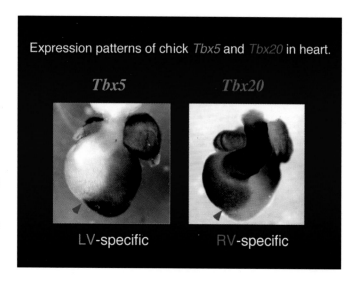

Expression patterns of chick *Tbx5* and *Tbx20* in heart.

Tbx5 *Tbx20*

LV-specific RV-specific

Plate 17 Expression patterns of Tbx5 and Tbx20. Tbx5 expression is restricted to the left ventricle, whereas Tbx20 is expressed in the right ventricle, making a complementary fashion of gene expression. Red arrowheads indicate the position of the ventricular septum.

Expression patterns of chick *Tbx20* and *Tbx5*

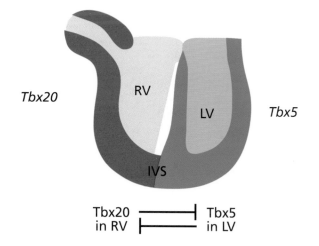

Tbx20 RV LV *Tbx5*

IVS

Tbx20 in RV ⊣ Tbx5 in LV

Plate 18 Establishment of the identities of the right and left ventricles. Tbx5 in the left ventricle and Tbx20 in the right exert their mutually repressive actions to establish a clear boundary of gene expression. Consequently, the ventricular septum develops at the position of this boundary. Tbx5 and Tbx20 act synergistically with other transcription factors, such as GATA4 and Nkx-2.5 to set up two different identities of developing ventricle.

Mutually repressive action in ventricles, but not in atria

Different modes of action in ventricles and atria??
Different signaling contexts affect Tbx5 and Tbx20??
GATA-4, Nkx-2.5 or others??

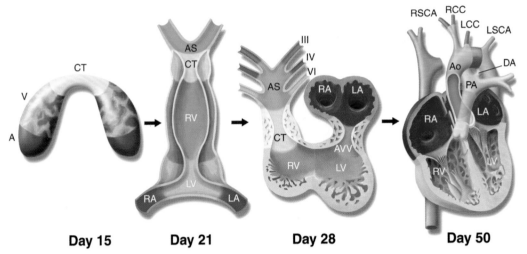

Day 15   **Day 21**   **Day 28**   **Day 50**

Plate 19 Schematic of cardiac morphogenesis. Illustrations depict cardiac development with color coding of morphologically related regions, seen from a ventral view. Cardiogenic precursors form a crescent (left-most panel) that is specified to form specific segments of the linear heart tube, which is patterned along the AP axis to form the various regions and chambers of the looped and mature heart. Each cardiac chamber balloons out from the outer curvature of the looped heart tube in a segmental fashion. Neural crest cells populate the bilaterally symmetric aortic arch arteries (III, IV, and VI) and aortic sac (AS) that together contribute to specific segments of the mature aortic arch, also color coded. Mesenchymal cells form the cardiac valves from the conotruncal (CT) and atrioventricular valve (AVV) segments. Corresponding days of human embryonic development are indicated. RV, right ventricle; LV, left ventricle; RA, right atrium; LA, left atrium; PA, pulmonary artery; Ao, aorta; DA, ductus arteriosus; RSCA, right subclavian artery; RCC, right common carotid; LCC, left common carotid; LSCA, left subclavian artery. Reprinted with permission from Srivastava and Olson.[1]

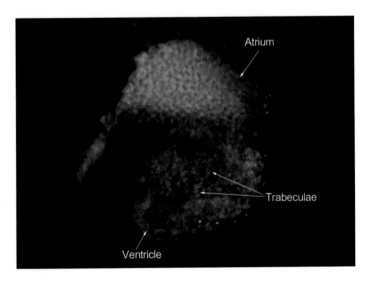

Plate 20 Expression of the HNK1 epitope (labeled by FITC) is found in the trabeculae of the ventricle; and almost the entire atrium of a 4-day-old zebrafish heart. The heart is rendered and deconvolved to show the 3-D structure.

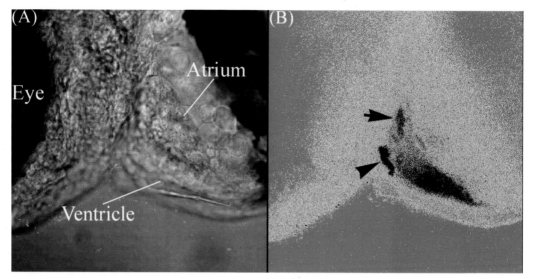

Plate 21 Projection of stacked confocal sections (2 μm apart) through the ventricular wall of a 3-day-old zebrafish. (A) Immunofluorescence localization of HNK1 (green) epitope of a 3-day zebrafish heart superimposed on the differential interphase contrast (DIC) image. (B) Sagittal section of the same heart with the intensity color code LUT shows the HNK1 epitope expressed extensively in the atrioventricular (arrow), outflow tract (arrowhead), and the ventricular regions.

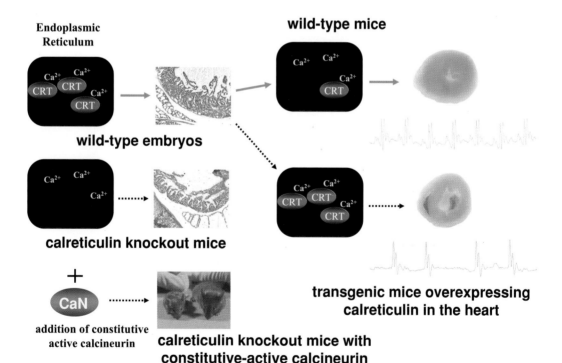

Plate 22 Summary of phenotype of calreticulin knockout mice and heart specific overexpression mice. Calreticulin is essential for heart development. Knockout mice is embryonic lethal because of decrease in ventricular wall thickness. The defect is rescued by additional expression of activated form of calcineurin in the heart. Calreticulin is abundant in embryonic heart. However, level of calreticulin expression is reduced in the newborn heart. Overexpression of calreticulin in the heart lead to arrhythmia and cardiac sudden death.

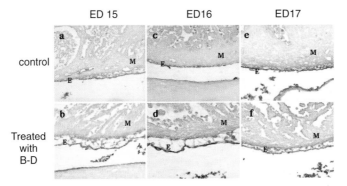

ED 15   ED16   ED17

control

Treated
with
B-D

Plate 23 Histological findings and VCAM-1 immunoexpressional patterns in control (a, c, e) and bis-diamine-treated hearts (b, d, f). The epicardium (E) approached and finally connected with the myocardium (M), and vascular plexuses, which were formed between the epicardium and ventricular myocardium, became thick and shortened in the control heart during these developmental stages (a, c, e). However, the epicardium stayed separate from the myocardium and the vascular plexus was loose and thin in the bis-diamine-treated heart (b, d, f). Note the thin ventricular myocardium in the bis-diamine-treated heart. VCAM-1 immunoreactivity was observed on the epicardium, vascular plexuses, and epicardial myocardium in both control and bis-diamine-treated hearts.

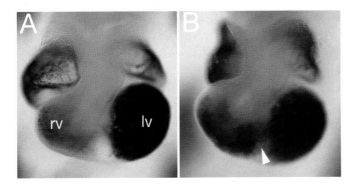

Plate 24 Whole-mount *in situ* hybridization for *ANF* in E10.5 wild-type (A) and *Tbx5*$^{del/+}$ embryos (B). Note increased expression in the *Tbx5*$^{del/+}$ RV and ectopic expression in the interventricular groove (arrowhead).

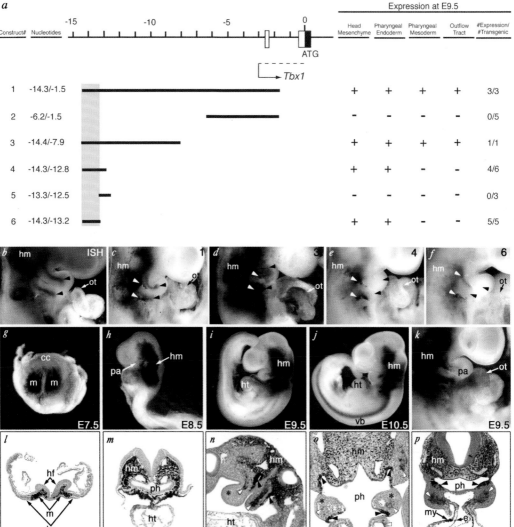

Plate 25 *Tbx1* expression is controlled by separable pharyngeal endoderm and mesoderm regulatory regions in transgenic mice. (a) Genomic organization of the 5' mouse *Tbx1* locus and flanking region. Boxes indicate exons and translation start site (ATG) is designated as nucleotide number zero. Construct number is indicated on the left, and the corresponding expression pattern of *lacZ* at E9.5 is summarized on the right. The far-right column indicates the fraction of F_0 transgenic embryos with *Tbx1*-like *lacZ* expression/*lacZ* gene positive embryos. (b) Endogenous expression of Tbx1 transcripts by whole-mount RNA *in situ* hybridization. (c)–(f) Right lateral views focusing on the pharyngeal arch of representative embryos obtained with each construct (indicated in upper right corner of each panel). Expression of *lacZ* in embryos with construct 1 (c) recapitulated endogenous *Tbx1* expression (b). *LacZ* expression in the head mesenchyme (hm) and pharyngeal endoderm (asterisks) was detectable in each embryo with construct 1 (c), 3 (d), 4 (e) and 6 (f), while that in the pharyngeal mesoderm (arrowheads) and cardiac outflow tract (ot) was only in embryos with construct 1 (c) or 3 (d). (g)–(p), Embryos from a stable transgenic line harboring the 12.8 kb fragment (construct 1) were analyzed at various times during mouse embryogenesis. (g)–(j) Whole-mount photographs of embryos from E7.5 to 10.5. (k) Right lateral view of embryo focusing on the pharyngeal arch and heart at E9.5. (l)–(p) Transverse (l,m,p), sagittal (n), or frontal (o) sections counterstained by Nuclear Fast Red from E7.5 to 9.5. (g),(l) *lacZ* was expressed in mesoderm cells (m) that give rise to head mesenchyme, but not in the cardiac crescent (cc) or lateral plate mesoderm (lm) at E7.5. (h),(m) Expression of *lacZ* was detectable in the head mesenchyme (hm) and pharyngeal arch (pa) at E8.5. (i),(n)–(p) *LacZ* expression was detectable in head mesenchyme, pharyngeal arch mesoderm (white arrowheads) and endoderm (black arrowheads), but not in neural crest-derived mesenchyme (asterisks) at E9.5. (j) Expression of *lacZ* extended to the primordia of vertebral bodies (vb). (k),(p) *LacZ* was expressed in both myocardial (my) and endocardial (e) layers of the ot at E9.5. hf, head fold; ht, heart; ph, pharynx.

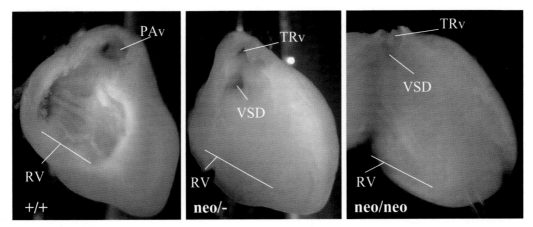

Plate 26 Intracardiac phenotype in *Tbx1⁺/⁺*, *Tbx1ⁿᵉᵒ/⁻*, and *Tbx1ⁿᵉᵒ/ⁿᵉᵒ* fetuses at E18.5. Frontal view after removal of the atria and free wall of the right ventricle (RV). The *Tbx1ⁿᵉᵒ/⁻* specimen has an intracardiac phenotype identical to that of *Tbx1⁻/⁻* fetuses. Note the very large ventricular septal defect (VSD) and the truncus originating entirely from the RV. In the *Tbx1ⁿᵉᵒ/ⁿᵉᵒ* specimen, the VSD is subvalvular. The truncus overrides the interventricular septum and communicates with the left and right ventricles. Pav, semilunar valves of pulmonary artery; TRv, truncal valve.

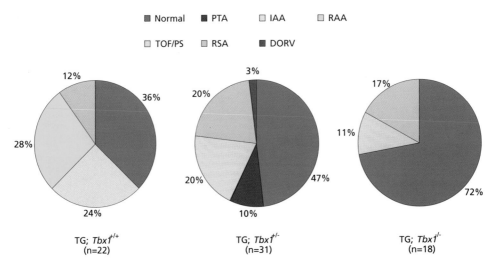

Plate 27 *Tbx1* overexpressing mice have higher incidence of cardiovascular anomalies: 64% of BAC transgenics in wild type background display various cardiovascular defects, compared with 28% of BAC transgenics in Tbx1 null background. This figure displays a detailed analysis of cardiovascular phenotype of BAC transgenics in wild type and Tbx1 null background.

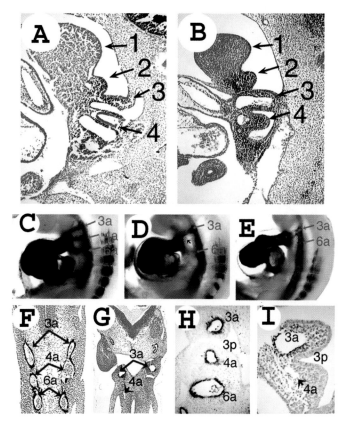

Plate 28 Fate mapping of neural crest cells was performed using P3proCre mice crossed with R26R lacZ reporter mice in wild type (A) and Lgdel/+ (B) embryos. Sagittal sections of E9.5 embryos (A, B) reveal neural crest cells (blue) surrounding the pharyngeal arch arteries in both wild type and Lgdel/+ embryos. Pharyngeal arches are numbered. SM22α-lacZ knockin mice were used to detect smooth muscle differentiation in wild type (C, F, H) and Lgdel/+ (D, E, G, I) embryos at E10.5. The aortic arch arteries are numbered. The 3rd aortic arch arteries are stained blue indicating smooth muscle differentiation in both wild type and Lgdel/+ embryo, while smooth muscle differentiation was severely deficient in the 4th and 6th aortic arch arteries of Lgdel/+ embryos. The black arrow in (D) points to a hypoplastic 4th aortic arch artery that is devoid of smooth muscle. In (E), there is minimal evidence of smooth muscle differentiation in the dorsal segment of the 6th aortic arch artery. Coronal sections (F, G) confirm β-galactosidase activity in the 3rd, 4th, and 6th aortic arch arteries bilaterally in wild type embryos, while no evidence of smooth muscle differentiation is present in the 4th arch artery of a Lgdel/+ embryo (G). The 6th arch artery is not visible in this section. Double staining of embryos to identify Sm22α-lacZ (blue) and smooth muscle actin (immunohistochemistry, dark brown) (H, I) confirms deficient smooth muscle differentiation in the 4th aortic arch of Lgdel/+ embryos (I) comparing to the wild type (H).

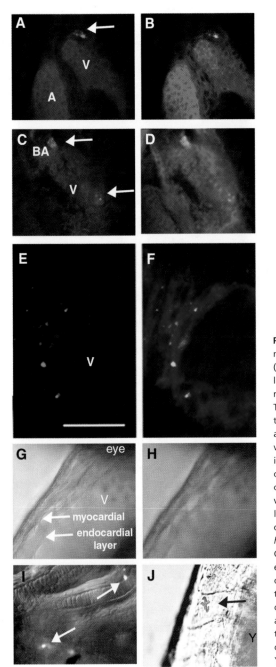

Plate 29 Three lineage-label approaches mark cardiac neural crest cells that form muscle cells in the myocardium. (A-F) Confocal cross sections of the green channel (lineage-labeled cells) shown in left panel, superimposed green and red (MF20) channels shown in right panel. (A-D) Transplanted neural crest cells transform into muscle cells in the myocardium at 3dpf. Cells in the ventricle (green label and arrow, panel A) and in the bulbus arteriosus (BA) and ventricle (V) (panel C) were also MF20-positive (yellow label in overlapped images, panel B and D). (E, F) Laser uncaging of DMNB-caged fluorescein dextran labeled neural crest cells at the 8-somite stage and confocal images of the ventricle of a 72hpf embryo were shown. By 72hpf, the lineage-labeling begins to appear punctate within the cytoplasm of lineage-labeled cells. (G, H) Laser activation of *hsp70-gfp* transgene in neural crest lineages resulted in GFP-labeled myocytes at 36hpf. Both myocardial layer and endocardial layer in the ventricle were detected in Nomarski optics (G). Three fluorescent-labeled cells were detected in the myocardial layer (H). (I, J) Cells labeled by laser uncaging or GFP-activation were also detected in (I) the pharyngeal arches and head cartilage and (J) a pigment cell, indicating that these techniques successfully labeled neural crest cells. Arrows indicate labeled cells. (Adapted from Sato and Yost.[19])

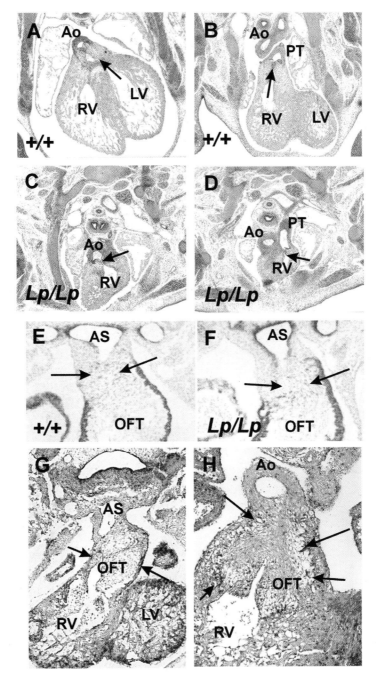

Plate 30 Defects in outflow tract remodeling in *Lp*, and expression pattern of the causative gene, *Vangl2*. (A), (B) Hematoxylin and eosin staining of transversely sectioned E13.5 *Lp*, shows that in wild-type fetuses, the aorta arises from the left ventricle, whereas the pulmonary trunk arises from the right ventricle (arrows). (C), (D) In *Lp/Lp* littermates, in contrast, both the aorta and the pulmonary trunk exit from the right ventricle (arrows). (E), (F) Immunohistochemistry, using an anti-α-smooth muscle actin antibody, visualizes neural crest cells in the outflow tract cushions at E11.5 (arrows). There are no apparent differences between +/+ and *Lp/Lp* littermates in the distribution of these cells. (G), (H) Expression of *Vangl2* in the myocardial wall of the outflow tract (arrows) and the ventricular myocardium at E11.5 and E12.5 suggests that *Vangl2* plays a primary role in outflow tract remodeling.

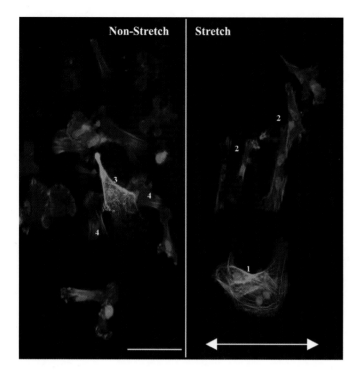

Plate 31 Representative image of 72 h non-stretched (left panel), and 48 h quiescent and 24 h stretched (right panel) embryonic ventricular cells stained for sarcomeric (green) and non-sarcomeric (red) α-actinin. Double arrows, principal stretch direction. 1, single populated cluster of cardiomyocytes (CM); 2, single populated cluster of noncardiomyocytes (NC); 3, cardiomyocytes connected to noncardiomyocytes (CM–NC); 4, noncardiomyocytes connected to cardiomyocytes (NC–CM). Scale bar = 20 μm.

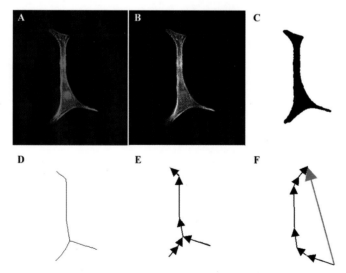

Plate 32 Measurement of cellular orientation. Either 8-bit green or red color channel was extracted from a captured RGB image (A). The extracted gray-scale image (B) was then binarised (C) and skeletanized (D). In each small segment the vector length and the angle to the principal stretch direction were measured (E). The average cellular orientation was then computed by summation of all segmental vectors (F, red arrows).

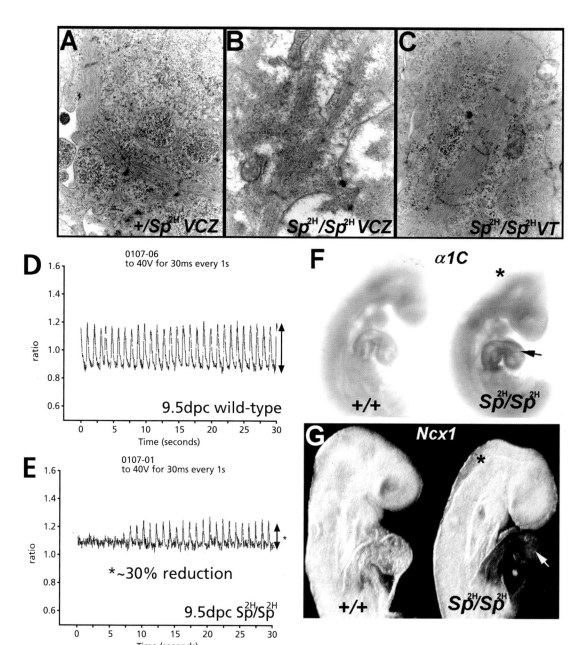

Plate 33 Cardiac failure in early homozygous Sp^{2h} embryos. (A)–(C) Transmission EM images of 10.0 dpc $+/Sp^{2h}$ control (A), ventricular compact zone (VCZ), Sp^{2h} homozygous ventricular compact zone (B) and Sp^{2h} homozygous (C) ventricular trabeculae (VT) at $\times 12\,500$ magnification. Note the myofilament deposition and parallel myofibril organization surrounding the forming Z-lines within both the normal control ventricular compact zone (A) and Sp^{2h} homozygous myocytes in the trabeculated wall of the common ventricular chamber (C), but that the Sp^{2h} homozygous ventricular compact zone myofibrils (B) are disorganized and surrounded by an abnormally sparse cytoplasm. The cellular membranes are intact, adherence junctions are present and there is no observable apoptosis within the homozygous Sp^{2h} ventricular compact zone. (D), (E) Examples of intracellular Ca^{2+} transients in 9.5 dpc wild type and homozygous Sp^{2h} freshly dissected heart tubes measured using 3 μm fura-2/AM. Ca^{2+} transients were elicited from the primitive ventricle by electrical field stimulation at 1Hz as described.[17,20] Note the reduction (~30%) of Ca^{2+} transients in homozygous mutant ($n = 6$) hearts. Basal Ca^{2+} concentration was not statically different between all three genotypes (average ~198 nM $[Ca^{2+}]_i$), but the peak $[Ca^{2+}]_i$ levels (not shown) and the times for the Ca^{2+} transients to decay by half of the peak magnitude peak within the Sp^{2h} homozygous 9.5 dpc hearts is significantly reduced (average ~228 nN in wild type; ~172 nM in heterozygotes; 108 nM in Sp^{2h} homozygous embryos). (F), (G) RNA whole mount *in situ* hybridization analysis α1-Ca^{2+}channel subunit (F) and of *Ncx1* (G) and expression within both control and homozygous Sp^{2H} mutant 9.5 (F) and 9.0 dpc (G). Note both Ca^{2+} handling genes are elevated within the mutant heart (arrows) when compared to the wild-type embryos. Both Sp^{2H} mutant embryos have exencephaly (*).

Holistic Molecular Genetic Medicine(HGM) and Collaborators

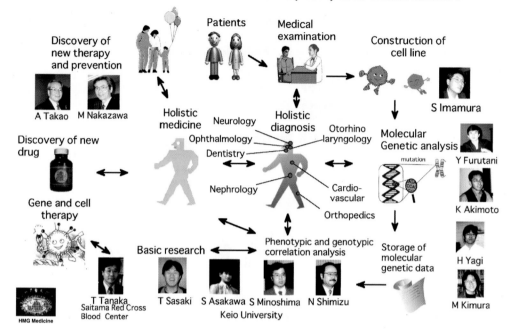

Plate 36 Holistic Molecular Genetic (HMG) medicine and collaborators. HMG is a new system of molecular genetic medical care, the aim of which is to clarify the molecular genetic pathogenesis of congenital and hereditary heart disease throughout life. HMG medicine was established in 1998. We have applied this system to conotruncal anomaly face syndrome (CAFS) and Holt–Oram syndrome patients.

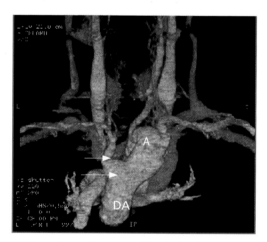

Plate 37 A posterior view of a 3-D CT image from a 30-year-old woman with deletion, a mother of a child with deletion and TOF, showing high cervical right arch (A), Kommerell's diverticulum (long arrow) and retro-esophageal left subclavian artery (short arrow). DA: descending aorta

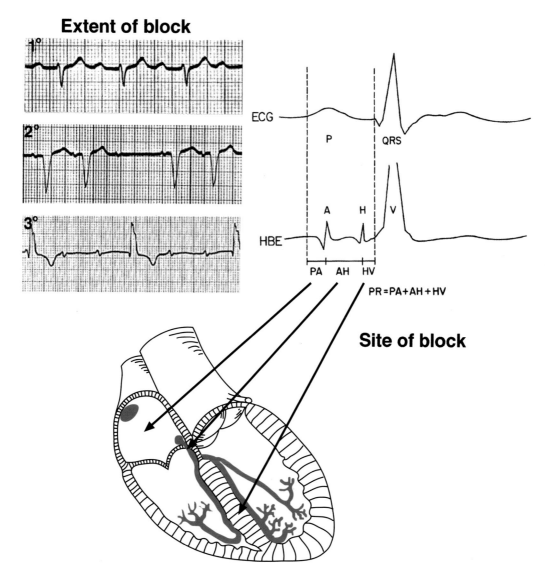

Extent of block

1°

2°

3°

Site of block

ECG

P   QRS

HBE

A   H   V

PA   AH   HV

PR = PA + AH + HV

Plate 38 Electroanatomic classification of AV conduction disturbances. Electrocardiographic traces depicting 1st, 2nd and 3rd degree AV block are shown. Sites of block, relative to intracardiac recording of the His bundle electrogram (HBE), are depicted. AH, conduction interval from onset of low septal atrial depolarization to His bundle spike (H) to onset of ventricular depolarization; HV, conduction interval from onset of His spike to onset of ventricular depolarization; PA, conduction interval from onset of P wave to low atrial septal depolarization.

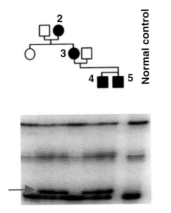

Normal

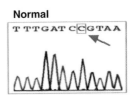

P121L Mutation

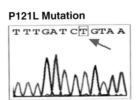

Plate 39 Left, SSCP analysis of one family with LVNC identifies an abnormal band (arrow) in affected members of this family. Right, automated sequencing identifies a point

mutation (C>T) at nucleotide 362 within exon 3 of a-dystrobrevin in affected individuals compared to the wild type normal sequence.

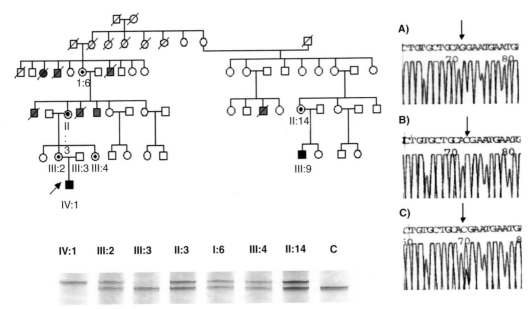

Plate 40 Left upper, Pedigree of the patients with isolated left ventricular noncompaction. Squares, males; circles, females; solid-filled squares, affected males; circles with dots, carrier females; slashes, dead individuals. The pedigree reveals a history of unexplained death during infancy and early childhood, indicated by hatched symbols. Arrow, proband (patient IV: 1). Left lower, SSCP analysis of exon 9 of

the proband (IV: 1), his mother (III: 2), father (III: 3), grandmother (II: 3), great grandmother (I: 6), aunt (III: 4), as well as the mother (II: 14) of the second patient (III: 9) and a normal unrelated control (C). Right, DNA sequence analysis of intron 8 and exon 9 of a normal control (panel A), the proband (panel B) and his mother, a heterozygous carrier (III: 2: panel C).

PART 8

Role of neural crest cells in cardiovascular development

Editorial perspective

Sachiko Miyagawa-Tomita, Makoto Nakazawa

During early vertebrate embryogenesis, neural crest cells are generated from the ectoderm at the border between the prospective neural plate and the epidermis. The neural crest, which is a population of pluripotent stem cells, undergoes an epithelial–mesenchymal transition[1] and migrates to various destinations through defined pathways,[2,3] finally giving rise to varieties of derivatives as they reach destinations.

Cardiac neural crest migration has been extensively investigated in avian species for the last two decades.[4] Kirby and co-workers, using ablated chick embryos and quail–chick chimeras, demonstrated that cardiac neural crest cells migrate to the developing pharyngeal arches and the conotruncal region, and differentiate into the smooth muscle of the aortic arches, thus contributing to septation of the outflow tract. Ablation of premigratory cardiac neural crest results in congenital cardiac abnormalities involving the outflow tract and great vessels, including persistent truncus arteriosus and double-outlet right ventricle.

Interestingly, Boot *et al.* show in this book that the early- and late-migrating cardiac neural crests play different roles. Using retroviral injection in the *in vitro* culture, they showed that the early-migrating cardiac

neural crest cells gave rise to mesenchymal cells with HNK1 expression, while late-migrating cardiac neural crest cells predominantly differentiated into smooth muscle cells with actin expression. Early migrating crest cells pass along the dorsolateral pathway to subdivide secondarily into each visceral arch,[5] and late migrating cells form the ganglionic crest because epithelialized somites inhibit the migrating crest cells during development. Environmental signals, such as the Eph-ephrin signaling pathway,[6] may affect the neural crest cell migration in a spatio-temporal manner.

Recently, several groups have performed fate-mapping experiments in the mouse using tissue-specific transgenes and Cre-lox technology (Table 1).[7–11] Sato *et al.* show in this book that the cardiac neural crest exists in zebrafish embryos, and gives rise to the myocardium in all segments of the heart, including the bulbus arteriosus, ventricle, atrioventricular junction, and atrium. The products of Cx43, Wnt1, and PlexinA2, which are markers of the cardiac neural crest, are expressed also in the left ventricle of mouse hearts.[7,10,12] Although we need more detailed data on the functions of these genes in the mouse ventricle, this evidence suggests that the cardiac neural crest affects myogenesis as demonstrated in neural crest-ablated chick embryos.[13]

Cardiac neural crest cells should require many envi-

Table 1 Cardiac neural crest markers

Transgene	References
Cx43-LZ	Lo et al. (1997)[7]; Waldo et al. (1999)[8]
P0-Cre	Yamauchi et al. (1999)[9]
Wnt1-Cre	Jiang et al. (2000)[10]
Pax3-Cre	Li et al. (2000)[11]

ronmental signals for specification, migration, proliferation, differentiation, and survival during their migration to the pharyngeal arches and the outflow tract of heart, as demonstrated in many gene-targeted knockout mice (Table 2).[14–28] These knockout mice show similar phenotypes to those seen in the chick with neural crest ablation, and, therefore, the anomalies of the pharyngeal arches and outflow tract in the mouse are very likely associated with the cardiac neural crest. Herein, Molin et al. examine the role of neural crest cells on pharyngeal arches development in the *Tgfβ2*-knockout mice using Wnt1-Cre-loxP reporter mice. They found that the number of neural crest cells

Table 2 Knockout mouse models for altered cardiac neural crest

Gene altered	Function	Expression	Cardiovascular phenotype*
Et-1 ko[14]	Endothelin 1 ligand	Epithelium of arch, endothelium of arch and oft Mesoderm core of arch	IAA, Arch anom, VSD
ECE-1 ko[15]	Endothelin converting enzyme-1	Epithelium and mesenchyme of arch Endocardium	IAA, Arch anom, VSD, DORV, PTA
ETA ko	Endothelin A receptor	Mesenchyme of arch and oft Myocardium	IAA, Arch anom, VSD, DORV, TGA, PTA
RAR / ko[17] RXR/RAR ko[18]	Retinoic acid receptor	RAR : myocardium† RAR : myocardium† RXR : ubiquitous	CoA, AP window, Arch anom, PTA, VSD, Common AVC
Sox4 ko[19,20]	Transcription factor	Mesenchyme of arch Endocardium of oft and AVC	Dysplastic semilunar valve, PTA, Infundibulum anom
Foxc1(mf1) ko[21,22]	Transcription factor	Mesenchyme of arch and cushions Endocardium of vent	IAA, CoA, VSD, Valve dysplasia
Foxc2(Mfh1) ko[23]	Transcription factor	Endothelium and mesenchyme of arch	IAA, VSD
Semaphorin3C ko[24]	Semaphorin3C receptor	Mesenchyme of arch and oft Oft myocardium	IAA, PTA, DORV
Neuropilin-1 ko[25]	Inhibitory axon guidance	Endothelium Endocardium	RAA, DAA, Arch anom, PTA
Tbx1 ko[26–28]	Transcription factor	Mesenchyme of arch Pharyngeal endoderm Dorsal wall of aortic sac	IAA, Arch anom, PTA, VSD

* Arch, pharyngeal arteries; Arch anom, aortic arch anomalies; AVC, atrioventricular canal; CoA, coarctation of the aorta; DAA, double aortic arch; DORV, double-outlet right ventricle; IAA, interruption of the aortic arch; Infundibulum anom, infundibulum anomalies; Oft, outflow tract; PTA, persistent truncus arteriosus; RAA, right aortic arch; TGA, transposition of the great arteries; VSD, ventricular septal defect.

† Immunohistochemical findings [unpubl. data]

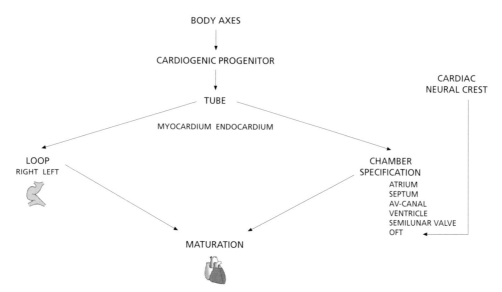

Fig. 1 Approach for understanding cardiac morphogenesis. The heart is the first organ to form during development. Mesodermal precursors are initially committed and specified to become cardiogenic cells, in response to inductive signals from the adjacent endoderm and other neighboring tissues. These cells, which form in bilaterally symmetrical regions near the anterior end of the embryo, converge at the midline to form a linear heart tube that initiates rhythmic contractions. The heart tube is subdivided along its length into segments and then undergoes right ward bending (ventricular D-heart looping), which positions the primitive atrial and ventricular chambers, morphologically. During chamber specification, the cardiac neural crest migrates to the pharyngeal arches and the outflow tract. Subsequent chamber maturation, formation of valves and septa, trabeculation, and formation of conduction system occur, to eventually give rise to the mature four-chambered heart.

is reduced along with apoptosis of these cells in the process of regression of the fourth arch artery. The nervus recurrence surrounding the aortic arch expressed Smad2, which is a member of the SMAD family of intracellular signal mediator proteins, and has been shown to transduce the Tgfβ signal from the cell membrane to the nucleus. Their data suggests that Tgfβ-Smad2 signaling, which is expressed in the arch artery and the nervus recurrence, might play an important role in the regression of the fourth arch artery.

Splotch mutant mouse, which is a spontaneous mutant mouse, shows heart anomalies specific to abnormality of the cardiac neural crest. This mouse has a deletion in the *Pax3* gene which encodes a DNA-binding transcription factor, and this functional defect is not intrinsic to the neural crest itself but seems to be inappropriate cell interactions during the emigration.[29] Using Splotch mutant mice, Maeda *et al.* show expression of the CXC chemokine, *Sdf1* ligand and *cxcR4* receptor, which is a transmembrane signaling. Although mice lacking *Sdf1* or *cxcR4* showed only ventricular septal defect, the *Sdf1/cxcR4* were reciprocally expressed along migration pathways of the cardiac neural crest in normal mouse and not in the Splotch mice. Since YY1, which is known to suppress the promoter activity of cxcR4, was over-expressed in the Splotch mice, they had inferred that the anomalous CXC chemokine pathway might lead to poor neural crest migration.

The neural crest plays a very important role in the development of the whole heart (Fig. 1), and its abnormalities in humans are also very likely to cause outflow tract anomalies, which are usually very severe and difficult to treat. Therefore, the precise role of the neural crest in the development of the heart should be extensively studied and clarified.

References

1 Bronner-Fraser M, Fraser SE. Cell lineage analysis reveals multipotency of some avian neural crest cells. *Nature* 1988; **335**: 161–4.

2 Le Douarin NM. *The Neural Crest.* London: Cambridge University Press, 1982.

3 Hall BK, Horstadius S. *The Neural Crest*. London: Oxford University Press, 1988.

4 Kirby ML, Gale TF, Stewart DE. Neural crest cells contribute to normal aorticopulmonary septation. *Science* 1983; **220**: 1059–61.

5 Shigetani Y, Aizawa S, Kuratani S. Overlapping origins of pharyngeal arch crest cells on the postotic hind-brain. *Dev Growth Diff* 1995; **37**: 733–46.

6 Smith A, Robinson V, Patel K, Wilkinson DG. The EphA4 and EphB1 receptor tyrosine kinases and ephrin-B2 ligand regulate targeted migration of branchial neural crest cells. *Curr Biol* 1997; **7**: 561–70.

7 Lo, C. W. *et al.* Cx43 gap junction gene expression and gap junctional communication in mouse neural crest cells. *Dev Genet* 1997; **20**: 119–32.

8 Waldo KL, Lo CW, Kirby ML. Connexin 43 expression reflects neural crest patterns during cardiovascular development. *Dev Biol* 1999; **208**: 307–23.

9 Yamauchi Y *et al.* A novel transgenic technique that allows specific marking of the neural crest cell lineage in mice. *Dev Biol* 1999; **212**: 191–203.

10 Jiang X, Rowitch DH, Soriano P, McMahon AP, Sucov HM. Fate of the mammalian cardiac neural crest. *Development* 2000; **127**: 1607–16.

11 Li J, Chen F, Epstein JA. Neural crest expression of Cre recombinase directed by the proximal Pax3 promoter in transgenic mice. *Genesis* 2000; **26**: 162–4.

12 Brown CB *et al.* PlexinA2 and semaphorin signaling during cardiac neural crest development. *Development* 2001; **128**: 3071–80.

13 Farrell MJ *et al.* FGF-8 in the ventral pharynx alters development of myocardial calcium transients after neural crest ablation. *J Clin Invest* 2001; **107**: 1509–17.

14 Kurihara Y *et al.* Aortic arch malformations and ventricular septal defect in mice deficient in endothelin-1. *J Clin Invest* 1995; **96**: 293–300.

15 Yanagisawa H *et al.* Dual genetic pathways of endothelin-mediated intercellular signaling revealed by targeted disruption of endothelin converting enzyme-1 gene. *Development* 1998; **125**: 825–36.

16 Clouthier DE *et al.* Cranial and cardiac neural crest defects in endothelin-A receptor-deficient mice. *Development* 1998; **125**: 813–24.

17 Mendelsohn C *et al.* Function of the retinoic acid receptors (RARs) during development (II). Multiple abnormalities at various stages of organogenesis in RAR double mutants. *Development* 1994; **120**: 2749–71.

18 Lee RY, Luo J, Evans RM, Giguere V, Sucov HM. Compartment-selective sensitivity of cardiovascular morphogenesis to combinations of retinoic acid receptor gene mutations. *Circ Res* 1997; **80**: 757–64.

19 Schilham MW *et al.* Defects in cardiac outflow tract formation and pro-B-lymphocyte expansion in mice lacking Sox-4. *Nature* 1996; **380**: 711–14.

20 Ya J *et al.* Sox4-deficiency syndrome in mice is an animal model for common trunk. *Circ Res* 1998; **83**: 986–94.

21 Winnier GE *et al.* Roles for the winged helix transcription factors MF1 and MFH1 in cardiovascular development revealed by nonallelic noncomplementation of null alleles. *Dev Biol* 1999; **213**: 418–31.

22 Kume T, Jiang H, Topczewska JM, Hogan BL. The murine winged helix transcription factors, Foxc1 and Foxc2, are both required for cardiovascular development and somitogenesis. *Genes Dev* 2001; **15**: 2470–82.

23 Iida K *et al.* Essential roles of the winged helix transcription factor MFH-1 in aortic arch patterning and skeletogenesis. *Development* 1997; **124**: 4627–38.

24 Feiner L *et al.* Targeted disruption of semaphorin 3C leads to persistent truncus arteriosus and aortic arch interruption. *Development* 2001; **128**: 3061–70.

25 Kawasaki T *et al.* A requirement for neuropilin-1 in embryonic vessel formation. *Development* 1999; **126**, 4895–902.

26 Jerome LA, Papaioannou VE. DiGeorge syndrome phenotype in mice mutant for the T-box gene, Tbx1. *Nat Genet* 2001; **27**: 286–91.

27 Lindsay EA *et al.* Tbx1 haploinsufficieny in the DiGeorge syndrome region causes aortic arch defects in mice. *Nature* 2001; **410**: 97–101.

28 Merscher S *et al.* TBX1 is responsible for cardiovascular defects in velo-cardio-facial/DiGeorge syndrome. *Cell* 2001; **104**: 619–29.

29 Epstein JA *et al.* Migration of cardiac neural crest cells in Splotch embryos. *Development* 2000; **127**, 1869–78.

CHAPTER 35

Sdf1/CxcR4 chemotaxis is disrupted within the *splotch* mouse mutant cardiovascular system

Manabu Maeda, Jian Wang, Rhonda Rogers, Nurul H. Sarker, Simon J. Conway

Cytokines are essential for cardiogenesis, hematopoiesis, and vasculogenesis during embryonic development, in addition to their involvement in chemotaxis of leukocyte subsets and endothelial cells. Transmembrane signaling of the CXC chemokine *stromal cell-derived factor-1 (Sdf1)* ligand which is exclusively mediated by *cxcR4*, a G-protein-coupled receptor initially identified in leukocytes and shown to serve as a co-receptor for the entry of HIV into lymphocytes.[1–3] *Sdf1* and *cxcR4* have been shown to modulate cell migration, differentiation, and proliferation and both are expressed in various tissues including the brain, embryonic hematopoietic system, and heart.[4] The *Xenopus* homologue *XcxcR4* is similarly expressed within brain and embryonic hematopoietic system, but as *XcxcR4* is absent from the heart anlage (but present in the neural crest), this has led to the suggestion that *XSdf1* is expressed in the heart to attract cardiac neural crest cells from the neural tube into the heart itself to regulate both septation of the cardiac outflow tract and differentiation of the myocardium during early heart development.[5] Studies, principally in the chick[6] and mouse,[7] have demonstrated that conotruncal defects and poor myocardial function can result from failure of the "cardiac" neural crest to colonize the developing aortic arch system and outflow tract. Mice lacking *Sdf1* (1) or *cxcR4*[8,9] die parentally and exhibit identical hematopoietic, neuronal, and cardiac defects (interventricular septal defect, VSD). Furthermore,

rat *Sdf1* mRNA was induced in permanent coronary artery occlusion model of myocardial infarction[10] and high *cxcR4* mRNA levels are present within both chronic failing and nonfailing human myocardium[11] indicative of its role in the inflammatory events in cardiovascular disease. Additionally, *Sdf1* has been shown to act as an attractive guidance cue for rats and mice neuronal migration[12] and that the *Sdf1/cxcR4* axis stimulates human *VEGF* secretion.[13] Although it is well documented that cardiomyopathy is an important cardiac complication in acquired immunodeficiency syndrome (AIDS) and that HIV has been detected in cardiac myocytes in AIDS,[1–3] there is little data regarding how HIV affects the developing embryonic/fetal heart. In order to begin to determine the role of *Sdf1/cxcR4* within the pathogenesis of the congenital heart defects, we analyzed the spatiotemporal expression of *Sdf1/cxcR4* mRNA within both normal and *Splotch* mutant mouse embryonic hearts mutant that have been shown to develop conotruncal defects, poor myocardial function, and VSDs.[6,7]

Splotch mutant alleles have long been known to disrupt neural crest development, resulting in defects of neural crest derivatives. By studying this heart defect in the *splotch* (*Sp2H*) mutant mouse (which has a mutation in the DNA-binding homeodomain of the *pax3* transcription factor), we have shown that the cardiac neural crest cells (which specifically express *pax3*) fail to migrate into the developing heart resulting in outflow tract defects and embryonic lethality at 14.0dpc.[14,15] Here we showed the *Sdf1/cxcR4* reciprocally expressed along the cardiac neural crest migration pathways in normal mouse and that there is a lack of *Sdf1/cxcR4* mRNA in *Sp²ᴴ* mutant embryos.

Initial RT-PCR analysis revealed that both Sdf1 and cxcR4 mRNA expression is reduced in 10.5 and 12.5dpc *Sp²ᴴ* mutant embryos when compared to normal control littermates (Fig. 35.1). Furthermore, as *Yin Yang-1* (a zinc finger-containing transcription factor) is known to suppress the promoter activity of *cxcR4* (16), we assessed the level of *YY1* expression to determine whether down-regulation of *Sdf1/cxcR4* expression was directly or indirectly due to lack of normal *pax3* expression. RT-PCR analysis demonstrated that *YY1* was over-expressed in *Sp²ᴴ* mutant embryos (Fig. 35.1). Knockout of *YY1* results in embryonic lethality around implantation and a subset of heterozygotes embryos are developmentally retarded and exhibit neurulation defects.[17] Thus, RT-PCR analysis demonstrated that while *YY1* was over-expressed, both *Sdf1/cxcR4* were under-expressed in *sp²ᴴ* mutants and that lack of normal *pax3* function results in a lack of upstream control of the CXC chemokine pathway.

Given the abnormalities in mRNA levels, we used *in situ* hybridization to determine where *Sdf1/cxcR4* expression was affected. *In situ* hybridization confirmed that there is reduced expression of both the reciprocally-expressed *Sdf1/cxcR4* along the neural crest cell migration pathway and within the pharyngeal arches and outflow tract itself and significantly that there is no *cxcR4* expression within the apex of

the aorticopulmonary septum (Fig. 35.2). While *cxcR4* mRNA was expressed within the neural tube, some myocardial elements (possibly the conduction system), atrioventricular cushion tissue, the endothelial cells lining the arteries and pharyngeal endoderm, *Sdf1* mRNA was absent from the neural tube but was expressed within the mesenchyme, most of the cardiomyocytes and in the periostium surrounding the skeletal elements (Fig. 35.2). As septation of the left and right ventricular chambers occurs by fusion of the membranous portion of the interventricular septum, the enlarging endocardial cushions and the proximal region of the truncus arteriosus – the lack of SDF1/CXCR4 signaling within *sp²ᴴ* mutants at these sites suggests that abnormal expression of these cytokines may be involved in the final pathway leading to the observed congenital heart defects. These data indicate that the elevation of *YY1* may repress *cxcR4* expression leading to a chemotatic deficiency and poor neural crest migration. What is currently unclear is whether *YY1* is directly or indirectly regulated by *pax3* and further studies are aimed at trying to determine the role of *pax3/YY1* regulation and the how *Sdf1/cxcR4* help to regulate cardiac neural crest migration, guidance, and/or proliferation.

Materials and methods

RT-PCR and *in situ* hybridization

Total RNA was prepared from 10.5 and 12.5 dpc wild type (+/+) and *Splotch* embryos in accordance with the manufacturer's instructions (Life Technologies,

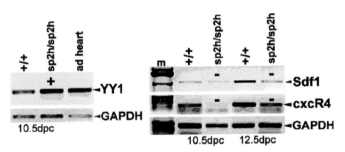

Fig. 35.1 RT-PCR analysis. mRNA was prepared from whole 10.5, 12.5 *dpc* wild-type (+/+) and mutant (*sp²ᴴ/sp²ᴴ*) littermates, plus adult hearts. cDNA was normalized using housekeeping gene *GAPDH* (18 PCR cycles). *YY1* (30 cycles) is significantly increased (+) within the *sp²ᴴ* mutants, while both *Sdf1* (20 cycles) and *cxcR4* (22 cycles) expression is significantly decreased (–) within 10.5, 12.5*dpc sp²ᴴ* embryos. Also note that *YY1* is highly expressed within the adult hearts, as are both *Sdf1/cxcR4* (not shown).

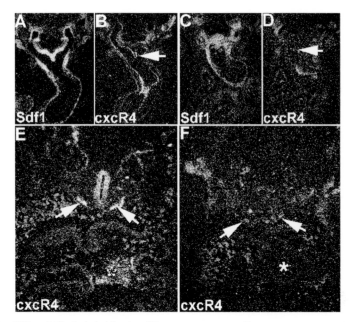

Fig. 35.2 Radioactive *Sdf1*, *cxcR4 in situ* hybridization. (A), (B) Control 10.0 dpc transverse sections. Note there are high levels of *Sdf1* within the mesenchyme surrounding the dorsal aorte, the pharyngeal arch region surrounding the 4th arch arteries and within the conotruncal myocardium. *CxcR4* is reciprocally expressed within the foregut endoderm and within the endothelial cells lining the dorsal aorta and conotruncal cushions, and a single cell layer covering the apex of the aorticopulmonary septum (arrow in B). (C, D) *Sp²ᴴ* 10.0 dpc transverse sections. Note the reduced expression of both *Sfd1* and *cxcR4* and that there is no cxcR4 expression within the apex of the aorticopulmonary septum (arrow in D). (E), (F) Control (E) and *sp²ᴴ* (F) 11.0dpc transverse sections. Note that the *cxcR4* expression within the 6th aortic arches is reduced within the *sp²ᴴ* mutant, as is the expression in the trachea and atrioventricuylar cushions (* in F).

Inc.). RNA was reverse-transcribed to cDNA using oligo(dT) primers and Superscript (Life Technologies, Inc.). PCR was performed using EX Taq DNA polymerase (Takara, Inc.) using published primers and PCR conditions.[1,8,19] Linearity of gene expression was established by cycle-based RT-PCR using the ubiquitously expressed GAPDH house-keeping gene. The PCR fragments were subsequently cloned and sequenced to confirm identity, and then used as radioactive *in situ* hybridization probes to determine whether there are any differences within the localization of the mRNAs within the mutant embryos.

References

1 Nagasawa T *et al*. Defects of B-cell lymphopoiesis and bone-marrow myelopoiesis in mice lacking the CXC chemokine PBSF/SDF-1. *Nature* 1996; **382**: 635–8.

2 d'Amati G, di Gioia CR, Gallo P. Pathological findings of HIV-associated cardiovascular disease. *Ann N Y Acad Sci* 2001; **946**: 23–45.

3 Barbaro G, Lipshultz SE. Pathogenesis of HIV-associated cardiomyopathy. *Ann N Y Acad Sci.* 2001; **946**: 57–81.

4 McGrath KE *et al*. Embryonic expression and function of the chemokine SDF-1 and its receptor, CXCR4. *Dev Biol* 1999; **213**: 442–456.

5 Braun M *et al. Xenopus laevis* stromal cell-derived factor 1: conservation of structure and function during vertebrate development. *J Immunol* 2002; **168**: 2340–7.

6 Creazzo TL *et al*. Role of cardiac neural crest cells in cardiovascular development. *Annu Rev Physiol* 1998; **60**: 267–86.

7 Conway SJ *et al*. Abnormal neural crest stem cell expansion is responsible for the conotruncal heart defects within the *Splotch (Sp²ᴴ)* mouse mutant. *Cardiovasc Res* 2000; **47**: 314–28.

8 Tachibana K *et al*. The chemokine receptor CXCR4 is essential for vascularization of the gastrointestinal tract. *Nature* 1998; **393**: 591–4.

9 Zou YR *et al*. Function of the chemokine receptor CXCR4 in haematopoiesis and in cerebellar development. *Nature* 1998; **393**: 595–9.

10 Pillarisetti K, Gupta SK. Cloning and relative expression analysis of rat stromal cell derived factor-1 (SDF-1)1:

SDF-1 alpha mRNA is selectively induced in rat model of myocardial infarction. *Inflammation* 2001; **25**: 293–300.

11 Damas JK *et al.* Myocardial expression of CC- and CXC-chemokines and their receptors in human end-stage heart failure. *Cardiovasc Res* 2000; **47**: 778–7.

12 Zhu Y *et al.* Role of the chemokine SDF-1 as the meningeal attractant for embryonic cerebellar neurons. *Nat Neurosci* 2002; **5**: 719–20.

13 Salcedo R *et al.* Vascular endothelial growth factor and basic fibroblast growth factor induce expression of CXCR4 on human endothelial cells: *in vivo* neovascularization induced by stromal-derived factor-1alpha. *Am J Pathol* 1999; **154**: 1125–35.

14 Conway SJ, Henderson DJ, Copp AJ. Pax3 is required for cardiac neural crest migration in the mouse: evidence from the splotch (Sp2H) mutant. *Development* 1997; **124**: 505–14.

15 Conway SJ *et al.* Neural crest is involved in development of abnormal myocardial function. *J Mol Cell Cardiol* 1997; **29**: 2675–85.

16 Ellis PD *et al.* Increased actin polymerization reduces the inhibition of serum response factor activity by Yin Yang 1. *Biochem J* 2002; **364**: 547–54.

17 Donohoe ME *et al.* Targeted disruption of mouse Yin Yang 1 transcription factor results in peri-implantation lethality. *Mol Cell Biol* 1999; **19**: 7237–44.

CHAPTER 36

Differences in migration and differentiation capacities of early- and late-migrating cardiac neural crest cells

Marit J. Boot, Adriana C. Gittenberger-de Groot, Robert E. Poelmann

Cardiac neural crest cells are considered as a contiguous group of pluripotent cells capable to differentiate into nerve tissue, smooth muscle cells of the pharyngeal arch arteries, and mesenchymal cells of the aorticopulmonary septum.[1–4] Studies in neural crest ablated chick embryos show that abnormal cardiac neural crest cell migration disturbs pharyngeal arch artery development and outflow tract septation.[5,6] Are these malformations related to subpopulations of the cardiac neural crest? Should the cardiac neural crest cells be subdivided in populations depending on the time point at which they emigrate from the neural tube?

We studied cardiac neural crest cell migration in chick embryos *in vivo* and *in vitro* at various developmental Hamburger and Hamilton stages.[7] Early-migrating cardiac neural crest cells were marked *in vivo* by injecting a *lacZ*-retrovirus into the neural tube lumen at HH10 as described by our group before,[2,3] and ablating the late cardiac neural crest at HH11 with a tungsten needle. Late-migrating cardiac neural crest cells were marked by injecting a *lacZ*-retrovirus into the neural tube lumen at HH12.

The migration pathways of the early- and late-migrating cardiac neural crest cells are very similar in the first days after retroviral injection. However, the differences between early- and late-migrating cardiac neural crest cells were distinct by HH30. The early-migrating cardiac neural crest cells massively target the condensed mesenchyme and prongs of the aorticopulmonary septum and the proximal and distal parts of the pharyngeal arch arteries. Ablation of late-migrating cardiac neural crest resulted in pharyngeal arch arteries with interrupted concentric layers. The late-migrating cardiac neural crest cells tend to be restricted to the proximal part of the pharyngeal arch arteries. This suggests that the early-migrating cardiac neural crest cells are indispensable for outflow tract septation, while the late-migrating cardiac neural crest cells are involved in pharyngeal arch artery remodeling.

To determine if there is only a difference in fate of the two subpopulations or if there is also a difference in developmental potential was studied *in vitro* by culturing neural tube explants. Neural tubes from the mesencephalon to the level of the fourth somites were excised from chick embryos, and after collagenase induced removal of the adhering tissues, placed in M199 medium on fibronectin coated glass and cultured for 48 h. The early neural tube explants taken from embryos HH10 gave rise to a high frequency of mesenchymal cells; these cells stained positive for HNK1. In the late neural tube explant cultures, taken from embryos HH12, the number of HNK1 stained cells was lower. Interestingly, after staining for actin with HHF35 we observed a low number of cells expressing actin in the early explant cultures (Fig. 36.1a) and a very high number of actin

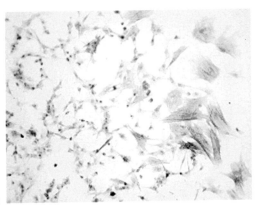
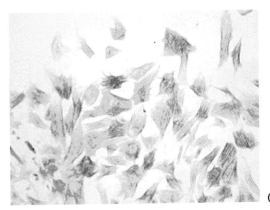

(a)

(b)

Fig. 36.1 Actin filaments stained with HHF35 in a low number of cells in the early (HH10) neural tube explant culture (a) and a high number of smooth muscle cells in the late (HH12) neural tube explant culture (b).

expressing cells in the late neural tube explants (Fig. 36.1b). This suggests that late-migrating cardiac neural crest cells predominantly differentiate into smooth muscle cells and are intrinsically different from early-migrating cells.

From our data we can conclude that cardiac neural crest cell migration patterns and differentiation potential strongly depend on the time at which the cardiac neural crest cells emigrate from the neural tube. This division in subpopulations was not reported before for the cardiac neural crest; however it had been described for the trunk. In trunk neural crest the early-migrating cells differentiate into many derivatives like pigment cells, neurons, and adrenergic cells, while late-migrating cardiac neural crest cells never show characteristics of adrenergic cells.[8] The specific behavior of the late-migrating cardiac neural crest cells might be partly due to intrinsic differences between the early- and late-migrating cardiac neural crest populations. Other important factors are the environment through which the cardiac neural crest cells migrate, but *in vivo* also guiding signals of the early-migrating cardiac neural crest cells will probably affect the behavior of the late-migrating cardiac neural crest cells. The effects that subpopulations of neural crest cells have on each other was described for the contribution of the mesencephalic crest to the cartilage of the jaw.[9]

The implications of subpopulations of cardiac neural crest cells involved in different developmental processes reflect upon cardiovascular malformations in which the focus should be pointed to a specific time window. By narrowing the developmental range in which congenital heart diseases arise we may exclude a number of supposed candidate genes involved in these diseases.

References

1 Kirby ML, Gale TF, Stewart DE. Neural crest cells contribute to normal aorticopulmonary septation. *Science* 1983; **220**: 1059–61.

2 Poelmann RE, Mikawa T, Gittenberger-de Groot AC. Neural crest cells in outflow tract septation of the embryonic chicken heart: differentiation and apoptosis. *Dev Dyn* 1998; **212**: 373–384.

3 Bergwerff M, Verberne ME, DeRuiter MC, Poelmann RE, Gittenberger-de Groot AC. Neural crest cell contribution to the developing circulatory system. Implications for vascular morphology? *Circ Res* 1998; **82**: 221–31.

4 Verberne ME, Gittenberger-de Groot AC, VanIperen L, Poelmann RE. Distribution of different regions of cardiac neural crest in the extrinsic and the intrinsic cardiac nervous system. *Dev Dyn* 2000; **217**: 191–204.

5 Bockman DE, Redmond ME, Kirby ML. Alteration of early vascular development after ablation of cranial neural crest. *Anat. Rec* 1989; **225**: 209–17.

6 Kirby ML, Turnage KL, Hays BM. Characterization of conotruncal malformations following ablation of "cardiac" neural crest. *Anat Rec* 1985; **213**: 87–93.

7 Hamburger V, Hamilton HL. A series of normal stages in the development of the chick embryo. *J Morphol* 1951; **88**: 49–92.

8 Artinger KB, Bronner-Fraser M. Partial restriction in the developmental potential of late emigrating avian neural crest cells. *Dev Biol* 1992; **149**: 149–57.

9 Baker CVH, Bronner-Fraser M, Le Douarin NM, Teillet MA. Early- and late-migrating cranial neural crest cell populations have equivalent developmental potential *in vivo. Development* 1997; **124**: 3077–87.

CHAPTER 37

TGFβ2 does not affect neural crest cell migration but is a key player in vascular remodeling during embryogenesis

Daniel G. M. Molin, Marco C. DeRuiter, Thomas Doetschman, Henry M. Sucov, Robert E. Poelmann, Adriana C. Gittenberger-de Groot

Transforming growth factor beta (TGFβ) belongs to the TGFβ superfamily of growth and differentiation factors. Only *Tgfβ2*-knockout mice present major cardiovascular abnormalities.[1–3] During normal development, the pharyngeal arch artery (PAA) system remodels from its initially symmetrical paired arch artery system into a left-sided aortic arch and ductus arteriosus by regression of several vascular segments. We previously showed that this process involves apoptosis, which was markedly altered in *Tgfβ2*-knockout mice.[3] Smooth muscle cells (SMCs) of the PAA are predominantly neural crest cell (NCC) derived and play an important role in the development of the PAA vasculature.[4,5] TGFβ has been proven to influence the differentiation of NCC into SMC as well as to enhance the expression of smooth muscle specific proteins.[6,7] Here we show that in *Tgfβ2*-knockout mice NCC are still capable to migrate to and populate the PAAs, and eventually differentiate into SMCs. Nonetheless, a clear reduction of NCC derived SMCs is apparent, being most outspoken for the 4th PAA. This reduction coincided with anomalous development of the 4th PAA, enhanced vascular apoptosis and aberrant *Tgfβ2*-SMAD2 signaling.

ISH was applied both to scrutinize the spatiotemporal vascular expression patterning of *Tgfβ1–3* and to reveal overlap of expression between the isoforms. The latter is important as the isoforms are capable of mimicking their function *in vitro* and as such might have redundant effects.[1] *In vivo* a positive correlation between TGFβ1 and arterial smooth muscle differentiation was found,[8] but knockout studies revealed only minor vascular defects.[9] *Tgfβ2* knockout mice develop vascular anomalies including hypoplasia and aortic arch interruptions (4th arch artery).[2,3] *Tgfβ1–3* are expressed in the vascular system. *Tgfβ1* is present in the vascular endothelium during E9.5–15.5. In the early embryo (E9.5–10.5), *Tgfβ2* shows a high expression in the media throughout the vascular system confined to SMC differentiation. The expression of *Tgfβ2* and *Tgfβ3* greatly overlap from E11.5 onwards, being present in the media and adventitia of the great arteries. When the expression patterns are taken into consideration the *Tgfβ* isoforms might have supplementary roles during vascular development.

Of special interest are NCCs, as they supply SMC precursors to the developing pharyngeal arch arteries.[10] To analyze the effect of *Tgfβ2* on NCC migration and differentiation *Tgfβ2*-knockouts were crossed with NCC (Wnt-1) Cre-loxP reporter mice.[5] The potential of NCC to migration and populate the PAAs as well as differentiate into SMC is unaltered. Nonetheless, a reduced number of NCC-derived SMCs (related to the degree of hypoplasia) are found in the PAAs of stage E14.5–17.5 knockouts. Especially the 4th arch artery is affected, presenting severe vascular hypoplasia, coinciding with a complete interruption of its midpoint in the most severe cases.

As regression of the 4th PAA can result from vascular apoptosis, we analyzed apoptosis in serial sections 9using TUNEL and HE staining) of E12.0–15.5 wild type and *Tgfβ2* -knockout mice. A high number of apoptotic cells was found in the mesenchyme surrounding the 4th PAA and in the vessel wall, being significantly higher for the knockout mice. To determine if the vascular segment of the 4th PAA that regresses relates to the segment reported to exhibit a poor α-SM-actin, elastin make-up,[11] and extended NCC-related CX43 expression,[12] we analyzed 4th PAA sections with antibodies against α-smooth muscle-actin (α-SM-actin;1A4) and neurofilaments (RMO-270). A SMAD2 antibody (to detect positive nuclei) was used to discriminate for *Tgfβ* signaling. The 4th PAA segment that regresses in *Tgfβ2* knockouts locates in close proximity to the nervus vagus and nervus recurrence overlaps with a poor α-SM-actin positive segment that highly expresses RMO-270 and contains cells that are SMAD2 (nuclei) positive. These data put forward a potential relationship between the morphologically distinct vascular segment of the 4th PAA, its interruption, and TGFβ2-SMAD2 signaling.

References

1 Sanford LP *et al.* TGFβ2 knockout mice have multiple developmental defects that are non-overlapping with other TGFβ knockout phenotypes. *Development* 1997; **124**: 2659–70.
2 Bartram U *et al.* Double-outlet right ventricle and overriding tricuspid valve reflect disturbances of looping, myocardialization, endocardial cushion differentiation, and apoptosis in TGFß2-knockout mice. *Circulation* 2001; **103**: 2745–52.
3 Molin DGM *et al.* Altered apoptosis pattern during pharyngeal arch artery remodelling is associated with aortic arch malformations in Tgfbeta 2 knockout mice. *Cardiovasc Res* 2002; **56**: 312–22.
4 Bergwerff M, Verberne ME, DeRuiter MC, Poelmann RE, Gittenberger-de Groot AC. Neural crest cell contribution to the developing circulatory system. Implications for vascular morphology? *Circ Res* 1998; **82**: 221–31.
5 Jiang X, Rowitch DH, Soriano P, McMahon AP, Sucov HM. Fate of the mammalian cardiac neural crest. *Development* 2000; **127**: 1607–16.
6 Topouzis S, Majesky MW. Smooth muscle lineage diversity in the chick embryo. Two types of aortic smooth muscle cell differ in growth and receptor-mediated transcriptional responses to transforming growth factor-β. *Dev Biol* 1996; **178**: 430–45.
7 Hautmann MB, Adam PJ, Owens GK. Similarities and differences in smooth muscle alpha-actin induction by TGF-beta in smooth muscle versus non-smooth muscle cells. *Arterioscler Thromb Vasc Biol* 1999; **19**: 2049–58.
8 Grainger DJ, Metcalfe JC, Grace AA, Mosedale DE. Transforming growth factor-β dynamically regulates vascular smooth muscle differentiation *in vivo. J Cell Sci* 1998; **111**: 2977–88.
9 Dickson MC, Slager HG, Duffie E, Mummery CL. RNA and protein localisations of TGFβ2 in the early mouse embryo suggest an involvement in cardiac development. *Development* 1993; **117**: 625–39.
10 Gittenberger-de Groot AC, DeRuiter MC, Bergwerff M, Poelmann RE. Smooth muscle cell origin and its relation to heterogeneity in development and disease. *Arterioscle Thromb Vasc Biol* 1999; **19**: 1589–94.
11 Bergwerff M, DeRuiter MC, Hall S, Poelmann RE, Gittenberger-de Groot AC. Unique vascular morphology of the fourth aortic arches: possible implications for pathogenesis of type-B aortic arch interruption and anomalous right subclavian artery. *Cardiovasc Res* 1999; **44**: 185–96.
12 Waldo KL, Lo CW, Kirby ML. Connexin 43 expression reflects neural crest patterns during cardiovascular development. *Dev Biol* 1999; **208**: 307–23.

CHAPTER 38

Neural crest cells contribute to heart formation and cardiomyogenesis in zebrafish

Mariko Sato, H. Joseph Yost

In birds and mammals, cardiac neural crest is essential for heart development, and contributes to conotruncal cushion formation and outflow tract septation.[1–9] The zebrafish prototypical heart lacks outflow tract septation,[10] raising the question of whether cardiac neural crest exists in zebrafish. Here, results from three distinct lineage-labeling approaches indicate that zebrafish neural crest cells have the ability to generate MF20-positive muscle cells in heart chambers during development. Fate-mapping demonstrates that cardiac neural crest cells originate both from neural tube regions analogous to those found in birds, as well as from a novel region rostral to the otic vesicle. In contrast to other vertebrates, zebrafish cardiac neural crest invades the myocardium in all segments of the heart, including the bulbus arteriosus, ventricle, atrioventricular (AV) junction, and atrium. Three distinct groups of premigratory neural crest along the rostrocaudal axis have different propensities to contribute to different segments in the heart and are correspondingly marked by unique combinations of gene expression patterns.

Three distinct experimental approaches were performed: (1) cell transplantation;[11] (2) caged-fluorescein dextran lineage labeling;[12–14] (3) laser activation of *hsp70-gfp* labeling.[15] The neural crest cells at the 8-somite stage were labeled and their cell fate followed. To identify muscle lineage in the heart, immunohistochemistry with MF20 was performed on the fixed embryos[13,16–18] and images were taken by confocal microscopy. With the first two methods, we found lineage-labeled neural crest cells were present in the bulbus arteriosus, ventricle, AV junction, and the atrium at 72 h postfertilization (hpf) and were double labeled with MF20 (Plate 29a–f). In addition, laser activated neural crest cells in *hsp70-gfp* transgenic fish were detected as cardiomyocytes in the ventricle at 36 hpf (Plate 29g,h). Other lineage-labeled cells contributed to the pharyngeal arches and cartilage (Plate 29i), and a pigment cell (Plate 29j), confirming that neural crest was successfully labeled by laser activation. These lineage labeling results indicate that zebrafish neural crest cells migrate to the developing heart and form myocytes in the functional myocardial layer of the heart.

In order to pursue a complete fate map of zebrafish cardiac neural crest, we performed a lineage-labeling experiment by labeling small patches of cells in the neural crest by laser activation of DMNB-caged fluorescein dextran. At the 8-somite stage, fluorescein dextran was uncaged in 15 cells within the neural crest by labeling each cell individually based on a subdivision map (Fig. 38.1a). Labeled neural crest cells in the heart structures were observed at 72 hpf in 398 labeled embryos. In contrast to the more limited domains of cardiac neural crest reported for avian embryos, cardiac neural crest arises from more extensive rostrocaudal regions, ranging from anterior of the midbrain/hindbrain boundary to the somite 6. Interestingly, lateral neural crest showed three distinct groups that made frequent contributions to the heart; divisions –5 to –4 (group A), divisions 1 to 3 (group B), and divisions 5 to S2 (group

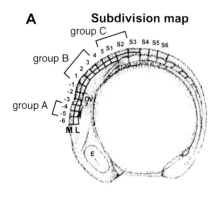

A   **Subdivision map**

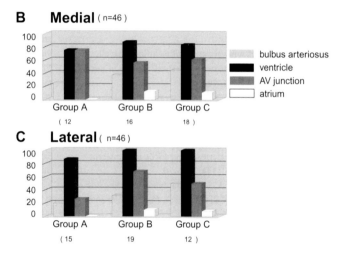

Fig. 38.1 Cardiac neural crest originates from a broad rostrocaudal region in zebrafish. (A) Topological map of an 8-somite embryo used for fate mapping (modified from [20]). Neural crest were divided rostrocaudally into 17 divisions designated –6 through S6. Each division was further subdivided into medial (M) and lateral (L) layers along the orthogonal axis. *Y: yolk, E: eye, OV: otic vesicle, M: medial, L: lateral subdivision.* (B) Medial and (C) lateral groups of cardiac neural crest (Group A, B, and C) make distinct contributions to heart segments. Lower numbers, in parenthesis, indicate the number of appropriately labeled embryos. In Group A, medial neural crest cells contributed to both the ventricle and AV junction (B), however, lateral neural crest cells contributed predominantly to the ventricle (C). There was no neural crest contribution to the atrium from Group A. The neural crest contribution to the bulbus arteriosus was statistically greater in Group C than in Group A ($P < 0.01$). (Adapted from Sato and Yost.[19])

C). Rostral group A has not been described in other vertebrates. Each neural crest group made distinct contributions to segments in the heart (Fig. 38.1b,c). The ventricle and AV junction received strong contributions from each group, but Group A did not contribute to the atrium. These results suggest that distinct neural crest contributions to cardiac segments indicate that the rostrocaudal positions of a particular neural crest cell before emigration biases the cardiac segment to which the crest cell will contribute. In addition, several differences between medial and lateral neural crest contribution were observed. These rostrocaudal and mediolateral specific constraints in cardiac neural crest cell fates have not been described in other vertebrate embryos.

We describe a developmental source of myocardial muscle cells that arises from outside the primary or the secondary heart fields: cardiac neural crest

cells form muscle cells in the zebrafish myocardium. The discovery of zebrafish cardiac neural crest provides a basis for analysis of the diverse contributions of neural crest cells in organogenesis and the mechanisms controlling vertebrate heart development. Analysis of mutations that disrupt the development of cardiac neural crest might reveal mechanisms underlying cardiac morphogenesis. Full details of our work was published in *Developmental Biology.*[19]

Acknowledgments

We thank A. Tsodikov for statistical analyses, D. Grunwald and M. Fishman for DNA clones, M. Halloran for transgenic fish. MS is an American Heart Association Postdoctoral Fellow. This research was supported by grants from the Huntsman Cancer Foundation and NHLBI.

CHAPTER 39

Outflow tract remodeling – a role for tissue polarity?

Deborah J. Henderson, Helen M. Phillips

The outflow tract initially forms as a single muscular vessel, connected to the common ventricle proximally and to the pharyngeal arch arteries distally. The myocardium of the outflow tract wall is distinct from that of the atria and ventricles, in that it arises from a secondary (or anterior) heart field.[1-3] It thus has a separate origin from the myocardium found in the rest of the heart, and therefore may be subject to an alternative developmental pathway to the chamber myocardium and the atrioventricular canal. This primitive outflow vessel is septated by the formation of mesenchymal endocardial cushions along its length, which grow towards each other, and with a contribution from the neural crest, fuse to separate the vessel into two separate channels – the aortic and pulmonary trunks. Concomitant with septation, the ventricular outlets remodel such that the aorta exits from the left ventricle, whereas the pulmonary trunk exits from the right ventricle. As a component of this remodeling, the initially mesenchymal proximal outflow tract cushions become muscularized to form the subpulmonary infundibulum,[4,5] which walls the aorta into the left ventricle. This 'myocardialization' of the endocardial cushion tissue only occurs in the outflow tract of the developing mouse heart, and is absent from the atrioventricular cushions. Abnormalities in outflow septation or remodeling can result in defects that include common arterial trunk, double outlet right ventricle, tetralogy of Fallot, and ventricular septal defect.

Loop-tail (*Lp*) is a naturally occurring mouse mutant that develops severe neural tube and axial rotation defects,[6] abnormalities that arise from mal-development of the embryonic midline. As a consequence of the known association between midline and congenital heart defects, we examined *Lp* litters for cardiovascular defects. Using hematoxylin and eosin staining of paraffin-embedded sections of E13.5–E18.5 *Lp* embryos, we found that *Lp/Lp* embryos develop fully penetrant cardiovascular defects. The most common of these were double outlet right ventricle, perimembranous ventricular septal defects, and abnormalities in remodeling of the aortic arch[7] (Plate 30a-d; data not shown), that were found in all *Lp/Lp* fetuses examined. Abnormalities in neural crest cell colonization of the outflow tract are frequently associated with these types of defects,[8,9] so we examined both the migration pattern of neural crest cells, using a digoxigenin-labeled riboprobe for *erbB3* (a gift from Dr Carmen Birchmeier, Berlin), in wholemount *in situ* hybridization,[7] and their colonization of the outflow tract cushions using an antibody raised against α-smooth muscle actin (clone 1A4, Sigma) as a marker in immunohistochemistry. In both cases, neural crest cells seemed to be normally distributed in *Lp/Lp* when compared with their wild type and heterozygote littermates[7] (Plate 30e,f). A correlation between cardiac looping abnormalities and the axial rotation defects that are found in *Lp* partially explains the malalignment of the ventriculoarterial connections, although the looping defects are most apparent before E10.5, becoming less evident from E11.5 onwards, when outflow tract remodeling takes place.[7] It is possible, however, that subtle abnormalities in cardiac positioning may be enough to prevent normal remodeling of this readily disrupted region of the developing heart.

The *Lp* gene (known as *Vangl2, strabismus-like, Ltap* or *Lpp1*) has recently been cloned[10,11] and shown to encode a protein related to *Drosophila Van gogh* (*Vang*). The Vangl2 protein contains four putative transmembrane domains and a PDZ domain, similar to *Vang*, consistent with shared functional properties. We examined the expression pattern of *Vangl2* during cardiac development using digoxigenin-labeled riboprobes for *in situ* hybridization on paraffin-embedded sections,[12] and showed that it is strongly expressed, from E11.5 to E15.5, in the outflow tract of the developing mouse heart, overlapping with the period when the outflow tract remodels. Moreover, *Vangl2* mRNA distribution correlated with the process of myocardialization (Plate 30g,h).[13] This suggests that *Vangl2* might play a primary role in the myocardialization process, and argues that the defects in outflow tract remodeling in *Lp/Lp* fetuses may not be simply due to abnormalities in cardiac looping, secondary to incomplete axial rotation.

Vang acts downstream in the frizzled/disheveled planar cell polarity pathway, which mediates changes in cell orientation, migration, and fate, via alterations in the cytoskeleton.[14] Similar pathways operate in vertebrate embryos, regulating such diverse activities as convergent extension movements during gastrulation (reviewed in ref. 15), and stereocilia organization in the inner ear (reviewed in ref. 16), and may well be operating in other tissues where polarized growth of cells is required. Indeed, targeted disruption of *disheveled* 2 (*Dvl2*) in the mouse results in double outlet right ventricle,[17] and *frizzled* 2 (*Fz2*) is strongly expressed in the outflow tract septum,[18] supporting a role for this pathway in outflow tract development. *Vangl2* may therefore play a role in determining cell polarity in the developing outflow tract in the mouse embryo. Expression of *Vangl2* in the myocardial cells that extend into the proximal outlet septum, suggests that it may play a role in polarized myocardial cell growth into the septum. The precise mechanism underlying the myocardialization process is unclear. It was initially proposed that myocardial cells completely colonize the septum from the outflow tract wall,[5] but more recently it has been suggested that interdigitating myocardial cells from the outflow tract wall induce trans-differentiation of adjacent mesenchymal cushion cells, into muscle cells.[19] These two ideas are not mutually exclusive, and both might occur to some degree. Vangl2 could be involved in the change

in cell polarity that is required for interdigitation with the septum. Alternatively, Vangl2 might play an essential role in extension of the myocardial cells into the septum. A third possibility is that Vangl2 could play a role in the cell fate changes that have been proposed for the trans-differentiation of mesenchymal cushion cells into muscle. Experiments to establish the precise role for Vangl2 in outflow tract remodeling are underway in our laboratory.

Acknowledgments

This research was funded by the British Heart Foundation (BS/99001 and PG/02/035).

References

1 Mjaatvedt CH, Nakaoka T, Moreno-Rodriguez R *et al.* The outflow tract of the heart is recruited from a novel heart forming field. *Dev Biol* 2001; **238**: 97–109.
2 Waldo KL, Kumiski DH, Wallis KT *et al.* Conotruncal myocardium arises from a secondary heart field. *Development* 2001; **128**: 3179–88.
3 Kelly RG, Brown NA, Buckingham ME. The arterial pole of the mouse heart forms from Fgf10-expressing cells in the pharyngeal mesoderm. *Dev Cell* 2001; **1**: 435–40.
4 Ya J, van den Hoff MJ, de Boer PA *et al.* Normal development of the outflow tract in the rat. *Circ Res* 1998; **82**: 464–72.
5 van den Hoff MJ, Moorman AF, Ruijter JM *et al.* Myocardialization of the cardiac outflow tract. *Dev Biol* 1999; **212**: 477–90.
6 Strong LC, Hollander WF. Hereditary loop-tail in the house mouse. *J Hered* 1949; **40**: 329–34.
7 Henderson DJ, Conway SJ, Greene ND *et al.* Cardiovascular defects associated with abnormalities in midline development in the Loop-tail mouse mutant. *Circ Res* 2001; **89**: 6–12.
8 Kirby ML, Gale TF, Stewart DE. Neural crest cells contribute to normal aorticopulmonary septation. *Science* 1983; **220**: 1059–61.
9 Conway SJ, Henderson DJ, Anderson RH, Kirby ML, Copp AJ. Development of a lethal congenital heart defect in the *splotch* (*Pax3*) mutant mouse. *Cardiovasc Res* 1997; **36**: 163–73.
10 Kibar Z, Vogan KJ, Groulx N *et al.* Ltap, a mammalian homolog of Drosophila Strabismus/Van Gogh, is altered in the mouse neural tube mutant Loop-tail. *Nat Genet* 2001; **28**: 251–5.
11 Murdoch JN, Doudney K, Paternotte C, Copp AJ, Stanier P. Severe neural tube defects in the loop-tail mouse result from mutation of *Lpp1*, a novel gene involved in floor plate specification. *Hum Mol Genet* 2001; **10**: 2593–601.

12 Breitschopf H, Suchanek G, Gould RM, Colman DR, Lassmann H. *In situ* hybridization with digoxigenin-labeled probes: sensitive and reliable detection method applied to myelinating rat brain. *Acta Neuropathol (Berl)* 1992; **84**: 581–7.

13 Phillips HM, Murdoch JN, Doudney K *et al. Vangl2*, the gene mutated in the loop-tail mouse mutant, is involved in remodelling of the outflow tract. *Circ Res* (In press).

14 Adler PN, Lee H. Frizzled signaling and cell-cell interactions in planar polarity. *Curr Opin Cell Biol* 2001; **13**: 635–40.

15 Darken RS, Scola AM, Rakeman AS *et al.* The planar polarity gene strabismus regulates convergent extension movements in *Xenopus. EMBO J* 2002; **21**: 976–85.

16 Friedman TB, Sellers JR, Avraham KB. Unconventional myosins and the genetics of hearing loss. *Am J Med Genet* 1999; **89**: 147–57.

17 Hamblet NS, Lijam N, Ruiz-Lozano P *et al.* Dishevelled 2 is essential for cardiac outflow tract development, somite segmentation and neural tube closure. *Development* 2002; **129**: 5827–38.

18 van Gijn ME, Blankesteijn WM, Smits JF, Hierck B, Gittenberger-de Groot AC. Frizzled 2 is transiently expressed in neural crest-containing areas during development of the heart and great arteries in the mouse. *Anat Embryol* 2001; **203**: 185–92.

19 van den Hoff MJ, Kruithof BP, Moorman AF, Markwald RR, Wessels A. Formation of myocardium after the initial development of the linear heart tube. *Dev Biol* 2001; **240**: 61–76.

CHAPTER 40

Hdf-affected gene fragment revealed by subtraction study of Hdf (heart defect) mouse

X. Zhang, T. Nakaoka, Corey H. Mjaatvedt,
Roger R. Markwald, N. Yamashita

The hdf mouse is a recessive lethal mouse strain that arose from a lacZ reporter-containing transgene insertional mutation.[1] Homozygous embryos die *in uteri* by embryonic 11.5 dpc and exhibit specific cardiac defects along the anterior–posterior cardiac axis. The future right ventricle and conus/truncus of the single heart tube fail to form, and consequently the portion of the heart comprising ventricle and atrium are highly dilated. The endocardial cushions in the atrioventricular are also absent. In addition to these cardiac abnormalities, hdf mice are smaller than their littermates and their bodies have turning defects; 10.5 dpc hdf mice remain unturned, while turning is normally completed by 9.5 dpc. As a result of chromosome mapping and the analysis of DNA sequences flanking the transgene, *Cspg2* was identified as a candidate gene disrupted by the transgene insertion in the hdf mouse line.[2] Thus, the *Cspg2* gene is thought to be required for the normal development of the endocardial cushion swellings and heart segments that give rise to the right ventricle and conus/truncus.

In order to further address the molecular mechanisms responsible for abnormal heart development in hdf mice, we performed subtraction analysis. Suppressive subtractive hybridization was performed using the PCR-Select cDNA subtraction kit (Clontech) essentially according to the manufacturer's instructions. Briefly, total RNA was extracted from 9.5 dpc embryos of either homozygous, hemizygous hdf mice or wild type littermates C57BL/6J

using Trizol Reagent (Invitrogen); 1 μg total RNA was used for synthesis and amplification of each cDNA fraction. In the SSH reaction, hemizygous hdf cDNA was used as a tester, while homozygous hdf cDNA served as a driver. Following subtraction, differentially expressed cDNA fragments were amplified by two rounds of PCR. After purification through a QIAquick PCR purification Kit (Qiagen), these fragments were cloned into pCR4-TOPO (Invitrogen), followed by an electrical transformation into *Escherichia coli* DH5α cells. The PCR-amplified inserts were blotted, duplicated onto Hybond XL nylon membrane (Amersham), and hybridized with the α-^{32}P-dCTP-labeled cDNA pools.

For real-time PCR, the cDNA fraction was constructed from 0.25 to 1 μg aliquots of total RNA with Superscript II (Invitrogen) using oligo-d(T)$_{12-18}$ as a primer. In some cases, cDNA fractions were constructed using a SMART PCR cDNA synthesis kit brought to the reaction. PCR product (typically 90–120 bp long) was confirmed by gel electrophoresis before the real-time reaction. The reaction, which was performed in triplicate using a QuantiTect™ SYBR Green PCR kit (Qiagen), was monitored in an iCycler iQ system (Bio-Rad). Crossover point values, where fluorescent signal exceeds a threshold set above background, were determined for each reaction. A threshold cycle difference of 1 approximates a 1.5- to 1.7-fold increase or decrease of cDNA. For Northern blotting, 20 μg total RNA was electrophoresed on a 1.2% formaldehyde agarose gel and blotted onto Hybond XL nylon membrane (Amersham). Hybridization was performed with a ^{32}P-labeled probe prepared using a Prime-It II Random Primer Labeling Kit (Stratagene). Whole mount *in situ* hybridization was performed essentially as described by Moorman *et al.*[3] A digoxigenin-labeled probe was synthesized with T7 RNA polymerase or T3 RNA polymerase using a DIG RNA Labeling Kit (Roche). Probe bound to the embryos was immunologically detected using sheep anti-digoxigenin-AP, Fab fragment, and NBT/BCIP stock solution (Roche).

From the subtracted cDNA pool, 600 clones were isolated, and the candidate clones were checked by a real-time PCR after screening through hybridization with the α-^{32}P-dCTP-labeled tester and driver cDNA, respectively. As a result, mRNA expression of one clone (hdf-affected gene 2, *hag-2*), was decreased in hdf homozygous mouse to the level of one-tenth the mRNA expression in their littermates. Northern analysis showed that hag-2 mRNA is c. 10 kb long and that its expression in the embryo starts to be detectable at 9.5 dpc, peaked at 10.5 dpc, and then gradually decreased thereafter. *hag-2* expression in adult mouse tissue was detected relatively abundantly in the uterus and less abundantly in heart, lung, and spleen. Sequence of the hag-2 fragment has not hit any known gene by blast search so far. Whole mount *in situ* analysis of 10.5 dpc normal mice showed *hag-2* expression in nasal process, branchial arches, both limb buds and segmentally in body trunk without any detectable signal in the heart. *hag-2* expression in the arches, which is robust at 10.5 dpc, seems to fade away at 11.5 dpc. On the other hand, its expression in limb buds remains at 11.5 dpc. Hdf mouse strain was generated by insertion of a LacZ containing transgene.

Extracardiac LacZ expression in *hdf* hemizygotes is seen in the anterior extension of maxillary and mandibular cartilages, and chondrogenic regions of the forming digit. This pattern of LacZ expression is similar to the expression pattern of Hag-2 in normal mouse embryo; although not identical, *hag-2* gene expression was significantly decreased in *hdf* homozygotes. It is intriguing that *hag-2* expression was not detected in the heart in normal mouse embryos. It is not known whether or how decreased expression of the *hag-2* gene is related to defective heart formation in the hdf phenotype as yet. A fundamental concept of heart development is that the early heart tube forms from two regions of lateral plate mesoderm. Meanwhile, it is known that neural crest cells contribute significantly to the formation of aortic arch and to some extent to conotruncus formation. It is also known that the cells from the transverse septum migrate to populate the epicardium of the heart. Therefore, the strong expression of *hag-2* in the branchial arches might suggest an involvement of *hag-2* in the formation of the outlet portion of the heart, despite a lack of its expression in the heart.

References

1 Yamamura H, Zhang M, Markwald R, Mjaatvedt C. A heart segmental defect in the anterior-posterior axis of a transgenic mutant mouse. *Dev Biol* 1997; **186**: 58–72.

2 Mjaatvedt CH, Yamamura H, Capehart T, Turner D, Markwald RR. The Cspg2 gene, disrupted in the hdf mutant, is required for right cardiac chamber and endocardial cushion formation. *Dev Biol* 1998; **202**: 56–66.

3 Moorman AF, Houweling AC, de Boer PA, Christoffels VM. Sensitive nonradioactive detection of mRNA in tissue sections: novel application of the whole-mount in situ hybridization protocol. *J Histochem Cytochem* 2001; **49**: 1–8.

PART 10

Imaging techniques
Editorial perspective

Michael Artman

With the number and types of murine mutants with defects in cardiovascular development, it becomes increasingly important to develop methods for the noninvasive analysis of cardiac form and function in embryonic mice. Magnetic resonance (MR) microscopy is a relatively new technique that holds promise as a means of studying embryonic cardiovascular development. MR microscopy may offer several advantages in that it can be used to study morphology, spectroscopy, blood flow (velocity, distribution, oxygenation, diffusion), and tissue or organ volumes. Furthermore, it is a noninvasive technique that makes it possible to perform repeated studies in a serial manner.

Hogers *et al.* explored the utility of MR microscopy for the study of living embryos. Previously published data confirm the usefulness of this approach in fixed images, but the application to living embryos remains elusive. Despite using techniques such as cooling to slow the heart rate, the major limitations of MR microscopy remain that of motion artifact and suboptimal spatial resolution. Although major advances have occurred in these techniques, further refinements are necessary before this approach will have a routine role in studies of embryonic cardiovascular development.

CHAPTER 41

Imaging of heart development in embryos with magnetic resonance microscopy

Bianca Hogers, Dieter Gross, Volker Lehmann,
Huub J. M. de Groot, Kees Erkelens,
Adriana C. Gittenberger-de Groot, Robert E. Poelmann

Traditional embryological studies are invasive; embryos are sacrificed and processed in order to reveal specific information such as morphology, histology, antigen distribution, gene expression patterns, or physiological parameters. Each objective requires a specific method, which excludes the use of one specimen for several questions, while it is impossible to perform a longitudinal study in one embryo as each study starts with killing the embryo. For temporal information it is common to repeat the experiments on other specimens at subsequent stages during development, which requires many animals without the final proof that a certain condition in an early stage will develop into a specific malformation.

Magnetic resonance (MR) microscopy is a new technique with two major advantages. At one hand it is a multi-image modality on its own, as morphology, angiography, spectroscopy, blood flow (velocity, distribution, oxygenation, diffusion), and tissue or organ volumes can be measured or calculated. On the other hand, it is a noninvasive technique that makes it possible to study, over an extended period, the subsequent stages of normal development in a single embryo, the course of congenital malformations and pathological processes in adult specimens, and even the effectiveness of therapeutic interventions. The value of MR imaging is now being explored for embryological studies. Fixed human, rat, mouse, chicken, and dolphin em-

bryos[1,2,3] are already imaged and several (3-D) datasets are available on the internet.[4]

We explored the usefulness of MR microscopy for living embryos with special emphasis on the development of the heart. Insufficient resolution could be the bottleneck for anatomical detail at the beginning of cardiac development. Therefore, we started our research to assess whether the early looped heart tube could be visualized under ideal circumstances. As motion is deleterious for MR imaging and embryos increase rapidly in size, we used fixed embryos. As resolution is proportional to the field strength, we repeated the same experiment at higher magnetic field strengths and compared the results. For living embryos we started by concentrating on one avian embryo inside an egg, and finally we visualized individual mouse embryos *in utero*.

We imaged fixed chicken embryos with vasculature that was contrast-enhanced with gadolinium with a 3D spin echo, with a resolution of 31–55 µm. In our youngest embryo (stage 15) the complete heart loop, the individual pharyngeal arch arteries, and the dorsal aorta were clearly discernable. For tissue contrast we imaged postseptated chicken embryos (stage 37) with the spin echo diffusion method, in which we obtained images almost similar to transverse 'microscopic' slides, with a resolution of 35 µm. The great arteries, the atrial septum, the ventricular septum, and the valves were visible with enough detail that a congenital heart malformation could be diagnosed.

We explored the use of an ultra high magnetic field (17.6 T, 750 MHz) for magnetic resonance microscopy (MRM), to increase image quality per image acquisition time. We compared both images (300 vs. 750 with identical parameters) made of the same embryo. We found a three times increase in SNR and a 3.5 times increase in the contrast to noise ratio.[5]

Our real challenge was imaging the living embryos. For the *in ovo* study we used quail embryos as the chicken egg was too large to fit in the probe. To avoid moving artifacts, the method needed to be very fast. From all imaging sequences multislice RARE[6] seemed to give the best anatomical detail, and we reached a resolution of 68 μm. We also performed a longitudinal study in which the eggs were scanned on embryonic day 4, 5, 11, and 12. The older embryos were sedated by hypothermia (room temperature) to prevent motion. After the experiments the embryonic weight of the MRM group was compared to that of a control group to test for any harmful effect of the magnetic field or the hypothermia, and no significant difference was found ($P = 0.95$). We obtained clear images of the heart during development without cardiac pacing (Fig. 41.1) and we

are planning the visualization of congenital malformations (avian models) at real time in the near future.

The technique of visualizing living mouse embryos is still in development. As the mother mouse has to fit in the resonator, the filling factor for the individual embryos is relatively poor. Although we obtained beautiful images of the embryos themselves (Fig. 41.2) the resolution is not high enough for anatomical detail at organ level. However, by combining the RARE method for obtaining a contrast-rich image of an embryo with fast gradient echo, we were able to obtain functional information in addition to the morphological image. By postprocessing, the flow information was converted into a color scale and superimposed on the RARE image, revealing blood flow through the heart and the vessels of the embryo. For abnormal heart development, as is pertinent in many transgenic mouse models, this method might reveal functional cardiac abnormalities well before anatomic defects can be detected.

Equipment

In our studies we used 89 mm vertical bore magnets, working at 300 MHz (7.0 T), at 400 Mhz (9.4 T)

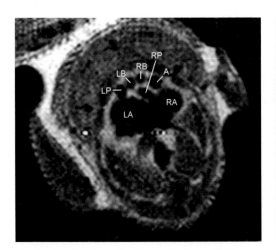

Fig. 41.1 Quail embryo, ED12, *in ovo*. Transverse MRM image of the heart at the level of the great arteries. Multislice RARE: TR/TE = 5000/9 ms, NEX = 2, resolution 59 μm. A, aorta; LA + RA, left and right atrium; LB + RB, left and right brachiocephalic artery; LP + RP, left and right pulmonary artery.

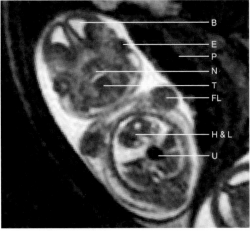

Fig. 41.2 Mouse embryo, ED14, *in utero*. Coronal MRM image of one of the embryos of a 14-days pregnant mother mouse. Multislice RARE: TR/TR = 10000/6 ms, NEX = 4, resolution 137 μm. B, brain; E, eye; FL, front leg; H, heart and lungs; N, nose; T, tongue; U, umbilicus.

(with AVANCE consoles) or at 750 MHz (17.6 T) (with a DSX-750 console). We used a gradient system of 100 G/cm (1 T/m) with the Micro2.5 probe with exchangeable rf-coils (4 mg solenoid coil, 10–15 mg birdcage coils) or a gradient system of 20 G/cm with the Mini0.5 probe with fixed 38 mg resonator. The ParaVision software was used for data acquisition and processing. All from Bruker BioSpin MRI GmbH, Rheinstetten, Germany.

References

1 Smith BR, Johnson GA, Groman EV, Linney E. Magnetic resonance microscopy of mouse embryos. *Proc Natl Acad Sci USA* 1994; **91**: 3530–3.

2 Smith BR, Linney E, Huff DS, Johnson GA. Magnetic resonance microscopy of embryos. *Comp Med Imag Graph* 1996; **20**: 483–90.

3 Marino L, Murphy TL, Gozal L, Johnson JI. Magnetic resonance imaging and three-dimensional reconstructions of the brain of a fetal common dolphin, *Delphinus delhis*. *Anat Embryol* 2001; **203**: 393–402.

4 <www.civm.mc.duke.edu/>; <www.mouseatlas.caltech.edu>

5 Hogers B, Gross D, Lehmann V *et al.* Magnetic resonance microscopy at 17.6-Tesla on chicken embryos *in vitro*. *J Magn Res Imaging* 2001; **14**: 83–6.

6 Henning J, Nauerth A, Friedburg H. RARE imaging: a fast imaging method for clinical MR. *Magnet Reson Med* 1986; **3**: 823–33.

7 Hogers B, Gross D, Lehmann V *et al.* Magnetic resonance microscopy of mouse embryos *in utero*. *Anat Rec* 2000; **260**: 373–7.

PART 11

Cardiovascular physiology during development

Editorial perspective

Michael Artman

It is clear that form and function are inextricably linked during embryonic cardiovascular development. What is less clear, however, are the molecular and cellular processes that link morphogenesis, cardiac function, and hemodynamics. This section contains a series of papers that address this important topic. Keller elegantly summarized the current state-of-the-art and challenges for the future. He defined a major challenge in integrating cell and molecular biology with physiology and biomechanics in order to fill the large gap that remains in translating altered genotype to phenotype. Furthermore, a strong case was made for directing additional attention to areas that have up to now been less intensively studied, such as defining maternal–embryo and maternal–fetal interactions; determining metabolic regulation of cardiovascular structural and functional maturation; and assessing the role of environmental imprinting on developmental processes.

A series of papers addressed the issue of the effects of mechanical forces on cellular and fiber orientation during development. Yoshigi *et al.* presented a new method to study actin fiber orientation in endothelial cells in response to stretch. This approach should prove valuable in future studies in that it allows a more quantitative assessment of the responses to various interventions.

Tobita *et al.* used cyclical stretch to study the orientation responses of embryonic noncardiac cells and cardiomyocytes. They demonstrated that noncardiomyocytes aligned perpendicular to the principal stretch direction but that early embryonic ventricular cardiomyocytes did not orient in response to mechanical stretch. However, embryonic cardiomyocytes acquired perpendicular orientation to mechanical stimulation after establishing contact with nonmyocytes. These new findings suggest that during early cardiogenesis, cardiomyocytes lack the ability to respond to mechanical stimulation and require signaling from noncardiac cells to orient properly in response to mechanical loading. This work lays the foundation for future studies to characterize the signaling pathways involved in these processes. Tobita *et al.* also reported the effects of reducing mechanical load on the ventricular fiber architecture in the intact heart, using a left atrial ligation model in the embryonic chick heart. Left atrial ligation resulted in alterations in the myofiber maturation process in the LV compact myocardium but not within the trabecular myocardium. Thus it seems that mechanical load modulates both local myofiber orientation and maturation in the developing compact myocardium.

Using a variety of complementary techniques, Poelmann *et al.* studied shear stress and the expression of several genes in response to shear stress during cardiovascular development. The underlying hypothesis is that changes in local shear stress, caused by alterations in contraction mode (from peristaltic to cyclic), geometry (looping and septation), and growth modulate expression patterns of a number of signaling molecules (TGFβ, PDGF) and vasoactive substances (endothelin, nitric oxide) that are involved in further development of heart and vessels. A mathematical model of fluid dynamics was applied to characterize shear stress in the stage 18 chicken embryo. This technique can be used to assess dynamic changes in shear stress during the cardiac cycle and is expected to provide important insights in both normal and abnormal cardiovascular development. Analysis of gene expression confirmed some of the predictions derived from the computational fluid model and demonstrated that specific regions of the atrioventricular junction and outflow tract express shear stress responsive genes.

Several papers in this section addressed excitation–contraction coupling and the regulation of contractile function in the developing heart. Mancarella *et al.* demonstrated differences in responses of the sodium–calcium exchanger to beta-adrenergic signaling in the immature rabbit heart that may have important implications in understanding modulation of contraction and relaxation in the developing heart. It has previously been shown that the sodium–calcium exchanger may play a more important role in the developing heart as compared to mature myocardium. Wang *et al.* provided further evidence of the essential role of the sodium–calcium exchanger during embryonic development by studying *Splotch* mice. Their results suggest that the sodium–calcium exchanger is upregulated in Sp^{2H} hearts to maintain intracellular Ca^{2+} homeostasis and promote survival.

Minimasawa and Matsuoka studied the potential role of sarcolipin as a modulator of atrial contractile function. It is proposed that atrial sarcolipin may be analogous to phospholamban in ventricular muscle. These studies demonstrated that sarcolipin is expressed selectively in murine and human atrial myocardium and is developmentally regulated. Although not yet proven, the results are consistent with the concept that sarcolipin may be involved in the regulation of calcium cycling in atrial tissue.

The cardiac responses to oxygen deprivation during early postnatal maturation have been characterized by Ostadal *et al.* These results demonstrate a complex temporal change in the responses during the first week of life. Furthermore, studies of expression of genes involved in mitochondrial energy metabolism and the responses to ischemic preconditioning and simulated intermittent high altitude suggest that the determinants of cardiac responses to hypoxia undergo developmental regulation. Future studies based upon these data are likely to provide additional insights into the cellular and molecular mechanisms that account for age-related changes in the tolerance to hypoxia and ischemia. These approaches have important implications for both the immature and adult heart.

CHAPTER 42

Shear stress in the developing cardiovascular system

Robert E. Poelmann, Adriana C. Gittenberger-de Groot,
Bianca C. W. Groenendijk, Beerend P. Hierck, Bianca Hogers,
Frans T. M. Nieuwstadt, Mathieu J. B. M. Pourquie,
Paul Steendijk, Sandra Stekelenburg-de Vos,
Nicolette T. C. Ursem, Jury W. Wladimiroff

Introduction

The development of the cardiovascular system depends on many interlocking mechanisms. It is evident that the temporal sequence of regulation of gene expression profiles dominates the differentiation of the heart fields in an early embryo as well as the ensuing phases including heart tube formation, looping, septation, chamber specification, valve development, differentiation of the conduction system, etc. It is equally evident that as soon as the tubular heart starts to contract, hemodynamic and mechanical factors have to be taken into account as well. The main focus of this study deals with the hemodynamic regulation of the expression of a subset of shear-stress responsive genes on cardiovascular development. Cardiac contraction propels the blood in a peristaltic fashion during early stages, followed later by the cyclic changes characteristic for the contraction–relaxation mode of the mature heart. Furthermore, as the heart becomes geometrically more complicated by looping and septation, the flow profiles, generating forces on the cardiac and vascular wall, become increasingly more complex. Finally, the cardiovascular system increases tremendously in size and force to provide for the equally increasing demands of the growing embryo. Experimental evidence exists that by changing flow patterns, the normal cardiovascular development is disrupted. Hogers *et al.*[1] demonstrated that flow in the early embryo (stages 10–17) is laminar and that blood from vessels joining a larger one does not mix, even when it passes through the pumping heart. Rerouting the blood from the yolk sac by blocking any of the larger vitelline veins resulted in increased mortality and in a specific set of cardiovascular malformations in the surviving embryos, predominantly in the outflow tract region and the pharyngeal arch arteries.[2] As cardiac function measured at stage 34, but not at stage 24 of development, was dramatically hindered,[3] we postulated that the induced alterations in flow and shear stress, and the emerging structural anomalies were mutually interactive.

Hypotheses

Proper cardiovascular development depends on self-generated hemodynamic forces, in particular flow-driven fluid shear stress. Changes in local shear stress, caused by alterations in contraction mode (from peristaltic to cyclic), by alterations in geometry (looping and septation), and by increase in diameter (growth), take care of modulation of gene expression patterns. Shear-stress responsive genes coding for important signaling molecules such as growth factors (TGFβ, PDGF) and vasoactive substances (endothelin, nitric oxide), are involved in further development of the heart and vessels.

Antitheses

As it is tremendously difficult to measure the influence of changes in shear stress upon development *in vivo* directly, we developed surrogate endpoints from which to move to different approaches. For this reason we combined physiological approaches studying flow and pressure, with molecular biological approaches, studying shear-stress responsive genes, and computational fluid dynamics, studying cardiac geometry to predict shear-stress patterns. We have to be aware of the translational difficulties when moving between these dissimilar approaches.

Hemodynamics

Chick embryos were used throughout the study because of accessibility to experimental manipulation. Fertilized eggs were incubated and used between stages HH16 and 30. Hemodynamic measurements were performed in stages 16–28 according to Ursem *et al.*[4] and Stekelenburg-de Vos *et al.*[5] In brief, blood velocity was measured in the dorsal aorta with a pulsed Doppler ultrasound (model 545C-4, Iowa Doppler Products), whereas pressure was measured inside the embryonic ventricle using the servo-null system. Pressure–volume loops were made by incorporating high-speed video recordings and subtracting the ventricular wall volume from the outer contour, revealing the ventricular volume. PV-loops (Fig. 42.1) were analyzed using custom-made software (see ref. 6). Using these approaches we performed a new set of acute experiments in which we analyzed the changes in volume flow in stage 17 during the first 5 h after clipping one of the vitelline veins. It was evident that hemodynamic parameters did not return to baseline in this period, whereas control embryos showed a continued increase, probably owing to growth of the embryo. During the first hours after clipping, the heart was not able to return to even base-level performance. One day (stage 21) after clipping, however, the hemodynamic parameters, including PV loops, no longer differed from control embryos. The hearts of the clipped embryos had apparently compensated for the earlier lack of performance. Nevertheless, at still later stages, a number of embryos were found dead and a high percentage of the living ones showed cardiac anomalies,[2] demonstrating that the stage 17 intervention

had not been fully met. We concluded, therefore, that the early temporary decrease in hemodynamic values must be responsible for the cardiovascular malformations, again fueling the hypothesis that shear stress is involved in cardiogenesis.

Computational fluid dynamics (CFD)

As shear stress cannot be measured directly, we decided to apply CFD on the geometry of a stage 18 chicken embryo (Fig. 42.2). A custom-made program was developed based on the force method allowing triangulation of the internal surface of the looped heart tube. Furthermore, the triangles could be changed in dimension to allow for a semirealistic movement of the heart tube, mimicking peristaltic or cyclic contraction as well as opening and closing of the atrioventricular (AV) and outflow tract (OFT) areas as surrogate for endocardial cushion function. The flow and shear stress were calculated giving representations of areas with low and high stress during all phases of contraction and relaxation. This means that we were handling a 4-D model of cardiac action, the fourth dimension being time. The model clearly showed that areas of changing shear stress occur during opening and closure of the AV and OFT endocardial cushions. The upstream slope of the constrictions showed larger changes compared with the downstream slope. Despite the curved geometry of the ventricular part of the heart tube, this segment was surprisingly devoid of changes in shear stress. The segment in the model comparable to the aortic sac, i.e. distal to the OFT constriction, showed considerable changes in shear stress as well. These patterns of shear stress changes are hypothesized to be related to expression patterns of the genes we wanted to study.

Expression of genes responsive to shear stress

Radioactive *in situ* hybridization protocols were used to study expression patterns in serial sections between stages 16 and 30 of genes responsive to shear stress. The latter comprise TGFβ2, KLF2, NOS3 (or eNOS) and genes in the endothelin-signaling cascade (endothelin1, the receptors ETA and ETB, and the endothelin converting enzyme1,

ECE1). Expression patterns of the functional antagonists ET1 (vascular contraction in adult vessels) and NOS3 (vascular relaxation) and the novel KLF2, which is reported to react proportional to changes in shear stress[7] were reconstructed three-dimensionally using the Amira software package (TGS Europe, Merignac, France). As ET1 is upregulated by low shear stress and NOS3 and KLF2 by high shear stress, alternating and excluding patterns were expected. As mentioned above, the most intense changes in shear stress were predicted for the narrow regions of the heart tube. In stage 18 and later embryos this general pattern was indeed observed. Where the sinus venosus meets the atrium, and also in the AV junction and the OFT area, we showed expression of genes responsive to shear stress. The atrial endocardium was negative, while the ventricular endocardium was negative for ET1 and KLF2 but positive for NOS3 (Fig. 42.3). The endothelium of the pharyngeal arch arteries and the dorsal aorta showed expression of the three genes in a patchy, partly overlapping, partly excluding pattern. The pattern in later stages became more complicated. For example, nonendocardial and nonendothelial tissues also demonstrated the expression of ET1 (particularly in the ectoderm, endoderm, and mesoderm of the pharyngeal arches surrounding the OFT and aortic sac). We expected that expression at these locations was not shear stress dependent, but was regulated by parallel pathways.

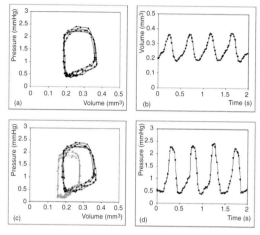

Fig. 42.1 Pressure-volume loop of a stage 21 chick embryo heart. (a) PV loop of an intact embryo as derived from the combination of volume readings (b) and pressure readings (d). (c) Normal loop and PV loop (grey) after hemorrhage of a small vitelline blood vessel, demonstrating the degree of adaptation to the decreased amount of circulating blood.

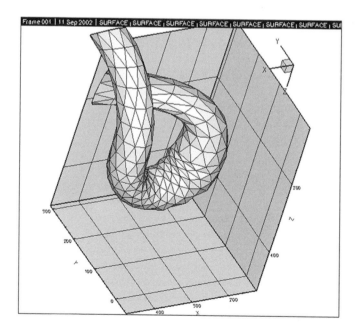

Fig. 42.2 Computational fluid dynamic model of a heart tube of a stage 18 chick embryo, demonstrating the tiled surface of the endocardial lumen.

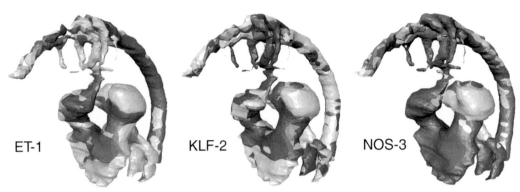

Fig. 42.3 Endothelial/endocardial expression patterns of three shear stress responsive genes (ET1, KLF2, NOS3) as projected on a lumen reconstruction of a stage 18 chicken embryo. Radioactive *in situ* hybridization using the appropriate probes has been applied on a serially sectioned heart. Consecutive sections were fed into the Amira program to allow for 3-D visualization. Note the lack of expression of all probes in the atrium, but the ventricular staining in the ventricle for NOS3 only. The patterns in the narrow areas of the heart tube (sinoatrial transition, AV canal and outflow tract) are patchy but mainly nonoverlapping. Although other than endothelial/endocardial expression patterns have also been observed (e.g. ET1 in the outflow tract mesenchyme) these were excluded from the 3-D reconstructions as these are not considered to be shear stress-related.

Conclusions

Although not all the approaches provided comparable "hard evidence," we have acquired reasonably reliable material on the influence of changes in shear stress on cardiovascular development. We used the combination of experimental embryology (venous clipping), computational fluid dynamics (4-D modeling of geometry and shear stress), flow measurements (using pulsed Doppler ultrasound) and the assessment of shear stress-dependent gene expression patterns (with *in situ* hybridization).

The combination of venous clipping and ultrasound revealed the acute drop in hemodynamics after clipping with a gradual restoration to normal. Nevertheless, as secondary effects, structural malformations emerged even resulting in embryonic death. Furthermore, *in situ* hybridization confirmed some of the predictions deduced from the computational fluid model. In particular, the upslopes of the AV and OFT regions proved to be prone to express genes responsive to shear stress. Other narrow regions of the cardiovascular system were also predicted to be shear stress responsive. The wall of the atrium, however, remained negative for most of the genes throughout development, suggesting that changes in shear stress have no influence in this segment, or do not take place.

ET1 and NO are established vasoactive substances in mature vessels (and also elsewhere), but their function during embryonic development is not yet elucidated. Likewise, the role of KLF2 (LKLF) has been postulated in embryonic development of the vascular media[8] and its function has been addressed in adult vessels only recently.[7] We need further research upon its role in development. We are currently studying the changed gene expression patterns after clipping and want to expand our predictions from computational fluid dynamics to later stages of development.

Acknowledgments

We express our gratitude to Madelon Fekkes, Liesbeth van Iperen, and Jan Lens for valuable support. This study has been sponsored by the Netherlands Heart Foundation (2000B016).

References

1 Hogers B, DeRuiter MC, Baasten AMJ, Gittenberger-de Groot AC, Poelmann RE. Intracardiac blood flow patterns related to the yolk sac circulation of the chick embryo. *Circ Res* 1995; **76**: 871–7.
2 Hogers B, DeRuiter MC, Gittenberger-de Groot AC, Poelmann RE. Unilateral vitelline vein ligation alters normal intracardiac blood flow patterns and morphogenesis in the chick embryo. *Circ Res* 1997; **80**: 473–81.

3 Broekhuizen MLA, Hogers B, DeRuiter MC *et al.* Altered hemodynamics in chick embryos after extra-embryonic venous obstruction. *Ultrasound Obstet Gynacol* 1999; **13**: 437–45.

4 Ursem NTC, Struijk PC, Poelmann RE, Gittenberger-de Grot AC, Wladimiroff JW. Dorsal aortic flow velocity in chick embryos of stage 16–28. *Ultrasound Med Biol* 2001; **27**: 919–24.

5 Stekelenburg-de Vos S, Ursem NTC, Hop WCJ *et al.* Acutely altered hemodynamics following venous obstruction in the early chick embryo. *J Exp Biol* 2003; **206**: 1051–7.

6 Maniar HS, Prasad SM, Gaynor SL *et al.* Impact of pericar-dial restraint on right atrial mechanics during acute right ventricular pressure load. *Am J Physiol Circ Physiol* 2003; **284**: H350–7.

7 Dekker RJ, van Soest S, Fontijn RD *et al.* Prolonged shear stress induces a distinct set of endothelial cell genes, most specifically lung Kruppel-like factor (KLF2). *Blood* 2002; **100**: 1689–98.

8 Kuo CT, Veselits ML, Barton KP *et al.* The LKLF transcription factor is required for normal tunica media formation and blood vessel stabilization during murine embryogenesis. *Genes Dev* 1997; **11**: 2996–3006.

CHAPTER 43

Quantitative analysis for stretch-induced cytoskeletal remodeling in endothelial cells

Masaaki Yoshigi, Edward B. Clark, H. Joseph Yost

Cells in the vascular wall experience complex mechanical forces *in vivo*. Pulsatile blood flow and pressure exert shear, stretch, and compression on endothelial cells, adventitial fibroblasts, and smooth muscle cells. The mechanical forces influence cell morphology, function, signaling, and gene expression of those cells in the vascular wall.[1] However, mechanisms by which cells in the vascular wall sense and respond to mechanical force are not fully elucidated, especially during embryonic angiogenesis.

In vivo and *in vitro* studies have examined the relationships between mechanical force and cell alignment.[1] Particularly, studies *in vitro* have shown that cells stimulated by cyclic stretch align cell orientation perpendicular to the stretch direction, regardless of the cell type. Comparisons of cell orientation in various culture environments, however, are difficult owing to lack of robust measures for cell shape and orientation. Manual determination of the cell axis could involve errors when the cell shape is diverse.

We assumed that actin fibers, a major cytoskeletal protein, determine the primary cell axis, and may be used to determine cell orientation. We then developed a quantitative system (see Methods) that calculates local orientation of actin fibers at the pixel level, using fluorescence microscopy and digital image processing techniques. This simple system allowed us to average orientation of local actin fibers for individual cells, any given regions of interest, or an entire image.

Using a custom cell stretch device, which stimulates cells with unidirectional strain, we analyzed stretch-induced actin remodeling to examine the relationships between stretch direction and actin fiber orientation (Fig. 43.1). Our system also provided a relative parameter of "actin fiber density" that allowed us to evaluate early phase of actin remodeling induced by cyclic stretch (Fig. 43.2).

The variance in stretch-induced morphological responses in previous studies[3–9] may be attributed to the following factors. First, most studies manually determined the cell axis based on cell shape, which could be triangular, cuboidal, or polygonal. Determining a cell axis for cell shapes that are complex introduces some intra- and inter-observer variance. Second, most studies used subconfluent cells to determine the cell axis for individual cells, where the cell density may vary among studies. Cell density also influences the phenotype and shape of cells, especially for smooth muscle cells, thus introducing some variance in the determination of the cell axis. Another reason may be the difference in stretch apparatus and culture scaffolds such as collagen or fibronectin which influences cell shape and signaling mechanisms.[10] Our analysis system has a potential to reduce the variance, which will allow us to define details of stretch-induced cytoskeletal remodeling in various culture conditions.

Use of these parameters should facilitate future studies using pharmacological and/or molecular blockades of mechano-induced signal transduction pathways. Another extension of our technique is a 3-D analysis of cytoskeletal fiber orientation. By increasing the dimension of the convolution kernels (See Eq. 43.1 and 43.2 in Methods), cytoskeletal fiber

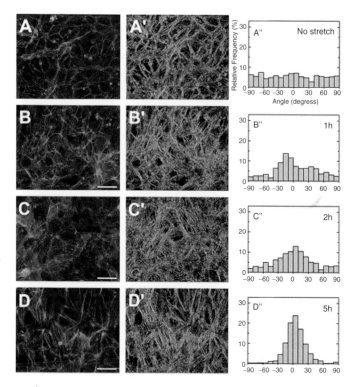

Fig. 43.1 (A)–(D) Actin fibers in control (A) and stretched cells [(B), 1 h, (C): 2 h; (D): 5 h]. Note increased actin fibers in (B)–(D), and perpendicular alignment in (D). (A')–(D') Color coding of actin fiber orientation. See to ref. 2 for color reproduction. (A")–(D") Histogram of actin fiber orientation. Note gradual alignment of actin fibers started in (C"), and more obvious alignment at 0° in (D"). Scale bar = 50 μm and stretch direction. Stretch axis is ±90° in histograms.

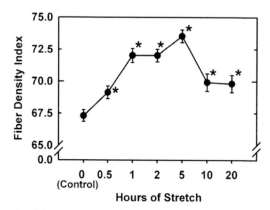

Fig. 43.2 Increase in actin fibers induced by cyclic stretch. Fiber density index demonstrated 30 minutes are enough to induce statistically significant ($P < 0.05$) changes.

orientation can be measured in the 3-D space.[11] Describing stretch-induced cytoskeletal remodeling in the 3-D system is a critical link to the "tensegrity" hypothesis of mechanosensing.[12] In addition, this method will lay the foundation for analyzing the relationships between orientation of actin fibers and orientation of extracellular matrix fibers during embryonic angiogenesis and cardiomyofibrilogenesis.[13]

Methods

The processing algorithm is based on a Sobel filter.[11] Two convolution kernels (i.e. matrix defining weighted sum of neighboring pixels) were defined to perform the Sobel filter as follows:

Horizontal kernel (K_h)

$$K_h = \begin{pmatrix} -1 & 0 & 1 \\ -2 & 0 & 2 \\ -1 & 0 & 1 \end{pmatrix} \qquad \text{(Eq. 43.1)}$$

Vertical kernel (K_v)

$$K_v = \begin{pmatrix} -1 & -2 & -1 \\ 0 & 0 & 0 \\ 1 & 2 & 1 \end{pmatrix} \qquad \text{(Eq. 43.2)}$$

A sample matrix $S_{(i,j)}$ was defined as 3×3 matrix surrounding pixel of interest. Then, two convolution values G_h and G_v were calculated as follows:

$$G_h(i,j) = \sum \left(K_h \cdot S_{(i,j)} \right) \qquad \text{(Eq. 43.3)}$$

$$G_v(i,j) = \sum \left(K_v \cdot S_{(i,j)} \right) \qquad \text{(Eq. 43.4)}$$

where G_h represents the amplitude of intensity variation along the *horizontal* direction, and G_v represents the amplitude of intensity variation along the *vertical* direction.

We calculated the angle (θ) of intensity variation in the sample matrix $S_{(i,j)}$ by:

$$\theta(i,j) = \tan^{-1} \frac{G_v}{G_h} \qquad \text{(Eq. 43.5)}$$

Then, amplitude (r) of the intensity variation in the sample matrix $S_{(i,j)}$ was calculated by:

$$r(i,j) = \sqrt{G_h^2 + G_v^2} \qquad \text{(Eq. 43.6)}$$

We designated color coding for each θ and r using HSI coding system.[11] For details, refer to ref. 2.

References

1 Frangos SG *et al.* The integrin-mediated cyclic strain-induced signaling pathway in vascular endothelial cells. *Endothelium* 2001; **8**: 1–10.

2 Yoshigi M, Clark EB, Yost HJ. Quantification of stretch-induced cytoskeletal remodeling in vascular endothelial cells by image processing *Cytometry* 2003; **55A**: 109–18.

3 Iba T, Sumpio BE. Morphological response of human endothelial cells subjected to cyclic strain *in vitro*. *Microvasc Res* 1991; **42**: 245–54.

4 Lundberg MS, Sadhu DN, Grumman VE, Chilian WM, Ramos KS. Actin isoform and alpha 1B-adrenoceptor gene expression in aortic and coronary smooth muscle is influenced by cyclical stretch. *In Vitro Cell Dev Biol Anim* 1995; **31**: 595–600.

5 Putnam AJ, Cunningham JJ, Dennis RG, Linderman JJ, Mooney DJ. Microtubule assembly is regulated by externally applied strain in cultured smooth muscle cells. *J Cell Sci* 1998; **111**: 3379–87.

6 Civelekoglu G, Tardy Y, Meister JJ. Modeling actin filament reorganization in endothelial cells subjected to cyclic stretch. *Bull Math Biol* 1998; **60**: 1017–37.

7 Zhao S *et al.* Synergistic effects of fluid shear stress and cyclic circumferential stretch on vascular endothelial cell morphology and cytoskeleton. *Arterioscler Thromb Vasc Biol* 1995; **15**: 1781–6.

8 Takemasa T, Sugimoto K, Yamashita K. Amplitude-dependent stress fiber reorientation in early response to cyclic strain. *Exp Cell Res* 1997; **230**: 407–10.

9 Wang JH, Goldschmidt-Clermont P, Yin FC. Contractility affects stress fiber remodeling and reorientation of endothelial cells subjected to cyclic mechanical stretching. *Ann Biomed Eng* 2000; **28**: 1165–71.

10 Yano Y, Geibel J, Sumpio BE. Cyclic strain induces reorganization of integrin alpha 5 beta 1 and alpha 2 beta 1 in human umbilical vein endothelial cells. *J Cell Biochem* 1997; **64**: 505–13.

11 Russ JC. *The Image Processing Handbook.* Boca Raton, FL: CRC Press, 2002.

12 Ingber DE. Tensegrity: the architectural basis of cellular mechanotransduction. *Annu Rev Physiol* 1997; **59**: 575–99.

13 Shiraishi I, Takamatsu T, Onouchi Z, Fujita S. In: Clark EB, Markwald RR, Takao, A, eds. *Developmental Mechanisms of Heart Disease.* New York: Futura, 1995.

CHAPTER 44

Differential effects of cyclic stretch on embryonic ventricular cardiomyocyte and non-cardiomyocyte orientation

Kimimasa Tobita, Jason B. Garrison, Bradley B. Keller

Introduction

Following the onset of heart beat, cardiovascular tissues are continuously subjected to various forms of cyclical mechanical stimulation. Studies have shown that alterations in mechanical load, such as wall stress, strain, and fluid shear, change developing embryonic heart function and structure resulting in cardiovascular malformations,[3,8] and that mechanical load is one of the major epigenetic factors regulating cardiovascular morphogenesis.[5]

At tissue and cellular levels, mechanical stretch influences cell orientation, shape, contractile protein turnover, and numerous biochemical signaling pathways. Terracio *et al.*[7] showed that neonate rat heart cells aligned perpendicular to the stretch direction when uniaxial stretch was applied while Vandenburgh *et al.*[9,10] showed that neonatal rat cardiomyocytes aligned parallel to the stretch direction and increased cell size. Kada *et al.*[4] showed that ED17 cardiomyocytes from mouse embryos changed cell orientation from parallel to perpendicular to the stretch direction in response to sustained stretch. Simpson *et al.*[6] reported that contractile protein turnover was influenced by the relation between myofibril orientation and stretch direction. Gopalan *et al.*[1] recently reported in an anisotropic neonatal rat cardiomyocyte stretch study that transverse stretch rather than longitudinal stretch to the cell has greater effects in regulating

sarcomere organization. However, relatively little is known about how mechanical stimulation influences embryonic cardiac cell orientation, shape, contractile protein turnover, and biochemical signaling pathways during early cardiovascular morphogenesis. In the present study we investigated the effects of cyclic stretch on cell orientation using acutely isolated ventricular cells from chicken embryos.

Method and results

Fertilized eggs from white leghorn chickens were incubated in a standard force-draft incubator to Hamburger-Hamilton stage 27, day 5 of a 21 day (46 stages) incubation period.[2] At stage 27, the embryonic chick heart contains primitive right and left ventricular chambers. Approximately 20 embryonic ventricles (including both primitive right and left ventricles) were excised from the embryo and were digested enzymatically using 0.05% trypsin. Suspension of isolated embryonic ventricular cells was then plated at 5×10^5 cells/mL in 35-mm diameter collagen type I, coated silicone membranes (BioFlex, Flexcell International Corp, PA). We applied quasi-uniaxial cyclic stretch (maximum 18% elongation at a rate of 0.5 Hz) using a Flexcell 4000T stretch system (Flexcell International) and custom made rectangular solid loading posts. Cells were cultured and stretched by the following protocols: protocol 1, 24 hour quiescent culture followed by cyclic stretch for 48 hours; protocol 2, 24-h quiescent culture, culture during cyclic stretch for 24 h, and then quiescent culture for next 24 h; protocol 3, quiescent culture for 48 h followed by cyclic stretch for 24 h; protocol 4, quiescent culture for 72 h (non-stretch). Cells were then fixed at the end of each protocol using standard methods and stained with sarcomeric and non-sarcomeric α-actinin using routine immunocytochemical staining techniques. We characterized cellular orientation in subgroups based on cell type and cell–cell connections, i.e. isolated or single populated cluster of cardiomyocytes (CM), isolated or single populated cluster of noncardiomyocytes (NC), CM connected to NC (CM–NC), and NC connected to CM (NC–CM). Cells forming a cluster, in which the majority of cells

were not adhered to the silicone membrane directly, were excluded from image analysis (Plate 31).

Cellular orientation was analyzed by segment vector accumulation. An 8-bit gray image was extracted from the captured RGB image. The extracted image was then binarised and skeletanized using Scion Image software (Scion Corporation, MD). In each small segment the vector length and the angle to the principal stretch direction was measured using LabVIEW software (National Instruments, TX). The principal cell orientation was then computed by summation of all segmental vectors (Plate 32).

In the absence of cyclic stretch, both CM and NC were randomly oriented (Fig. 44.1). After cyclic stretch stimulation, NC and NC–CM cells oriented

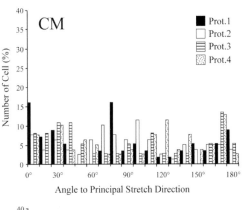

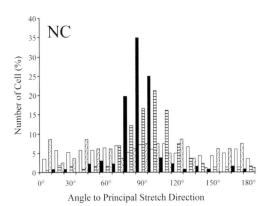

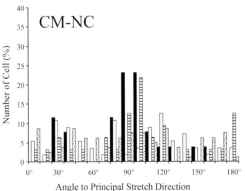

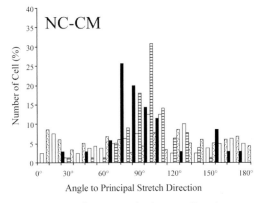

Fig. 44.1 Distribution of cellular orientation to principal stretch direction. Note that cardiomyocytes (CM) did not acquire a preferential orientation in response to cyclic stretch in the absence of attachment to noncardiomyocytes. Noncardiomyocytes aligned perpendicular to the principal stretch direction (NC, $P < 0.05$ in protocol 1 and 3). Initiation and duration of stretch stimulation did not influence non-cardiomyocyte orientation (protocol 1 vs. protocol 3).

However, noncardiomyocytes that became aligned perpendicular to the principal stretch direction lost this orientation after 24 h without stretch (NC, protocol 2). Both cardiomyocytes attached to noncardiomyocytes and noncardiomyocyte attached to cardiomyocytes aligned perpendicular to the principal stretch direction (CM–NC and NC–CM). * $P < 0.05$, directionality test; § $P < 0.05$ vs. non-stretch.

perpendicular to the principal stretch direction ($P <$ 0.05, Rayleigh test; Fig. 44.1). Single populated CM did not acquire a preferential orientation in response to cyclic stretch while CM–NC oriented perpendicular to the stretch direction similar to NC ($P <$ 0.05). Preferential NC orientation was lost within 24 h after removal of cyclic stretch stimulation.

We also tested the relationship between CM contraction and cell orientation in response to cyclic stretch. Cells were cultured without stretch for 48 h and then treated with high potassium (15 mM K$^+$) containing culture medium 20 min prior to stretch stimulation. Contraction arrest of CM was confirmed by visual inspection before stretch. We then cultured cells for 24 h during cyclic stretch. Contractile arrest using high potassium solution did not alter either NC or CM cell orientation in response to cyclic stretch.

Discussion

Our findings in the present study are: (1) noncardiomyocytes aligned perpendicular to the principal stretch direction; (2) maintenance of noncardiomyocyte alignment required persistent mechanical loading; (3) isolated early embryonic ventricular cardiomyocytes did not orient in response to mechanical stretch; (4) embryonic cardiomyocytes acquired perpendicular orientation to mechanical stimulation only after establishing contact with nonmyocytes; (5) myocyte contraction had no effect on cell orientation in response to stretch stimulation. Our results in the present study differ from previous studies in which CM from later developmental stage embryos and/or neonate CM, oriented either parallel or perpendicular to the principal stretch direction. We speculate that nascent and functionally immature cardiomyocytes during early cardiogenesis lack a primary response to mechanical stimulation and therefore require direct signaling from NC in order to reorient in response to mechanical stimulation. In contrast to immature CM, NC such as cardiac fibroblasts and endocardial cells have already acquired the ability to sense external mechanical stimulation during early cardiogenesis. Thus, we conclude that noncardiomyocytes play a critical role in coordinating the cellular response to external mechanical stimulation within the embryonic myocardium during cardiogenesis, and that altered mechanical stimulation changes cellular orientation and associated intracellular and cell to cell signaling in the developing embryonic myocardium.

References

1 Gopalan SM, Flaim C, Bhatia SN *et al.* Anisotropic stretch induced hypertrophy in neonatal ventricular myocytes micropatterned on deformable elastomers. *Biotechnol Bioeng* 2003; **81**: 578–87.

2 Hamburger V, Hamilton HL. A series of normal stages in the development of the chick embryo. *J Morphol* 1951; **88**: 49–92.

3 Hove JR, Koster RW, Forouhar AS *et al.* Intracardiac fluid forces are an essential epigenetic factor for embryonic cardiogenesis. *Nature* 2003; **421**: 172–7.

4 Kada K, Yasui K, Naruse K *et al.* Orientation change of cardiocytes induced by cyclic stretch stimulation: time dependency and involvement of protein kinases. *J Mol Cell Cardiol* 1999; **31**: 247–59.

5 Keller BB. Function and biomechanics of developing cardiovascular systems. In: Tomanek RJ, Runyan RB, eds. *Formation of the Heart and Its Regulation*. Boston: Birkhauser, 2001: 251–72.

6 Simpson DG, Majeski M, Borg TK, Terracio L. Regulation of cardiac myocyte protein turnover and myofibrillar structure *in vitro* by specific directions of stretch. *Circ Res* 1999; **85**: e59–69.

7 Terracio L, Miller B, Borg TK. Effects of cyclic mechanical stimulation of the cellular components of the heart: in vitro. *In Vitro Cell Dev Biol* 1988; **24**: 53–8.

8 Tobita K, Keller BB. Right and left ventricular wall deformation patterns in normal and left heart hypoplasia chick embryos. *Am J Physiol Heart Circ Physiol* 2000; **279**: H959–69.

9 Vandenburgh HH, Solerssi R, Shansky J *et al.* Response of neonatal rat cardiomyocytes to repetitive mechanical stimulation in vitro. *Ann NY Acad Sci* 1995; **752**: 19–29.

10 Vandenburgh HH, Solerssi R, Shansky J, Adams JW, Henderson SA. Mechanical stimulation of organogenic cardiomyocyte growth in vitro. *Am J Physiol* 1996; **270**: C1284–92.

CHAPTER 45

Physiology and biomechanics of developing cardiovascular systems: expanding frontiers

Bradley B. Keller

Our investigation of the interaction between biomechanical load and cardiovascular (CV) morphogenesis has shown that the embryonic heart adapts both structure and function to maintain cardiac output to the embryo. Acute adaptive mechanisms in the embryo include the redistribution of blood flow within the heart, dynamic adjustments in heart rate and developed pressure, and beat to beat variations in vascular resistance. Chronic adaptive mechanisms include alterations in myocardial cell growth and death and both regional and global changes in myocardial architecture. These adaptive mechanisms allow the embryo to survive epigenetic stresses (environmental, maternal) and to compensate for developmental errors (genetic). Recent work from numerous laboratories shows that a subset of these adaptive mechanisms is present in every developing multicellular organism with a "heart" equivalent structure.

Developmental cardiovascular physiology and biomechanics – general concepts

The function and biomechanics of developing cardiovascular systems have been of interest to scientists for centuries and "normal" development occurs within a definable range of functional parameters.[1-7] Due to variations in the environment in which embryos develop (vertebrate and invertebrate) adaptive mechanisms allow the developmental process to vary morphogenesis in order to optimize embryo survival. Stated another way, any event which alters the function of a developing CV system beyond a developmental stage- and species-specific "threshold" will produce an altered CV structural phenotype at the completion of morphogenesis. Failed adaptation to this stressor may result in embryo death prior to completion of morphogenesis. These deviations from normal developmental pathways have been described by W. Burggren as "altered developmental trajectories."

Several general concepts are relevant for developing CV systems. First, structural maturation occurs during cardiac morphogenesis so that increasing cardiac output matches increasing embryonic metabolic demand. As the structure and function of the heart expands, the ratio of heart to body weight decreases in most species suggesting increasing CV efficiency. While the early embryo can receive metabolic support via diffusion from surrounding tissues in the absence of CV function,[8] rapid embryo growth requires expanded CV supply without interruption to support morphogenesis. Thus, for practical purposes one goal of successful CV morphogenesis is the establishment of an adequate and effective CV system to deliver nutrients to the developing embryo and to respond to acute and chronic changes in metabolic demand.

The second general concept is that all CV systems (developing and mature) can vary "pump function" acutely within a range of operational parameters to optimize "work" performed by the system. Embryonic CV systems can adjust functional parameters including preload (determined by circulating volume, venous capacitance, and filling time),[3] pump function (cycle length, contractility defined as the pressure generated in response to a set preload),[9] and afterload (vascular resistance and impedance).[10] Embryos also release vasoactive substances and alter neural CV regulation during this process).[11] However, all systems have limits and when these limits are exceeded during CV morphogenesis embryo death occurs. The ability of the immature myocardium to acutely adapt CV function in response to a range of environmental "stressors" has been noted in every species studied to date. For mammalian embryos, this adaptive process actively involves the placental circulation and altered placental function can be either adaptive or maladaptive. Of note, adaptation within the mammalian placenta can preferentially benefit the mother, the fetus, or both and in general, maternal survival occurs at the expense of fetal survival.[12–14]

The next general concept is that structural morphogenesis of developing CV systems is dynamically influenced by CV function (and vice versa) such that the final structural phenotype can vary depending upon the functional "history." For example, numerous experiments in the developing chick embryo have shown that the developing heart requires specific mechanical loading conditions to accomplish "normal" CV morphogenesis. If venous return to the heart is impaired by unilateral vitelline vein ligation,[15] or more selectively, left ventricular filling is reduced by left atrial ligation,[16] CV morphogenesis is altered so that defects occur in myocardial growth, ventricular septation, and septation of the developing outflow track. It is interesting to note that the developing myocardium adapts to increased mechanical load by accelerating growth and preserving CV function[17] while reduced mechanical loading during critical periods of development leads to impaired function.[18,19] The mechanisms by which changes in mechanical load are transduced by the developing CV system into changes in morphogenesis remain an area of intense investigation. While there are numerous examples of isolated experimental interventions that result in dramatic changes in CV phenotype there are likely a very large number of much more subtle interactions that are additive in determining the phenotypic variation present in "normal" populations.

Experimental models and methods to investigate CV functional maturation

Our investigation of CV structural and functional maturation requires reproducible, accessible, and affordable experimental models and technically feasible and reproducible experimental methods. Fortunately, the perseverance of generations of scientists has produced a wide spectrum of experimental models for the investigation of CV morphogenesis (from fly to man) and the ingenuity of these scientists has produced a comparable spectrum of experimental methods. The selection of a specific experimental model (for example, the chick embryo) and a specific experimental method (for example, the measurement of intraventricular blood pressure using a fluid-filled glass cannula and a servo-null pressure system while varying heart rate by thermal probe application to the cardiac pacemaker region) must be matched to a specific question (for example, defining the relationship between cardiac time intervals, filling volumes, and developed pressure) while recognizing the experimental limitations (accuracy of pressure measurement, variation in vascular resistance in response to altered stroke volume, etc.).

The embryonic left-atrial ligation (LAL) model of chronically reduced left ventricular (LV) filling produces a left-heart hypoplasia phenocopy of hypoplastic left heart syndrome and provides insight into both acute and chronic CV adaptation to altered mechanical load.[20,21] LAL produces immediate changes in intracardiac blood flow patterns and immediate changes in regional myocardial deformation patterns consistent with redistributed mechanical load between the LV and RV. Following load redistribution, LV and RV growth become disparate with subsequent LV "hypoplasia" relative to stage-matched controls. LAL induced LV hypoplasia is associated with regional changes in myocardial architecture at both the trabecular and myofiber levels and is associated with altered myocardial passive properties. Regulation on cardiomyocyte microtubule synthesis is increased in the LV following LAL and the LAL associated increase in passive stiffness can be reversed by microtubule depolymerization with colchicine.[22] We are now beginning to understand the relationship between mechanical load and cardiomyocyte differentiation and proliferation at the local level.

The investigation of embryonic CV function in the mammalian embryo presents unique technical challenges and offers the opportunity for unique insights for the human embryo and fetus.[23–26] It is well established that CV function is directly influenced by sedation, instrumentation, and restraint in the adult mouse, and each of these issues impacts the embryo as well.[18,24] The murine embryo is extremely sensitive to changes in maternal oxygenation and placental perfusion.[13,18] Screening mouse embryos for altered CV phenotypes is possible but requires significant dedicated resources. Numerous gene-targeted mice have embryonic CV phenotypes and a small subset of these animals may be valuable models for congenital CV malformations. Murine models of intrauterine growth restriction and "toxemia" are under development in order to better understand embryonic adaptation.

The availability of targeted genetic models in a wide range of species provides a unique opportunity to define the "molecular" regulation of structure-function relationships during CV development.[27] The first level of sophistication in this approach has been the targeted deletion of single genes and/or transcription factors from flies to mice with the subsequent characterization of altered CV phenotypes and survival. Genetic errors have been created via environmental mutagenesis protocols utilizing rapidly developing experimental models (*Drosophila, Xenopus,* zebrafish, mouse, to name a few) coupled with altered phenotype detection strategies (behavior, external phenotype, transparent embryo, bulk screening). These genetic approaches provide an almost unlimited source of unique experimental models for further characterization. While the initial focus in this field was on the generation of homozygous deletions the field is now shifting to focus on selective reductions in gene and protein number (heterozygotes or hypomorphs) with subtler changes in structure and function that may be more representative of biological adaptation and disease. Once again, specific molecular "model" animals are under investigation to define specific molecular pathways with respect to CV structural and functional maturation. Fortunately, many of the molecular pathways are conserved across a wide range of species (e.g. the tinman gene specifies dorsal vessel cells in Drosophila, and genetic homolog to NKX2.5 regulates cardiomyocyte fate in every species studied to date). It is important to note that single gene errors are associated with phenotypic variation within strains of the same species and across species due to the distribution of modifier genes as well as environmental influences during development.

Mathematical models of developing CV systems

While we can measure numerous aspects of CV structure and function acutely and can generate longitudinal trends related to developmental changes in these parameters during morphogenesis, there are aspects of biologic processes which can only be described by mathematical models (such as mechanical "stress") and other processes which reflect the integration of numerous simultaneous processes such that mathematical models can be used to estimate or predict these interactions. The description of "growth" within developing tissues is one example where mathematical models can integrate numerous interactions (physical, genetic, environmental) in order to predict normal processes or the adaptive response to altered interactions. With respect to developing CV systems, mathematical methods have been developed to describe the mechanical forces that influence the developing myocardium[28,29] and that remodel the developing vasculature[30] including the calculation of regional variations in hemodynamic shear stress in the developing zebrafish embryo.[31] Models have also been proposed to predict changes in CV structure in response to differential growth and mechanical loading conditions.[32] We also use numerical methods to integrate measures of blood pressure and blood velocity to describe the impedance of the developing vasculature.[10]

The challenge ahead: integrating cell and molecular biology with physiology and biomechanics

Despite the geometric expansion of available information (novel genetic organisms and animals, novel genetic and imaging reagents, novel experimental methods for structural and functional phenotyping) related to developmental biology, a large gap still exists in the translation of altered genotype to phenotype. Deconstructing the complex molecular regulatory architecture of a developing organism does not necessarily provide evidence of the interactive regulation of the developmental process or the mechanisms for adapting morphogenesis in response to genetic or environmental events. With respect to the role of mechanical load in the regulation of CV morphogenesis, much work needs to be done to define the specific regulation of altered cell function (gene expression, energy production, protein synthesis and assembly) that results in the adaptive response. Of course, we cannot assume that adaptive mechanisms present in the very immature embryonic heart (e.g. prior to cardiac septation) will be the same as those present in the fetal heart (following the completion of cardiac morphogenesis) or mature heart, but we can assume that the processes are related. However, one specific example of how these adaptive processes differ is the ability of the developing myocardium to alter cell number (hyperplasia) in response to altered mechanical load while the mature myocardium is restricted to altering cell size (hypertrophy). The regulation of cell proliferation, differentiation, and death during CV morphogenesis remain central themes as our field moves forward. The investigation of CV morphogenesis in a wide range of species and experimental paradigms has become the rule rather than the exception.

Defining maternal–embryo and maternal–fetal interactions

Maternal–embryo and maternal–fetal interactions clearly impact both on the developmental trajectory of the embryo and fetus and on both maternal and fetal outcomes. Developmental maternal imprinting occurs immediately following fertilization and persists throughout life. As technology evolves to allow the simultaneous investigation of embryonic and maternal physiology we will be able to investigate novel paradigms of maternal–embryo interactions that alter both embryo and maternal fate. These paradigms may result in adaptive strategies that target either the fetus or mother,[33] or both in order to optimize developmental outcome.

Defining the metabolic regulation of CV structural and functional maturation

When we state that developing systems operate within an optimal range one of the critical operational states must relate to energy availability and utilization. Methods are available to quantify energy availability and energy utilization in developing organisms however much less is known about how subtle variations in energy balance directly influence developmental processes. Specifically, little is known how changes in energy balance altered the molecular regulation of developmental and adaptive processes that impact on "final trajectory." Due to the adaptive interaction on many system components (cell to cell, ventricle to vasculature, embryo to placental to mother) the investigation of the "integrated" metabolic regulation of CV development will reveal fascinating biology and will likely provide insights into some of the events that alter CV development and embryo fate.

Defining environmental imprinting on developmental processes

While the impact of altered environment on CV morphogenesis has been well established, the specific mechanisms that regulate these interactions are now under intense investigation. The availability of defined genetic pathways responsible for basic developmental sequences provides new paradigms to assess the regulation of development by changes in energy state and by external compounds (inert or biologically active) that can alter biologic processes. It is important to note that in addition to the sequencing of the human genome, a recent sub-project has completed the characterization of a subset of human genes recognized to be sensitive to altered environmental forces. These "environmentally-responsive" genetic pathways become obvious targets for investigation related to adaptive developmental processes.[34]

In summary, we have made outstanding progress in our understanding of the adaptive interaction between CV structure and function during morphogenesis in a broad range of species. Many mechanisms are conserved while others are distinct.[35] Our knowledge remains quite immature with respect to the many remaining questions available and with the proper support *and talented young investigators* the future remains without limit.

The investigation of developing CV systems is rapidly expanding in a large number of laboratories (www.biol.unt.edu/developmentalphysiology). Unique examples of adaptive CV strategies are present across a wide spectrum of organism size and complexity. As with the genetic insights gained from simpler organisms, conserved adaptive mechanisms to altered biomechanical load in simpler organisms will provide insights into CV adaptation in mammals.

References

1 Clark EB, Hu N. Developmental hemodynamic changes in the chick embryo from stages 18 to 27. *Circ Res* 1982; **51**: 810–15.

2 Nakazawa M, Miyagawa S, Ohno T, Miura S, Takao A. Developmental hemodynamic changes in rat embryos at 11 to 15 days of gestation: normal data of blood pressure and the effect of caffeine compared to data from chick embryo. *Pediatr Res* 1988; **23**: 200–5.

3 Keller BB. Functional maturation and coupling of the embryonic cardiovascular system. In: Clark EB, Markwald RR, Takao A, eds. *Developmental Mechanisms of Heart Disease.* Mount Kisco, NY: Futura, 1995: 367–86.

4 Keller BB. Embryonic cardiovascular function, coupling, and maturation: a species view. In: Burggren W, Keller BB, eds. *Development of Cardiovascular Systems: Molecules to Organisms.* New York: Cambridge University Press, 1996: 65–87.

5 Burggren WW, Fritsche,R. Amphibian cardiovascular development. In: Burggren W, Keller BB, eds. *Development of Cardiovascular Systems: Molecules to Organisms.* New York: Cambridge University Press, 1997: 166–83.

6 Warburton SJ, Fritsche R. Blood pressure control in a larval amphibian, *Xenopus laevis. J Exp Biol* 2000; **203**: 2047–52.

7 Hu N, Sedmera D, Yost HJ, Clark EB. Structure and function of the developing zebrafish heart. *Anat Rec* 2000; **260**: 148–57.

8 Burggren WW, Warburton SJ, Slivkoff MD. Interruption of cardiac output does not affect short-term growth and metabolic rate in day 3 and 4 chick embryos. *J Exp Biol* 2000; **203**: 3831–8.

9 Casillas CB, Tinney JP, Keller BB. Influence of acute alterations in cycle length on ventricular function in the chick embryo. *Am J Physiol* 1994; **267**: H905–11.

10 Yoshigi M, Hu N, Keller BB. Dorsal aortic impedance in the stage 24 chick embryo following acute changes in circulating blood volume. *Am J Physiol* 1996; **270**: H1597–606.

11 Hu N, Hansen AL, Clark EB, Keller BB. Atrial natriuretic peptide reduces diastolic filling in the stage 21 chick embryo. *Pediatr Res* 1995; **37**: 465–8.

12 Kohl T, Sharland G, Allan LD *et al.* World experience of percutaneous ultrasound-guided balloon valvuloplasty in human fetuses with severe aortic valve obstruction. *Am J Cardiol* 2000; **85**: 1230–3.

13 Adamson Sl, Lu Y, Whiteley KJ *et al.* Interactions between trophoblast cells and the maternal and fetal circulation in the mouse placenta. *Dev Biol* 2002; **250**: 358–73.

14 Gluckman PD, Pinal CS. Maternal-placental-fetal interactions in the endocrine regulation of fetal growth: role of somatotrophic axes. *Endocrine* 2002; **19**: 81–9.

15 Hogers B, DeRuiter MC, Gittenberger-de Groot AC, Poelmann RE. Unilateral vitelline vein ligation alters intracardiac blood flow patterns and morphogenesis in the chick embryo. *Circ Res* 1997; **80**: 473–81.

16 Tobita K, Keller BB. Right and left ventricular wall deformation patterns in normal and left heart hypoplasia chick embryos. *Am J Physiol* 2000: **279**: H959–69.

17 Clark EB, Hu N, Frommelt P, Vandekieft JL, Dummett JL, Tomanek RJ. Effect of increased ventricular pressure on heart growth in chick embryo. *Am J Physiol* 1989; **257**: H55–61.

18 Tobita K, Tinney J, Keller BB. Cardiovascular phenotype analysis of murine embryos. In: Hoit BD, Walsh RA, eds. *Cardiovascular Physiology in the Genetically Engineered Mouse,* 2nd edn. New York: Kluwer Academic Publishers, 2002: 353–76.

19 Tobita K, Schroder EA, Tinney JP, Garrison JB, Keller BB. Regional passive ventricular pressure-strain relations during development of altered loads in the chick embryo. *Am J Physiol* 2002; **282**: H2386–96.

20 Sedmera D, Pexieder T, Rychterova V, Hu N, Clark EB. Remodeling of chick embryonic ventricular myoarchitecture under experimentally changed loading conditions. *Anat Rec* 1999; **254**: 238–52.

21 Tobita K, Garrison JB, Liu LJ, Tinney JP, Keller BB. Three dimensional myofiber architecture of the embryonic left ventricle during normal and development of altered mechanical loads. *Anat Rec* 2004 (in press).

22 Schroder EA, Tobita K, Tinney JP, Keller BB. Microtubule involvement in the adaptation to altered mechanical load in the developing chick myocardium. *Circ Res* 2002; **91**: 353–9.

23 Gui YH, Linask KK, Khowsathit P, Huhta JC. Doppler echocardiography of normal and abnormal embryonic mouse heart. *Pediatr Res* 1996; **40**: 633–642.

24 Keller BB. Analysis of murine embryonic structural and functional phenotype. In: Hoit BD, Walsh RA, eds. *Cardio-*

vascular *Physiology in the Genetically Engineered Mouse.* New York: Kluwer Academic Publishers, 1998: 259–83.

25 Phoon CK, Aristizabal O, Turnbull DH. 40 MHz Doppler characterization of umbilical and dorsal aortic blood flow in the early mouse embryo. *Ultrasound Med Biol* 2000; **26**: 1275–83.

26 Zhou YQ, Foster FS, Qu DW, Zhang M, Harasiewicz KA, Adamson SL. Applications for multifrequency ultrasound biomicroscopy in mice from implantation to adulthood. *Physiol Genomics* 2002; **10**: 113–26.

27 Srivastava D. Genetic assembly of the heart: implications for congenital heart disease. *Annu Rev Physiol* 2001; **63**: 451–69.

28 Taber LA, Keller BB, Clark EB. Cardiac mechanics in the stage 16 chick embryo. *J Biomech Eng* 1992; **114**: 427–34.

29 Taber LA. Biomechanics of cardiovascular development. *Annu Rev Biomed Eng* 2001; **3**: 1–25.

30 Ling P, Taber LA, Humphrey JD. Approach to quantify the mechanical behavior of the intact embryonic chick heart. *Ann Biomed Eng* 2002; **30**: 636–45.

31 Hove JR, Koster RW, Forouhar AS *et al.* Intracardiac fluid forces are an essential epigenetic factor for embryonic cardiogenesis. *Nature* 2003; **421**: 172–7.

32 Lin IE, Taber LA. A model for stress-induced growth in the developing heart. *J Biomech Eng* 1995; **117**: 343–9.

33 Ursem NTC, Clark EB, Keller BB, Hop WCJ, Wladimiroff JW. Assessment of fetal heart rate and velocity variability by Doppler velocimetry of the descending aorta at 10–20 weeks of gestation. *Ultrasound Obstet Gynecol* 1999; **14**: 397–401.

34 Cunningham ML, Bogdanffy MYS, Zacharewski TR, Hines RN. Workshop overview: use of genomic data in risk assessment. *Toxicol Sci* 2003; **73**: 209–15.

35 Gittenberger-de Groot A. Principles of abnormal cardiac development. In: Burggren WW, Keller BB, eds. *Development of Cardiovascular Systems: Molecules to Organisms.* New York: Cambridge University Press, 1996; 259–67.

CHAPTER 46

Three-dimensional fiber architecture of the embryonic left ventricle during normal development and reduced mechanical load

Kimimasa Tobita, Jason B. Garrison, Bradley B. Keller

Introduction

Mechanical load is one of the major exogenous factors that play an important role in regulating embryonic ventricular function and structure during cardiac morphogenesis.[1,2] Recent studies in chick embryonic heart showed that reduced left ventricular (LV) mechanical loads change LV chamber architecture, myocardial material properties, protein expression, and cell proliferation patterns of the developing embryonic LV.[2,3–6] However, little is known regarding how the embryonic LV myocardium acquires a mature 3-dimensional (3-D) fiber architecture distribution and how reduced mechanical load influences the LV myofiber maturation process. We tested the hypothesis that reduced mechanical load alters the local 3-D fiber architecture of the embryonic LV myocardium. Our results showed that reduced mechanical load changed both 3-D myofiber angle distribution and maturation patterns of outer compact myocardium while inner trabecular myocardium was similar to normal development.

Material and methods

White leghorn chick embryos were studied at Hamburger-Hamilton stages 27 (5 day), 31 (7 days), and 36 (10 days) of a 46-stage (21 days) incubation period.[7] To reduce LV mechanical load, we performed left atrial ligation at stage 21 using a 10–0 nylon suture. The left atrial ligation reduces LV preload and redistributes intracardiac flow to the right ventricle (RV) resulting in LV hypoplasia.[2,4,8] The heart was arrested at end-diastolic phase by injecting chick ringer solution containing 60 mM potassium, 0.5 mM verapamil, and 0.5 mM EGTA.[4,6] The embryo was fixed in 4% paraformaldehyde for 12 h. The embryonic heart was excised from the embryo and then placed in a dorsoventral orientation within a 13% polyacrylamide gel that was immediately polymerized with 2% ammonium persulfate.[9] Polyacrylamide embedded hearts were sectioned at 200 μm thickness with a standard vibrotome. Sections representing LV myocardium were stained for f-actin with FITC-conjugated phalloidin. LV myocardium at the midventricular level was examined using a standard laser scanning confocal microscopy system. Z-serial optical sectioning was performed on 50 to 100 μm thick specimens with a z-depth of 1 μm at 1-μm intervals.

Reconstruction of 3-D fiber architecture and fiber orientation measurement

From the acquired images (resolution, 1024 × 1024 pixels in each section), we digitally reconstructed myofiber images in either transverse or coronal orientation to the LV longitudinal axis. For transverse sections we described myofibril angle with reference to the local epicardial tangential plane as viewed from above. For coronal sections we described myofibril angle with 0° assigned to the dorsoventral circumferential direction and 90° assigned to the apico-basal longitudinal direction, respectively. To determine the myofiber orientation of the compact myocardium, we then analyzed subregions [50 μm width] × [50 μm depth] × [compact myocardium thickness] of the reconstructed sections. Local myofiber angle was determined by examining local intensity gradients in small regions of interest (ROI) within each subregion (20–30 pixel-square, 100–225 ROIs per section). The dominant local

orientation was determined in subregions using an accumulator scheme. A 180-element array A_θ represented the possible angles (θ) 0 to 179° in subregions quantitated in 1° interval. Each accumulator bin value was determined using the following equation;[10]

$$A_\theta = \Sigma_{(i,j)}\, G_{(i,j)} * [(Exp(2\cos(2(\theta - \phi_{(i,j)})))/Exp(2)],$$
$$0° \le \theta < 180°$$

where, $G_{(i,j)}$ is sum of squares of horizontal and vertical gradients of ROI, $\phi_{(i,j)}$ is inverse tangent of the ratio of vertical to horizontal components of ROI, respectively.

Dominant local myofiber angle in the subregion was determined by the largest accumulator bin value

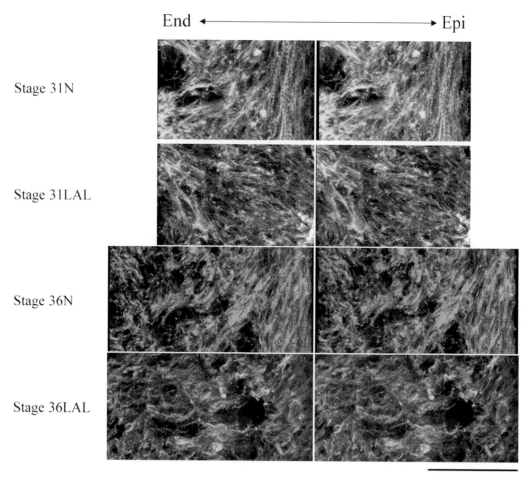

Fig. 46.1 Developmental changes in 3-D LV fiber architecture during normal development (N) and following left atrial ligation (LAL, stereo images). End; endocardium side, Epi; epicardial side. Scale bar = 50 μm.

and converted to range from -89° to +90°. All calculations were performed using a LabVIEW based custom made program. Calculated local fiber angles were then inspected visually in each image. Mean fiber orientation and circular standard deviation were calculated using circular statistics.[11] The mean orientation was computed by treating each measurement as a unit vector and averaging the vector components.

$$C = \Sigma(i)\cos(2\theta i), S = \Sigma(i)\sin(2\theta i), \theta i: \text{individual fiber angle,}$$

$$R^2 = C^2 + S^2,$$

$$\cos(2\theta_{mean}) = C/R, \sin(2\theta_{mean}) = S/R, \theta_{mean}: \text{mean fiber angle.}$$

The circular standard deviation (δ) is expressed as,

$$\delta = 0.5[-2\log(R_{mean})]^{0.5}, R_{mean} = R/n, n: \text{number of measurement.}$$

To test myofiber orientation directionality, the Rayleigh test was performed in each image.[1] We performed a nonparametric ranking test to determine differences in mean fiber angle throughout the compact myocardium in normal and LAL hearts.[11]

Three dimensional myofiber architecture and mean fiber orientation

Figure 46.1 shows representative 3-D fiber architecture of the outer compact myocardium during normal development and the development following LAL. Mean myofiber angles in transverse sections were distributed uniformly through the entire LV wall in both normal and LAL groups during development ($-10°$ to $+10°$, $P < 0.001$, Rayleigh test). In coronal sections (Fig. 46.2), mean fiber angles were distributed uniformly until stage 27 ($-5°$ to $+10°$, $P < 0.001$) in both normal and LAL hearts. At stage 31, the mean fiber angles at the outer 30% of the wall significantly increased ($+30°$ to $+60°$, $P < 0.05$) and extended to 40% at stage 36 during normal development. Following LAL, mean fiber angles in coronal sections were distributed uniformly until stage31 (-5 to $+5$, $P < 0.001$) and those of the outer 20% of the wall increased at stage 36 ($+15°$ to $+20°$, $P < 0.05$). In the inner trabecular myocardium mature myofibers were seen and the myofiber orientation was primarily parallel to the longitudinal axis of each trabecular segment. LAL did not appear to alter trabecular myofiber maturation and orientation (Fig. 46.3).

Summary

The present study suggests that: (1) transmural myofiber angle distribution in the LV compact myocardium changed from uniform to regionally unique non-uniform patterns during normal development; (2) reduced mechanical load produced by LAL altered the myofiber maturation process in the LV compact myocardium; (3) LV hypoplasia was associated with an 'immature' transmural variation of myofiber angle until stage 36; (4) reduced mechanical load produced by LAL did not effect local myofiber orientation within trabecular myocardium. In conclusion, reduced mechanical load modulates both local myofiber orientation and maturation in the developing compact myocardium.

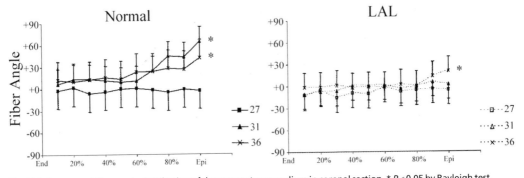

Fig. 46.2 Transmural fiber angle distribution of the compact myocardium in coronal section. * $P < 0.05$ by Rayleigh test. Horizontal axis represents transmural coordinate of compact myocardium from endocardium (0%) to epicardium (100%).

Normal LAL

Stage 27

Stage 31

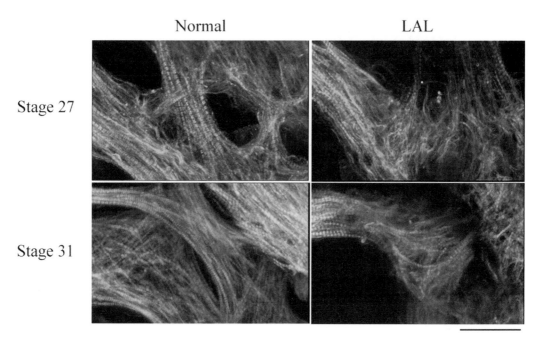

Fig. 46.3 Developmental changes in myofiber architecture of trabeculae. Scale bar = 25 μm.

Acknowledgments
Supported by the NIH (BBK).

References

1 Keller BB. Function and biomechanics of developing cardiovascular systems. In: Tomanek RJ, Runyan RB, eds. *Formation of the Heart and Its Regulation* Boston: Birkhauser, 2001: 251–72.

2 Tobita K, Keller BB. Right and left ventricular wall deformation patterns in normal and left heart hypoplasia chick embryos. *Am J Physiol Heart Circ Physiol* 2000; **279**: H959–69.

3 Schroder EA, Tobita K, Tinney JP, Folder JK, Keller BB. Microtubule involvement in the adaptation to altered mechanical load in developing chick myocardium. *Circ Res* 2002; **91**: 353–9.

4 Sedmera D, Pexieder T, Rychterova V, Hu N, Clark EB. Remodeling of chick embryonic ventricular myoarchitecture under experimentally changed loading conditions. *Anat Rec* 1999; **254**: 238–52.

5 Sedmera D, Hu N, Weiss K *et al*. Cellular changes in experimental left heart hypoplasia *Anat Rec* 2002; **267**: 137–45.

6 Tobita K, Schroder EA, Tinney JP, Garrison JB, Keller BB. Regional passive ventricular stress-strain relations during development of altered loads in chick embryo. *Am J Physiol Heart Circ Physiol* 2002; **282**: H2386–96.

7 Hamburger V, Hamilton HL. A series of normal stages in the development of the chick embryo. *J Morphol* 1951; **88**: 49–92.

8 Harh JY, Milton PH, Gallen WJ, Friedberg DZ, Kaplan S. Experimental reduction of hypoplastic left heart syndrome in the chick embryo. *Am J Cardiol* 1973; **31**: 51–6.

9 Nakagawa M, Price RL, Chintanawonges C *et al*. Analysis of heart development in cultured rat embryos. *J Mol Cell Cardiol* 1997; **29**: 369–79.

10 Karlon WJ, Covell JW, McCulloch A, Hunter JJ, Omens JH. Automated measurement of myofiber disarray in transgenic mice with ventricular expression of *ras*. *Anat Rec* 1998; **252**: 612–25.

11 Fisher NI. *Statistical Analysis of Circular Data.* Cambridge: Cambridge University Press, 1993.

CHAPTER 47

Changes in cardiac excitation–contraction coupling during mammalian development: implications for regulation of contractile function

Salvatore Mancarella, Shekhar Srivastava, Anita Go,
Ying-Ying Zhou, William A. Coetzee, Michael Artman

Cardiac contraction and relaxation depend on Ca^{2+} cycling to and from the myofibrils. In mature mammalian ventricular myocardium, the sarcoplasmic reticulum (SR) is the major source of Ca^{2+} for contraction and the major Ca^{2+} uptake mechanism during relaxation.[1] The release of a large amount of Ca^{2+} from the SR is triggered by a relatively small amount of Ca^{2+} entering the cell, predominately through sarcolemmal L-type Ca^{2+} channels. Relaxation occurs primarily from reuptake of Ca^{2+} into the SR by an ATP-dependent Ca^{2+} pump with efflux of a small amount of Ca^{2+} across the sarcolemma (mainly through the Na^+–Ca^{2+} exchanger).

Regulation of cytosolic Ca^{2+} concentration is very precisely controlled to maintain normal contractile function and to respond to changes in demand. Graded control of contractile force and relaxation are achieved through a variety of cellular processes, but the β-adrenergic signaling pathway is perhaps the best characterized. In mature myocytes, activation of β-adrenergic receptors (predominately $β_1$-AR) results in stimulation of adenylyl cyclase, generation of cAMP, activation of PKA, and phosphorylation of several key regulatory proteins involved in Ca^{2+} transport.[1,2] $β_1$-AR stimulation of contraction and relaxation occurs primarily from increases in L-type Ca^{2+} current, greater SR Ca^{2+} release, and enhanced SR Ca^{2+} reuptake.

Mechanisms for modulating contractile function in the developing heart have not been fully defined. Activation of the β-AR pathway in immature ventricular myocytes increases contractility, but the cellular processes that mediate this response are unclear. The major targets involved in the β-AR response in adult myocardium seem to play only a minor role in the developing heart. In distinct contrast to adult myocardium, the immature mammalian heart is much less dependent upon L-type Ca^{2+} channels and SR Ca^{2+} fluxes for contraction and relaxation. Instead, neonatal rabbits depend largely on the Na^+–Ca^{2+} exchanger for directly regulating Ca^{2+} concentration at the contractile proteins.[3–6] Therefore, we postulated that graded modulation of contractile events in the immature heart would occur primarily through alterations of the functional activity of the Na^+–Ca^{2+} exchanger. Specifically, we hypothesized that the β-AR response in neonatal ventricular myocytes is due to a β-AR mediated increase in Na^+–Ca^{2+} exchange activity.

We compared the effects of β-AR agonists on Na^+–Ca^{2+} exchange currents in freshly isolated ventricular myocytes from adult (AD) and newborn

(NB; 1- to 5-day-old) rabbits using the whole-cell, patch-clamp method. Previous studies have shown that β_2-AR stimulation by zinterol (specific agonist for β_2-AR) increases contraction amplitude in neonatal rat myocytes, but had little or no effect in adult cells.[7] Thus, we studied the effects of both isoproterenol (nonselective β-AR agonist) and zinterol in adults and neonates.

As shown in Fig. 47.1, isoproterenol significantly increased both inward and outward Na$^+$–Ca^{2+} exchange currents in adult and neonatal ventricular myocytes. In contrast, zinterol, a selective β_2-AR

agonist, increased Na$^+$–Ca^{2+} exchange currents only in neonatal myocytes (Fig. 47.2). These results demonstrate that the inotropic and lusitropic responses to β-AR agonists in immature ventricular myocytes may be mediated by increases in Na$^+$–Ca^{2+} exchange current, resulting in greater Ca^{2+} cycling to and from the contractile elements. Furthermore, these effects in neonatal cells appear to be mediated predominately by β_2-ARs.

In summary, cellular mechanisms for regulating contractile function and determining the responses to β-adrenergic receptor stimulation undergo major

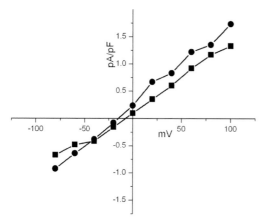
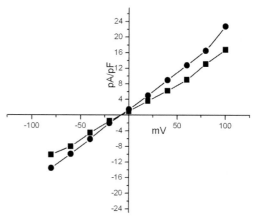

Fig. 47. 1 Effects of the non-selective β-adrenergic receptor agonist isoproterenol (1 µM) on I_{NaCa} recorded from adult (left panel) and newborn (right panel) ventricular myocytes.

Squares indicate control currents and circles indicate currents in the presence of isoproterenol.

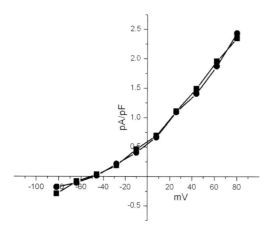
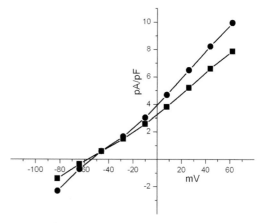

Fig. 47. 2 Effects of the selective β_2-adrenergic receptor agonist zinterol (100 nM) on I_{NaCa} recorded from adult (left panel) and newborn (right panel) ventricular myocytes.

Squares indicate control currents and circles indicate currents in the presence of zinterol.

changes during perinatal maturation. These new findings have important implications for understanding signal transduction pathways and regulation of cardiac contraction and relaxation in the developing heart.

Materials and methods

Single ventricular myocytes were isolated from the hearts of adult and newborn (1–5 days old) New Zealand white rabbits (either sex) using a collagenase-based digestion technique described previously.[5] Myocytes were transferred to a recording chamber and continuously superfused at 37 °C with Tyrode's solution composed of (mmol L^{-1}): NaCl, 140; KCl, 4; $CaCl_2$, 2.5; $MgCl_2$, 1; HEPES, 5; and glucose, 10, titrated to a pH of 7.4 with 4 mmol L^{-1} NaOH. Whole cell currents were measured by the patch-clamp technique. Patch pipettes were pulled to resistances of 3–5 MΩ. Pipettes were filled with internal solution containing (in mmol L^{-1}): Cs-aspartate, 70; CsCl, 40; HEPES, 10, KH_2PO_4, 2.5; NaCl, 20; $CaCl_2$, 1; tetraethylammonium, 20; BAPTA (1,2-bis(2-aminophenoxy)ethane-N,N,N',N'-tetraacetic acid), 10; MgATP, 4 (pH 7.2). To measure Na^+–Ca^{2+} exchange current (I_{NaCa}), the normal Tyrode's solution was changed to a K-free solution, which also contained 10 μmol L^{-1} strophanthidin to inhibit the Na^+–K^+ pump and 10 μmol L^{-1} nifedipine to block L-type Ca^{2+} current. I_{NaCa} was measured as the current sensitive to the addition of 5–10 mmol L^{-1} external Ni^{2+}. Currents were normalized to cell capacitance to account for differences in cell size.

References

1 Bers DM. Cardiac excitation–contraction coupling. *Nature* 2002; **415**: 198–205.

2 Steinberg SF. The molecular basis for distinct β-adrenergic receptor subtype actions in cardiomyocytes. *Circ Res* 1999; **85**: 1101–11.

3 Artman M, Ichikawa H, Avkiran M, Coetzee WA. Na^+–Ca^{2+} exchange current density in cardiac myocytes from rabbits and guinea pigs during postnatal development. *Am J Physiol* 1995; **268**: H1714–22.

4 Balaguru D, Haddock PS, Puglisi JL *et al.* Role of the sarcoplasmic reticulum in contraction and relaxation of immature rabbit ventricular myocytes. *J Mol Cell Cardiol* 1997; **29**: 2747–57.

5 Haddock PS, Coetzee WA, Artman M. Na^+–Ca^{2+} exchange current and contractions measured under Cl^- free conditions in developing rabbit hearts. *Am J Physiol* 1997; **273**: H837–46.

6 Haddock PS, Coetzee WA, Cho E *et al.* Subcellular $[Ca^{2+}]_i$ gradients during excitation–contraction coupling in newborn rabbit ventricular myocytes. *Circ Res* 1999; **85**: 415–27.

7 Kuznetsov V, Pak E, Robinson RB, Steinberg SF. $β_2$-adrenergic receptor actions in neonatal and adult rat ventricular myocytes. *Circ Res* 1995; **76**: 40–52.

CHAPTER 48

Role of the sodium–calcium exchanger (*Ncx-1*) within *Splotch* (*Sp²ᴴ*) myocardial failure

Jian Wang, Andrew Lindsley, Tony Creazzo,
Srinagesh V. Koushik, Simon J. Conway

The *Splotch* (*Sp²ᴴ*) mutant mouse is a radiation-induced strain that contains a 32-bp deletion in the homeodomain of the *Pax-3* transcription factor. *Pax3* mRNA is expressed within the neural tube, somites, and early migratory neural crest cells[1] and *Sp²ᴴ* embryos exhibit defects within neural tube closure (spina bifida and exencephaly), pigmentation, skeletal development, and a lack of limb musculature.[2,3] Additionally, there are wide-ranging defects within neural crest-derivatives (such as the melanocytes, thymus, thyroid, dorsal root ganglia, and elements of the aortic arch arteries and outflow tract septum) in *Sp²ᴴ* homozygotes.[4] It has also previously been shown that homozygous *Sp²ᴴ* embryos die *in utero* ~14.0 dpc owing to cardiac insufficiency and conotruncal outflow tract defects with obligatory perimembranous interventricular septal defect.[5–8] However, it is currently unclear as to why the homozygous *Sp²ᴴ* embryos die as conotruncal outflow tract defects are not usually thought to be lethal because separation of the systemic and pulmonary circulations is carried out at the maternal–embryonic interface/placenta *in utero*. In humans, *PAX3* mutations lead to Waardenburg syndrome, an autosomal dominant disorder that consists of defects in neural crest-derived tissues and is characterized by pigmentation, and hearing and facio-skeletal anomalies.[9] Cardiac defects have also been reported in some Waardenburg children.[10,11]

Molecular characterization of *Sp²ᴴ* mutants has demonstrated that the cardiac neural crest initiate migration but do not reach the pharyngeal arches or outflow tract in sufficient numbers for normal remodeling or outflow tract septation to occur.[6,12,13] Furthermore, we have shown that this lack of colonizing cardiac neural crest is due to abnormal neural crest stem cell expansion.[14] We have also shown that there is low level *Pax3* expression in normal 9.5 dpc hearts[6] and that 100% of the homozygous mutant embryos die by 14.0 dpc solely owing to the presence of conotruncal anomalies[6,7] and not the neural tube defects. Deficiencies in myocardial function further compromise cardiac function, as there is abnormal excitation-contraction (EC) coupling in the *Sp²ᴴ* mutants[7] resulting in *in utero* lethality by ~14 dpc. It has been proposed that this myocardial defect is an indirect consequence of the reduced numbers of migrating neural crest,[15] because neural crest cells are not thought to contribute directly to the myocardium.[16] However, Kirby and colleagues have shown that premigratory neural crest-ablation in chick results in myocardial dysfunction prior to the arrival of the cardiac neural crest within the heart, and have suggested that these early effects on the heart are due to a prolonged release of factors (FGFs, etc.) by the pharyngeal endoderm, which are normally involved in the induction of cardiac mesoderm.[17]

In order to determine when the *Sp²ᴴ* mutant hearts are affected, we initially analyzed the morphology, histology, and structure of the *Sp²ᴴ* embryos throughout development prior to lethality. Histological analysis using previously published methods[8] of the developing *sp²ᴴ* myocardium (8.0–13.5 dpc) revealed that morphologically the *Sp²ᴴ* myocardium is normal. This is in contrast to that reported for the *Sp* allele (that functions like a null allele), in which a thinned myocardium lacking the compact zone is evident from 11.5 dpc onwards and may be owing to upregulation and ectopic expression of *p57Kip2* (a cyclin-dependent kinase inhibitor of the p21 family) in *Sp* hearts.[18] However, our gene chip, RT-PCR, *in situ* hybridization and Western analysis using published methods[6,7,19] showed that the spatiotemporal expression of *p57Kip2* is normal within *Sp²ᴴ* mutants (data not shown), but that detailed transmission electron microscopy using published methods[20] revealed some myocytes in the *Sp²ᴴ* mutant ventricular compact zone and atria (not shown) are very abnormal (Plate 33b). The 10.0 dpc *Sp²ᴴ* mutant compact zone contained numerous cardiomyocytes that seemed to have undergone "cytoplasmic clearing" or degradation but not apoptosis; however, this was specific to the compact zone and atria as myocytes within the bulbus cordis (not shown) and trabeculae (Plate 33c) were unaffected. These differences in *splotch* phenotypes are interesting and could indicate that *Pax3* in *Sp²ᴴ* mutants (which has still has normal paired domain but non-functional homeodomain) is partially active and may constitute a hypomorphic (dominant negative?) allele.

Subsequent functional analysis of ventricular cardiac function of fura-2/AM-loaded heart tubes using published methods[20] revealed that Ca^{2+} transients (a functional measure of EC-coupling) are reduced within 9.5dpc *Sp²ᴴ* mutant hearts (Plate 33d,e). Furthermore, using a candidate gene approach we also determined that both the Na^+/Ca^{2+} exchanger (*Ncx1*) and the Ca^{2+} channel ($\alpha 1C$) Ca^{2+}-handling genes were misexpressed (higher) in early 9.0–9.5 dpc *Sp²ᴴ* hearts. Interestingly, *calmyrin* (an EF-hand Ca^{2+}-binding protein) has been shown to interact with *Pax3 in vitro* suggesting that Ca^{2+} itself can alter the DNA-binding activity and subsequent transcriptional activity of *Pax3*.[21] Thus, these combined data indicate that the aortic arch remodeling, outflow tract and interventricular septation defects (occurring ~11.0 dpc) are preceded by a defect in EC-coupling caused by a reduction in Ca^{2+} transients within the *Sp²ᴴ* hearts – almost from the first heartbeat (~9.0 dpc).

Ncx1 (a plasma membrane bound protein that catalyzes the electrogenic exchange of one intracellular Ca^{2+} ion for three extracellular Na^+ ions in all adult mammalian tissues) is one of the earliest functional genes to be expressed in the embryonic mouse heart[22] and there is a rapid upregulation of human *Ncx1* in response to pressure overload, end-stage heart failure, and senescence.[23] Overexpression has been thought to play a cardioprotective role (i.e. to maintain normal cardiac function and intracellular Ca^{2+}-levels). In order to try to determine whether the overexpression of *Ncx1* is beneficial or detrimental within *Sp²ᴴ* homozygotes, we generated a *lacZ* reporter knockin–knockout of *Ncx1*. *Ncx1* null embryos die ~11.5 dpc as they fail to generate a heartbeat and have a completely disorganized contractile apparatus.[20] Following the crossing of *Ncx1* and *Sp²ᴴ* heterozygotes, our results using published methods[20] indicate that *Sp²ᴴ–Ncx1* double homozygous mutants die earlier than +/*Sp²ᴴ–Ncx1* nulls (~9.0 dpc in Plate 34a; see Table 48.1). Interestingly, the lack of one copy of *Ncx1* (~50% reduction in *Ncx1* mRNA) does not adversely affect *Sp²ᴴ*/+ adults or embryos (Plate 34b,c). These data indicate that the *Sp²ᴴ* hearts are upregulating *Ncx1* expression to maintain intracellular Ca^{2+} homeostasis and survive, suggesting that *Ncx1* plays a cardioprotective role in *Sp²ᴴ* hearts and may provide novel insights into how the *in utero* heart functions and adapts to failure.

Acknowledgments
We thank Rhonda Roger and Hongmei Chen for their excellent technical assistance. This work is supported by NIH grants HL60714/HL60104 and

Table 48.1 Embryonic outcomes in various crossing strategies

Genotype – pax3	+/Sp²ᴴ	+/Sp²ᴴ	Sp²ᴴ/Sp²ᴴ	Sp²ᴴ/Sp²ᴴ
– Ncx1ˡᵃᶜᶻ	+/–	–/–	+/–	+/+
13.5 dpc	5	X	3	X
(Litters n = 2)				
9.5 dpc	17	19*	4	X
(Litters n = 5)				

Notes: X = not found; *Ncx1*ˡᵃᶜᶻ +/+ / +/+ & +/+ / +/– are not included in table; * some +/*Sp²ᴴ* x *Ncx1*ˡᵃᶜᶻ nulls have excencephaly (n = 5)

AHA/Southeast grant #0255460B (SJC) and a T32-NIH Integrative Cardiovascular Post-doctoral Research Fellowship (SVK).

References

1 Goulding M, Sterrer S, Fleming J *et al*. Analysis of the *Pax-3* gene in the mouse mutant *splotch*. *Genomics* 1993; **17**: 355–63.

2 Dickman ED, Rogers R, Conway SJ. Abnormal skeletogenesis occurs coincident with increased apoptosis in the *Splotch (Sp²ᴴ)* mutant – putative roles for *Pax3* and *PDGFRα* in rib patterning. *Anat Rec* 1999; **255**: 353–61.

3 Schubert FR, Tremblay P, Mansouri A *et al*. Early mesodermal phenotypes in *splotch* suggest a role for *Pax3* in the formation of epithelial somites. *Dev Dyn* 2001; **222**: 506–21.

4 Creazzo TL, Godt RE, Leatherbury L, Conway SJ, Kirby ML. Role of cardiac neural crest cells in cardiovascular development. *Annu Rev Physiol* 1998; **60**: 267–86.

5 Franz T. Persistent truncus arteriosus in the *Splotch* mutant mouse. *Anat Embryol (Berl)* 1989; **180**: 457–64.

6 Conway SJ, Henderson DJ, Copp AJ. *Pax3* is required for cardiac neural crest migration in the mouse: evidence from the (*Sp²ᴴ*) mutant. *Development* 1997; **124**: 505–14.

7 Conway SJ, Godt RE, Hatcher C *et al*. Neural crest is involved in development of abnormal myocardial function. *J Mol Cell Cardiol* 1997; **29**: 2675–85.

8 Conway SJ, Henderson DJ, Kirby ML, Anderson RH, Copp AJ. Development of a lethal congenital heart defect in the *splotch (Pax3)* mutant mouse. *Cardiovasc Res* 1997; **36**: 163–73.

9 Tassabehji M, Newton VE, Liu XZ *et al*. The mutational spectrum in Waardenburg syndrome. *Hum Mol Genet* 1995; **4**: 2131–7.

10 Banerjee AK. Waardenburg's syndrome associated with ostium secundum atrial septal defect. *J R Soc Med* 1986; **79**: 677–678.

11 Mathieu M, Bourges E, Caron F, Piussan C. Waardenburg's syndrome and severe cyanotic cardiopathy. *Arch Fr Pediatr* 1990; **47**: 657–9.

12 Serbedzija GN, McMahon AP. Analysis of neural crest cell migration in *Splotch* mice using a neural crest-specific *LacZ* reporter. *Dev Biol* 1997; **185**: 139–47.

13 Epstein JA, Li J, Lang D *et al*. Migration of cardiac neural crest cells in *Splotch* embryos. *Development* 2000; **127**: 1869–78.

14 Conway SJ, Bundy J, Chen J *et al*. Abnormal neural crest stem cell expansion is responsible for the conotruncal heart defects within the *Splotch (Sp²ᴴ)* mouse mutant. *Cardiovasc Res* 2000; **47**: 314–28.

15 Kwang SJ, Brugger SM, Lazik A *et al*. *Msx2* is an immediate downstream effector of *Pax3* in the development of the murine cardiac neural crest. *Development* 2002; **129**: 527–3.

16 Jiang X, Rowitch DH, Soriano P, McMahon AP, Sucov HM. Fate of the mammalian cardiac neural crest. *Development* 2000; **127**: 1607–16.

17 Waldo K, Zdanowicz M, Burch J *et al*. A novel role for cardiac neural crest in heart development. *J Clin Invest* 1999; **103**: 1499–507.

18 Kochilas LK, Li J, Jin F, Buck CA, Epstein JA. p57Kip2 expression is enhanced during mid-cardiac murine development and is restricted to trabecular myocardium. *Pediatr Res* 1999; **45**: 635–42.

19 Kruzynska-Frejtag A, Machnicki M, Rogers R, Markwald RR, Conway SJ. *Periostin* (an osteoblast-specific factor) is expressed within the embryonic mouse heart during valve formation. *Mech Dev* 2001; **103**: 183–88.

20 Koushik SV, Wang J, Rogers R *et al*. Targeted inactivation of the sodium-calcium exchanger (*Ncx1*) results in the lack of a heartbeat and abnormal myofibrillar organization. *FASEB J* 2001; **15**: 1209–11.

21 Hollenbach AD, McPherson CJ, Lagutina I, Grosveld G. The EF-hand calcium-binding protein calmyrin inhibits the transcriptional and DNA-binding activity of Pax3. *Biochim Biophys Acta* 2002; **1574**: 321–8.

22 Koushik SV, Bundy J, Conway SJ. Sodium-calcium exchanger is initially expressed in a heart-restricted pattern within the early mouse embryo. *Mech Dev* 1999; **88**: 119–22.

23 Philipson KD, Nicoll DA. Sodium-calcium exchange: a molecular perspective. *Annu Rev Physiol* 2000; **62**: 111–33.

CHAPTER 49

Sarcolipin, a novel regulator of calcium cycling, is preferentially expressed in the murine and human atrium

Susumu Minamisawa, Rumiko Matsuoka

Sarcolipin (SLN) is a 31-amino acid proteolipid in the sarcoplasmic reticulum (SR)[1] and is known to be expressed most abundantly in fast-twitch skeletal muscle, to a lesser extent in slow-twitch skeletal muscle, and to an even lesser extent in human and rabbit cardiac muscle.[2] This tissue distribution corresponds to that of the fast-twitch skeletal muscle SR Ca^{2+} ATPase (SERCA1), and SLN interacts with SERCA1 to modulate its activity.[3,4] By contrast, phospholamban (PLN), an integral membrane protein in the SR, is abundantly expressed in cardiac and slow-twitch skeletal muscle, where SERCA2a is the predominant SERCA isoform.[5] Thus, SLN expression is complementary to PLN expression. SLN's structure and protein sequence are similar to those of PLN.[2] Therefore, SLN and PLN may belong to the same family and SLN could be an analog of PLN in skeletal muscle.

PLN is an endogenous inhibitor of SERCA2 and plays a prime role in cardiac contractility and relaxation.[6,7] The expression of PLN is regulated by developmental, hormonal, and hemodynamic changes.[7] In the heart, PLN is predominantly expressed in the ventricles and to a lower extent in the atria.[8] The different levels of PLN expression in the heart are in part responsible for differences in the contractile parameters between the atrium and the ventricle. In contrast to PLN, the role of SLN in the heart remains unknown, even though SLN may play an important role in skeletal muscle contraction.[9] Since SLN expression is complementary to PLN expression, we hypothesized that SLN expression in the heart is higher in the atrium and is regulated in a developmental stage-specific manner.

We analyzed the distribution of SLN mRNA in various mouse tissues by Northern blot using the PCR-amplified full-length sarcolipin cDNA probe. The probe hybridized to a single transcript of 0.9 kb. SLN mRNA expression was most abundant in the atrium of the heart and to a lesser extent in esophageal muscle and to an even lesser extent in skeletal muscle and bladder (Plate 35a). In the murine myocardium, the expression of SLN mRNA was restricted to the atrium and was not found in the ventricle by Northern blot analysis. In skeletal muscle, the same levels of SLN mRNA expression were detected in fast-twitch skeletal muscle (extensor digitorum longus muscle) and slow-twitch skeletal muscle (soleus muscle). In smooth muscle, SLN mRNA expression was much greater in esophagus than in bladder. SLN mRNA was not expressed in brain, kidney, liver, spleen, thymus, or lung (liver, spleen, thymus, and lung: data not shown) by Northern blot analysis. Although a previous study showed that SLN mRNA expression was weak in the human heart,[2] its chamber-specific localization has remained undetermined. We found that SLN transcripts were highly expressed in the human atrium and were undetectable in the ventricle (data not shown). In contrast to mice, the expression of SLN mRNA in the atrium was weaker than in skeletal muscle in human.

In situ hybridization analysis using the antisense SLN RNA probe also demonstrated that SLN mRNA was expressed only in the atrium, but not in the ventricle of the heart (Plate 35b). The localization of SLN transcript in the atrial myocardium was ubiquitous in the right and left atria.

The developmental changes of SLN mRNA in the atrium were determined by Northern blot analysis using the above probes. Figure 49.1(a) shows that the expression of SLN and SERCA1 mRNA was increased over time in the atria and was not detected in the ventricle of any developmental stage. We examined the developmental changes of SLN mRNA ex-

pression in detail. No SLN transcript was found in embryos at embryonic day 10.5 and the expression of SLN transcript became detectable in the murine atrium at embryonic day 12.5 (Fig. 49.1b). After embryonic day 16.5, the expression of SLN mRNA was suddenly increased and was developmentally upregulated in the atria.

In conclusion, we found that SLN, a counterpart of PLN, was expressed selectively in the murine and human atrial myocardium. The expression of SLN mRNA was developmentally increased in the murine atrium, and was undetectable in the ventricle at any developmental stage. The present study suggests that SLN is likely to be an important regulator of Ca^{2+} cycling in the atrium.

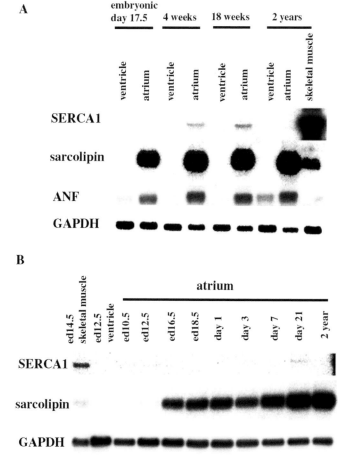

Fig. 49.1 Developmental upregulation of sarcolipin mRNA in the atrial myocardium. (A) The developmental change in the expression of SLN, SERCA1, and ANF mRNA in the atrial and ventricular myocardium. Northern blot analysis revealed that these transcripts are upregulated during development in the atrium. It should be noted that the expression of ANF transcript was also detected in the ventricle of embryos at embryonic day 17.5 and elder mice at 2 years old. (B) The developmental changes in the atrial expression of SLN and SERCA1 mRNA in detail. No SLN transcript was found in embryos at embryonic day 10.5 and the expression of SLN transcript started to be detected in the murine atrium at embryonic day 12.5. After embryonic day 16.5, the expression of SLN mRNA was abruptly increased. These data have been previously published elsewhere.[10]

References

1 Wawrzynow A, Theibert JL, Murphy C *et al.* Sarcolipin, the "proteolipid" of skeletal muscle sarcoplasmic reticulum, is a unique, amphipathic, 31-residue peptide. *Arch Biochem Biophys* 1992; **298**: 620–3.

2 Taschner PE, Scherer SW *et al.* Characterization of the gene encoding human sarcolipin (SLN), a proteolipid associated with SERCA1: absence of structural mutations in five patients with Brody disease. *Genomics* 1997; **45**: 541–53.

3 Odermatt A, Becker S, Khanna VK *et al.* Sarcolipin regulates the activity of SERCA1, the fast-twitch skeletal muscle sarcoplasmic reticulum Ca^{2+}-ATPase. *J Biol Chem* 1998; **273**: 12360–9.

4 Asahi M, Kurzydlowski K, Tada M, MacLennan DH. Sarcolipin inhibits polymerization of phospholamban to induce superinhibition of sarco(endo)plasmic reticulum Ca^{2+}-ATPases (SERCAs). *J Biol Chem* 2002; **277**: 26725–8.

5 Tada M, Toyofuku T. SR Ca(2+)-ATPase/phospholamban in cardiomyocyte function. *J Card Fail* 1996; **2**: S77–85.

6 Luo W, Grupp IL, Harrer J *et al.* Targeted ablation of the phospholamban gene is associated with markedly enhanced myocardial contractility and loss of beta-agonist stimulation. *Circ Res* 1994; **75**: 401–9.

7 Koss KL, Kranias EG. Phospholamban: a prominent regulator of myocardial contractility. *Circ Res* 1996; **79**: 1059–63.

8 Koss KL, Ponniah S, Jones WK, Grupp IL, Kranias EG. Differential phospholamban gene expression in murine cardiac compartments. Molecular and physiological analyses. *Circ Res* 1995; **77**: 342–53.

9 Tupling AR, Asahi M, MacLennan DH, Kurzydlowski K, Tada M. Sarcolipin overexpression in rat slow twitch muscle inhibits sarcoplasmic reticulum Ca^{2+} uptake and impairs contractile function. *J Biol Chem* 2002; **277**: 44740–6.

CHAPTER 50

Developmental aspects of cardiac sensitivity to oxygen deprivation: protective mechanisms in the immature heart

Bohuslav Ostadal, Ivana Ostadalova, Libor Skarka,
Frantisek Kolar, Jan Kopecky

Oxygen deprivation is the main pathophysiological feature of the hypoxemic congenital heart disease; in addition, the immature heart of children who have undergone open-heart surgery is subjected to acute ischemic arrest. It follows that understanding the mechanisms by which cyanotic congenital heart disease modifies the tolerance of the immature heart and how those modifications impact on the possible protective mechanisms during ischemia may provide insight into the therapeutic strategies limiting myocardial damage.[1] Furthermore, ischemic heart disease is no more the disease of the fifth and older decades of life, but its origin and consequences may be essentially influenced already prenatally by genetic factors as well as by risk factors acting during early postnatal development.[2] Accordingly, the experimental studies of the pathogenetic mechanisms of cardiac ischemia/hypoxia must shift to the early ontogenetic periods.

What are the developmental specificities of hypoxic/ischemic injury? Oxygen deprivation is a result of disproportion between the amount of oxygen supplied to the cardiac cell and the amount actually required by the cell. However, the degree of ischemic injury depends not only on the intensity and duration of the hypoxic stimulus but also on the level of cardiac tolerance to oxygen deprivation. This variable is determined by the relationship between myocardial oxygen supply and demand, i.e. myocardial

blood flow and oxygen carrying capacity of blood on the one hand, and the functional state of the cardiac muscle (level of contractile function, systolic wall tension, heart rate, and external work) and basal metabolism on the other. Because most of these determinants change significantly during development, it is understandable that marked ontogenetic changes also underline their common consequence, cardiac tolerance to oxygen deprivation.[3]

Our results have shown that cardiac tolerance to ischemia changes during the early phases of ontogenetic development. Detailed analysis in isolated rat hearts has revealed a significant decrease of tolerance to global ischemia (expressed as postischemic recovery of developed force) from postnatal day 1 to 7; ischemic tolerance remained lower even on day 10.[4,5] Riva and Hearse[6] and Awad *et al.*[7] have observed that the age dependent changes in resistance to global ischemia in the isolated rat heart showed a biphasic pattern, with increasing tolerance from the end of the first postnatal week up to the weaning period, followed by a decline to adulthood. The results, therefore, suggest a possible triphasic pattern of the ontogenetic development of cardiac sensitivity to oxygen deprivation, with a decrease during the first week of life.

The mechanisms of the high resistance of the newborn heart have not yet been satisfactorily clarified. As the mammalian fetus lives at an oxygen partial pressure corresponding to an altitude of 8000 m, newborn mammals exhibit a number of physiologic reactions similar to adaptive mechanisms known from hypoxia-tolerant individuals. The explanation may reflect not a only lower energy demand and greater anaerobic glycolytic capacity, but also higher glycogen reserves, decreased free fatty acid uptake, decreased production of reactive oxygen species, decreased sensitivity to acidosis, and decreased sensitivity to calcium overload.[3] Importantly, mitochondrial oxidative phosphorylation is not completely developed in the rat heart at birth and its maturation is associated with increasing content and specific activity of cytochrome-c oxidase[8] and increasing flux of adenine nucleotides across the inner mitochondrial membrane.[9] However, the mechanisms that modulate the efficiency of mitochondrial energy conversion and might affect myocardial sensitivity to oxygen deprivation during ontogeny require further characterization.

In order to assess changes in the composition of cardiac mitochondria during ontogeny, their content of cytochromes a + a$_3$ was quantified.[10] The specific content of cytochromes in mitochondria increased twofold between birth and postnatal day 30 and declined in older rats (Fig. 50.1). These results indicate that mitochondria of one-month-old rats have a higher content of cytochrome-c oxidase, the terminal part of respiratory chain, compared to animals of other ages. Further experiments were

focused on the ontogeny of uncoupling proteins (UCP2, UCP3) which may be involved in the modulation of coupling between oxidation and phosphorylation in cardiac mitochondria, as well as on the levels of transcripts for adenine nucleotide translocase (ANT1, ANT2) which may modulate mitochondrial energy conversion. Postnatal activation in the expression of UCP2, UCP3, and ANT1 genes resulted in the expression maxima between days 20 and 30. The expression declined following day 20 (UCP2, UCP3) or 30 (ANT1), while the expression of ANT2 decreased continuously during the first month of life. In order to characterize the status of the mitochondrial energy-converting machinery, cardiac mitochondria were isolated and mitochondrial membrane potential (MMP) was evaluated using flow cytometry. In mitochondria isolated on prenatal day 20 (i.e. 2 days before birth) and on postnatal days 1, 2, 5, and 10 only a single population of mitochondria with a relatively high MMP was found. Starting with postnatal day 28, a second population with significantly lower MMP appeared; the proportion between the low- and high-MMP populations of mitochondria steadily increased up to adulthood. Ultrastructural developmental studies indicate[11,12] that the originally chaotic organization of mitochondria and muscle fibers in the immature heart becomes gradually regular and two populations of mitochondria, subsarcolemmal and interfibrillar, typical of the adult myocardium, occur

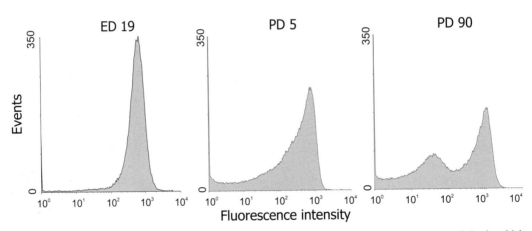

Fig. 50.1 Ontogenetic changes of mitochondrial membrane potential in the rat heart. Measurements were made by flow cytometry in mitochondria isolated from 19-day-old rat embryos (ED19), and from 5-day-old (PD5) and 90-day-old rats (PD90). x-axis, fluorescence intensity (mitochondrial membrane potential); y-axis, number of mitochondria. Data from Skarka et al.[10]

at the weaning period. Our study suggests that both fractions differ in MMP; unfortunately, distinct structural marker and isolation procedure for each population has not yet been identified.[13] Our results point to complex developmental changes in the cardiac mitochondrial energy conversion and ATP/ADP transport across the inner mitochondrial membrane and suggest the involvement of UCP3 and/or ANT1 in controlling this process. UCP3 and ANT1 are thus possible candidates for the determination of cardiac resistance to oxygen deprivation.[10]

Can we protect the highly tolerant immature heart? While a substantial amount of data is available concerning the protection of the adult myocardium, information on whether protective phenomena can be induced also in immature heart is inadequate. In this regard, the two most potent protective mechanisms have been described: long-lasting adaptation to chronic hypoxia,[14] and short–lasting adaptation, called 'ischemic precon-ditioning'.[15] We have observed that ischemic pre-conditioning (IP) induced in isolated perfused rat heart (three 3-min periods of global ischemia followed by 40-min ischemia and 30-min reperfusion) failed to improve recovery of developed force on postnatal day 1 but significant protective effect was observed on days 7 and 10.[4] Prenatal exposure to intermittent high altitude (IHA), simulated in barochamber (5000 m, 8h/day, 5 exposures) failed to increase cardiac tolerance to ischemia in one-day-old hearts, similarly as IP. In contrast, postnatal exposure to IHA significantly improved the recovery

of developed force after ischemia on day 7 and 10; the degree of protection was similar to the effect of IP (Fig. 50.2).[5] It seems, therefore, that decreasing tolerance to oxygen deprivation during early post-natal life is counteracted by the development of en-dogenous protection; both protective phenomena alone failed to improve ischemic tolerance just after birth but their protective effects developed during the early postnatal period.

In this connection the question arises whether is-chemic tolerance of the heart adapted to chronic hy-poxia can be further increased by IP. The clinical relevance of this question is obvious: in children suf-fering from cyanotic congenital heart disease the myocardium is chronically perfused with hypoxic blood which may influence the degree of protection, e.g. during cardiac surgery. We have observed[5] that combination of exposure to simulated IHA and IP induced higher protective effects as compared with both phenomena separately in all age groups under study (i.e. postnatal days 1, 7, and 10). Surprisingly, this effect was significant even on postnatal day 1, where both interventions applied separately failed to improve cardiac tolerance to oxygen deprivation.

The precise mechanism of cardioprotection by adaptation to chronic hypoxia and IP in the adult myocardium is still unclear and the same is true for the immature heart.[16,17] It has been shown that long-term adaptation to chronic hypoxia results in en-hanced activation of mitochondrial K_{ATP} channels in the heart of adult rats,[18,19] as well as in the myocardium of immature rabbits.[20] Similarly, in-creasing evidence has accumulated in support of

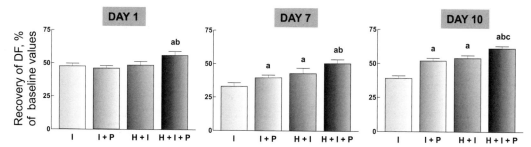

Fig. 50.2 Protection by ischemic preconditioning, adaptation to chronic hypoxia and combination of the two phenomena. Cardiac tolerance to ischemia (expressed as the recovery of developed force – DF – after 40 min ischemia), postnatal days 1, 7, and 10. Effect of ischemia (I), ischemia and preconditioning (I + P) in normoxic animals, and ischemia (H + I) and ischemia with preconditioning (H + I + P) in hypoxic animals. a, significant difference (P < 0.01) from the ischemic group (I); b, from the I + P group; c, from the H + I group. Data from Ostadalova et al.[5]

mitochondrial K_{ATP} channels as a trigger, mediator, and effector of cardioprotection by IP, again both in adult[21] and immature[22] hearts. Furthermore, mediators derived from the endothelium, particularly NO, have been suggested to play a role in the cardioprotective effect of IP in adult dogs[23] as well as adaptation to chronic hypoxia in immature rabbits.[24] We have observed[5] that neither the mitochondrial K_{ATP} channel blocker, 5-hydroxydecanoates nor the NOS inhibitor, L-NAME, abolished the protection by IP in normoxic rats but they decreased significantly the protection by IHA; the final recovery was even lower than the corresponding normoxic values.

In conclusion, ontogenetic development of cardiac sensitivity to oxygen deprivation exhibits a triphasic pattern with a decrease during the first postnatal week. It has been suggested that developmental changes of mitochondrial energy conversion may be involved in the mechanisms of the high resistance of the immature heart. IP and IHA failed to increase hypoxic tolerance of the newborn rat heart; their protective effect develops, however, during the early postnatal period. Combination of exposure to IHA and IP induced higher protective effects as compared with both phenomena separately in all age groups under study, even on postnatal day 1, where both interventions applied separately failed to improve cardiac tolerance to oxygen deprivation. It seems likely that protective mechanisms may differ during ontogenetic development, particularly in neonates. Mitochondrial K_{ATP} channels and NO may be involved in the protective mechanisms of adaptation to chronic hypoxia but not in IP, at least in neonates. It is, however, too soon to reach a definitive conclusion as to whether the mechanisms involved in the protection of the immature heart differ from those in the adult myocardium.

References

1 Baker EJ, Boerboom LE, Olinger GN, Baker JE. Tolerance of the developing heart to ischemia: impact of hypoxemia from birth. *Am J Physiol* 1995; **268**: H1165–73.

2 Fejfar Z. Prevention against ischemic heart disease: a critical review. In: Oliver MF, ed. *Modern Trends in Cardiology*. Boston: Butterworth-Heinemann, 1975: 465–99.

3 Ostadal B, Ostadalova I, Dhalla NS. Development of cardiac sensitivity to oxygen deficiency: comparative and ontogenetic aspects. *Physiol Rev* 1999; **79**: 635–59.

4 Ostadalova I, Ostadal B, Kolar F, Parratt JR, Wilson, S. Ischaemic preconditioning in neonatal rat hearts. *J Mol Cell Cardiol* 1998; **30**: 857–65.

5 Ostadalova I, Ostadal B, Jarkovska D, Kolar, F Ischemic preconditioning in chronically hypoxic neonatal rat heart. *Pediatr Res* 2002; **52**: 561–7.

6 Riva E, Hearse DJ. Age-dependent changes in myocardial susceptibility to ischemic injury. *Cardioscience* 1993; **4**: 85–92.

7 Awad WI, Shattock MJ, Chambers DJ. Ischemic preconditioning in immature myocardium. *Circulation* 1998; **98**: II-206–13.

8 Schagger H, Noack H, Halangk W, Brandt U, Von Jagow G. Cytochrome-c oxidase in developing rat heart. Enzymic properties and amino-terminal sequences suggest identity of the fetal heart and the adult liver isoform. *Eur J Biochem* 1995; **230**: 235–41.

9 Schonfeld P, Schild L, Bohnensack R. Expression of ADP/ATP carrier and expansion of the mitochondrial (ATP + ADP) pool contribute to postnatal maturation of the rat heart. *Eur J Biochem* 1996; **241**: 895–900.

10 Skarka L *et al*. Expression of mitochondrial ucoupling protein 3 and adenine nucleotide tranlocase 1 gene in developing rat heart: putative involvement in control of mitochondrial membrane potential. *J Mol Cell Cardiol* 2003; **35**: 321–30.

11 Ostadal B, Schiebler TH. The development of the capillaries in the rat heart. An electron microscopic study. *Z Anat Entwicklungsgesch* 1971; **133**: 288–304.

12 Palmer JW, Tandler B, Hoppel CL. Biochemical properties of subsarcolemmal and interfibrillar mitochondria isolated from rat cardiac muscle. *J Biol Chem* 1977; **252**: 8731–9.

13 Skarka L, Ostadal B. Mitochondrial membrane potential in cardiac myocytes. *Phys Res* 2002; **51**: 425–34.

14 Poupa O, Krofta K, Prochazka J, Turek Z. Acclimatization to simulated high altitude and acute cardiac necrosis. *Fed Proc* 1966; **25**: 1243–6.

15 Murry CE, Jennings RB, Reimer KA. Preconditioning with ischemia: a delay of lethal cell injury in ischemic myocardium. *Circulation* 1986; **74**: 1124–36.

16 Kolar F. Cardioprotective effects of chronic hypoxia: relation to preconditioning. In: Wainwright CL, Parratt JR, eds. *Myocardial Preconditioning*. Berlin: Springer-Verlag, 1996: 261–75.

17 Ostadal B, Kolar F. *Cardiac Ischemia: From Injury to Protection*. Dordrecht: Kluwer Academic, 1999.

18 Asemu G, Papousek F, Ostadal B, Kolar F. Adaptation to high altitude hypoxia protects the rat heart against ischemia-induced arrhythmias. Involvement of mitochondrial K_{ATP} channel. *J Mol Cell Cardiol* 1999; **31**: 1821–31.

19 Neckar J *et al*. Effects of mitochondrial K_{ATP} modulators on cardioprotection induced by chronic high altitude hypoxia in rats. *Cardiovasc Res* 2002; **55**: 567–75.

20 Eells JT, Henry MH, Gross GJ, Baker JE. Increased mitochondrial K_{ATP} channel activity during chronic myocardial hypoxia: is cardioprotection mediated by improved bioenergetics? *Circ Res* 2000; **87**: 915–21.

21 Baines CP, Wang L, Cohen MV, Downey JM. Myocardial protection by insulin is dependent on phosphatidylinositol 3-kinase but not protein kinase C or K_{ATP} channels in the isolated rabbit hearts. *Basic Res Cardiol* 1999; **94**: 188–98.

22 Baker JE, Holman P, Gross GJ. Preconditioning in immature rabbit heart. Role of K_{ATP} channels. *Circulation* 1999; **99**: 1249–54.

23 Vegh A, Komori S, Szekeres L, Parratt JR. Antiarhythmic effects of preconditioning in anaesthetized dogs and rats. *Cardiovasc Res* 1992; **26**: 487–95.

24 Baker JE *et al.* Nitric oxide activates the sarcolemmal K_{ATP} channel in normoxic and chronically hypoxic hearts by a cyclic GMP-dependent mechanism. *J Mol Cell Cardiol* 2001; **33**: 331–41.

PART 12

Patent ductus arteriosus

Editorial perspective

Toshio Nakanishi

The ductus arteriosus is a large vessel normally present in the fetus, connecting the pulmonary artery with the aorta and allowing blood ejected by the right ventricle to bypass the unexpanded lungs. At birth, the ductus constricts and within several hours functional closure of the ductus occurs. The factors that have been considered to function to maintain potency of the ductus in the fetus are:

1 exposure to low P_{O_2},
2 circulating and locally produced prostaglandin E2, and
3 nitric oxide.

Factors that have been considered to cause postnatal closure of the ductus are:

1 increases in P_{O_2},
2 increases in endothelin-1,
3 decreases in prostaglandin E2, and
4 decreases in the effect of nitric oxide.

Prostaglandins are produced mainly in the ductus and the placenta by the enzyme cyclooxygenase (COX) from arachidonic acid. The ductus in the immature fetus is more sensitive to relaxant effect of prostaglandin E2 than in the mature fetus, for unknown reasons.[1] In animal studies, ductus constriction in response to indomethacin and oxygen is weak in the premature fetus, compared to that in the mature fetus. Nevertheless, in the immature fetus, the constrictive effect of nonspecific inhibitors of COX such as in-

domethacin is greater than that of oxygen.[1] There are two isozymes of COX, COX-1 and COX-2. Gestational changes in the role of COX isozymes in maintaining ductal patency have not been investigated. Toyoshima *et al.* and Momma *et al.* in this part show that both COX-1 and COX-2 play a minor role in dilating the ductus in premature rat fetus and COX-2 plays a more important role in dilating the ductus in the mature rat fetus.

Administration of steroids increases the sensitivity to indomethacin and oxygen in the immature fetus. Takami and Momma show that in both the preterm (19th day) and near-term (21st day) rat fetus, the ductus constricted more with combined administration of dexamethasone and indomethacin than with dexamethasone or indomethacin alone. The mechanisms of ductal constriction induced by steroids remain to be studied.

Previous studies showed that nitric oxide synthase (NOS) exists in the endothelium of the ductus in the late-gestation fetal lamb, but the ductal constriction by a NOS inhibitor was minimal, suggesting that the role of NO in maintaining ductal patency in the mature fetus is minimal.[2,3] Gestational changes in the role of NO in maintaining ductal patency have not been investigated. Momma showed that nitric oxide (NO) plays the major role and PG has a minor role in dilating the ductus in premature fetal rats. In contrast, prostaglandins play the major role and NO plays a minor role in dilating the ductus in the mature fetal rat. Whether this is true in other species remains to be studied.

Changes in Po_2 play an important role in ductal closure after birth. However, the mechanisms of the oxygen-induced ductal constriction remain unclear. Coceani et al.[4,5] hypothesized that endothelin-1 mediates oxygen-induced ductal constriction. Fineman et al.,[6] however, showed that in the fetal lamb endothelin-1 does not mediate oxygen-induced ductal constriction. At least in the rat, mouse, and rabbit, however, previous studies suggest that endothelin plays a significant role in ductal constriction. Furthermore, Momma showed in the rat that endothelin receptor blockers inhibited indomethacin-induced ductal constriction, indicating that pharmacological ductal constriction also depends on endothelin.

In addition to endothelin, Nakanishi et al. hypothesized that oxygen may increase tissue ATP concentration and its increase may close ATP-dependent K channel (K_{ATP}), resulting in the membrane depolarization and ductal constriction. Their study shows that K_{ATP} was underdeveloped in the ductus of the premature fetal rats, supporting the hypothesis that K_{ATP} is one of the O_2 sensors in the ductus.

Oxygen-sensitive voltage-gated K channels (Kv) exist in the ductus and the pulmonary artery. It has been shown that oxygen opens Kv in the pulmonary artery and it closes Kv in the ductus. The mechanisms for this difference remain unclear. Kv is a tetramer of four alpha and four beta subunits. There are many members in the family of Kv and alpha and beta subunits specifically expressed in the ductus have not been detected.[7] Archer and his group hypothesized that

changes in tissue concentrations of reactive oxygen species including H_2O_2 during oxygenation may alter functional characteristics of Kv. The precise mechanisms of regulation of Kv by reactive oxygen species including H_2O_2 in the ductus and the pulmonary artery remains undetermined. Physiological importance of K_{ATP} and Kv in the constriction of the ductus also remains to be clarified. Better understanding of the mechanisms of ductal patency during fetal life and ductal closure after birth are important to develop better management of fetus and newborn with abnormal cardio-pulmonary anatomy and physiology.

References

1 Rudolph AM. The ductus arteriosus and persistent patency of the ductus arteriosus. In *Congenital Diseases of the Heart*. Futura, New York, 2001: 155–96.

2 Fox JJ, Ziegler JW, Ivy DD et al. Role of nitric oxide and cGMP system in regulation of ductus arteriosus tone in ovine fetus. *Am J Physiol* 1996; **40**: H2638–45.

3 Clyman RI, Waleh N, Black SM et al. Regulation of ductus arteriosus patency by nitric oxide in fetal lambs: The role of gestation, oxygen tension, and vasa vasorum. *Pediatr Res* 1998; **43**: 633–44.

4 Coceani F. Control of the ductus arteriosus- a new function for cytochrome p450, endothelin and nitric oxide. *Biochem Pharmacol* 1994; **48**: 1315–18.

5 Coceani F, Liu YA, Kelsey L et al. Endothelin A receptor is necessary for O_2 constriction but not closure of ductus arteriosus. *Am J Physiol* 1999; **277**: H1521–31.

6 Fineman JR, Takahashi Y, Roman C, Clyman RI. Endothelin-receptor blockade does not alter closure of the ductus arteriosus. *Am J Physiol* 1998; **275**: H1620–6.

7 Michelakis E, Rebeyka I, Baterson J, Olley P, Puttagunta L, Archer S. Voltage-gated potassium channels in human ductus arteriosus. *Lancet* 2000; **356**: 134–7.

CHAPTER 51

A comprehensive model for O_2 constriction in the human ductus arteriosus

Evangelos D. Michelakis, Bernard Thébaud, Xi-Chen Wu,
Kyoko Hashimoto, Rohit Moudgil, Gwyneth Harry,
Ivan M. Rebeyka, Stephen L. Archer

Introduction

Closure of the ductus arteriosus (DA) is initiated by an increase in P_{O_2} within minutes of birth. Vasoconstriction of the DA causes *functional closure* and forces blood through the newly expanded lungs. This vasomotor-mediated functional closure is usually complete in 1–3 days after birth and precedes anatomical closure, which results from cell proliferation. Thus O_2-induced DA constriction is a crucial step in the newborn's transition to an air-breathing organism. Failure to achieve early functional closure results in a cardiac shunt, cyanosis, and failure to thrive. The response of the normal term DA to O_2 is robust and rarely fails. However, ~70% of preterm DAs do not close despite adequate oxygenation, resulting in a common form of congenital heart disease, persistent DA. Almost half of preterm infants born before 28 weeks of gestation require either medical or surgical closure of patent DA. Surgical closure of an isolated patent DA can be accomplished with low mortality rates and prostaglandin H synthase inhibitor therapy can now be accomplished using agents such as ibuprofen.[1] Nonetheless, both medical and surgical treatments are associated with complications, especially in small preterm infants. Conversely, PGE is often used to maintain DA patency in certain congenital lesions as a bridge to surgical correction (e.g. single ventricle). Although highly effective, PGE has numerous com-

plications, most notably apnea. Thus there is a need for new therapies to allow one to close the preterm and occasionally to open the term DA. Recently we found that the type 5 phosphodiesterase inhibitor sildenafil (Viagra®) is highly effective in inhibiting DA constriction and perhaps promoting patency.[2] The constrictor response to O_2 is modulated by the endothelium (reinforced by endothelin and inhibited by vasodilator prostanoids and nitric oxide, NO)[3] but is intrinsic to the DA smooth muscle cell (DASMC).[4] O_2 constriction persists *ex vivo*, following endothelial denudation, and in the presence of inhibitors of prostaglandin H synthase, nitric oxide synthase, and endothelin-A receptors.[5,6] We have recently demonstrated that the sequence of events in functional closure of human DA is: alteration of a *redox sensor* (the DASMC's proximal mitochondrial electron transport chain, P-ETC), production of a diffusible *redox messenger* (H_2O_2), and inhibition of an *effector Kv channel*. Kv channel inhibition depolarizes the membrane potential (E_M), and activates L-type Ca^{2+} channels leading to vasoconstriction[7] (Fig. 51.1).

Endothelin modulates DA tone

O_2 induces endothelin synthesis in the DA and this contributes to constriction in near-term sheep DA.[8,9] However, Fineman *et al.* found in the same model that effective endothelin receptor blockade

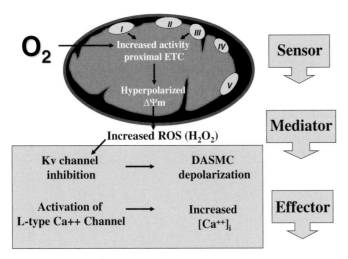

Constriction

Fig. 51.1 Schematic of the mechanism of O_2 constriction in the ductus arteriosus.

does not impair DA constriction to O_2.[10] Although acute O_2 constriction is reduced in mice lacking endothelin-A receptors, they manifest normal DA closure.[11] Our group has shown that *effective* inhibition of endothelin-A receptors and ET converting enzyme does not prevent O_2 constriction in human DA.[6] Since endothelin synthesis is slower to onset (~30 min) than O_2-induced DA constriction, this mechanism may serve to reinforce the early phase of O_2 constriction. Preliminary data suggest that while term DA use the Kv pathway almost exclusively, this mechanism is underdeveloped in preterm DAs (data not shown).

K+ channels and constriction of the DA

O_2- and/or redox-sensitive K+ channels are involved in the acute responses to changes in P_{O_2} of the pulmonary circulation,[12] the type 1 cell of the carotid body,[13] adrenomedullary cells,[14] and the neuroepithelial body.[3] Although this effector mechanism is widely conserved, the type of K+ channel and downstream response to channel inhibition varies amongst species, between tissues, and with maturation. Roulet and Coburn first demonstrated that O_2-induced DA constriction is associated with depolarization of the DASMC membrane potential (E_M) from −55 to −32 mV.[15] Nakanishi *et al.* suggested a role for K_{ATP} channels in this mechanism

based on the concordant effects of glyburide and O_2 in the rabbit DA.[16] However, in term rabbit DAs, we find that O_2 reversibly inhibits a Kv channel, without altering K_{ATP} activity.[7] Furthermore the Kv inhibitor 4-AP causes constriction of similar magnitude to O_2 and there is no additional effect of O_2 when added to 4-AP.[6,7] In addition, both 4-AP and O_2 constriction are completely inhibited by blockers of the L-type Ca^{2+} channel. In contrast, we find that glyburide causes minimal DA constriction. The basis for discordant results between groups is unclear; although glyburide can inhibit Kv channels at the dose Nakanishi used. However, both groups agree that the Ca^{2+} needed for O_2-induced DA constriction enters the cell via the L-type Ca^{2+}.

O_2 sensing, mitochondria and redox sensitive K+ channels in the DASMC

Although the pulmonary artery (PA) and the DA are contiguous, their response to O_2 is reversed. Hypoxia causes pulmonary vasoconstriction vs. DA relaxation. It is intriguing that similar 4-AP sensitive Kv channels are present in PA and DA SMCs.[6,7,17,18] The fact that the Kv inhibitor 4-AP constricts both DA and PA, suggests that the Kv channels setting E_M in the two tissues may be similar and by extension implies that the differential response of the tissues may relate to differences in either the O_2 sensor or the response of the K+ channels to the messenger produced by a common sensor. P-ETC inhibitors (e.g. rotenone and antimycin) mimic hypoxia better than any other class of drugs causing pulmonary vasoconstriction, systemic and DA vasodilatation and carotid body activation, consistent with our hypothesis that mitochondria are widely involved in cardiovascular O_2 sensing.[7,18] Furthermore, mitochondrial membrane potential ($\Delta\Psi$m), a major determinant of the amount of reactive O_2 species (ROS, radicals and peroxides) produced by the mitochondria, changes over a physiological range of Po_2 in the type I cell of the carotid body[19] and the rabbit DA.[7] The effects of P-ETC inhibitors on tone, whole cell K^+ current (I_K), $\Delta\Psi$m, and ROS generation is rapid (onset in 1–2 min), reversible, and initially is not associated with a loss of ATP or a change in Po_2.[7] $\Delta\Psi$m is less sensitive to complex IV inhibition by cyanide in DASMCs than in many other cell types, including cardiac myocytes, perhaps explaining the relative lack of effect of cyanide on DA tone.[7]

What then is the messenger linking the mitochondria to ion channel function and ultimately to vascular tone? Mitochondria are a major source of ROS and H_2O_2 and both hypoxia and P-ETC inhibitors decrease ROS production.[7,18] Most ROS are produced at complex I and III.[20,21] The contribution of various complexes can be dissected using well-validated, specific inhibitors. For example, complexes I–IV are inhibited by rotenone, thenoyltrifuoroacetone (TTFA), antimycin, and cyanide. In addition, complex III can be considered to have proximal and distal components, which are inhibited by myxothiazole and antimycin, respectively.

We postulate that manganese superoxide dismutase (MnSOD) converts superoxide anion, generated at complex I and III,[22] to a ROS with a long effective radius of diffusion (e.g. H_2O_2). H_2O_2 then enters the cytoplasm and, directly or indirectly, alters the function of redox sensitive membrane K^+ channels. Not all K^+ channels are susceptible to redox regulation and not all ROS produce the same effects on channels (i.e. peroxides and superoxide may have different effects).[23] Redox-sensitive channels have critically placed, sulfhydryl groups, usually associated with cysteines or methionines, the redox status of which controls channel gating.[24,25] The redox theory[26] holds that an endogenous sensor (NAD(P)H oxidase or the mitochondrial P-ETC)

delivers a redox messenger (e.g. H_2O_2) to the K^+ channels, in proportion to Po_2. However, there may be important heterogeneity in the type of O_2 sensors, K^+ channels and even in the effect of redox messengers amongst vascular beds. For example, while PASMC K^+ channel are activated by oxidants, oxidants inhibit K^+ channels in other tissues/models. In both the DA and the PA, O_2 increases H_2O_2 production.[7,18] However, in DASMC this increase in endogenous H_2O_2 inhibits I_K;[7,27] whereas in the PAMSC it increases I_K. Furthermore, in the DASMC, removal of endogenous H_2O_2 with intracellular catalase increases normoxic I_K and hyperpolarizes E_M.[27] Conversely, intracellular H_2O_2 (100 nM) and extracellular t-butyl hydroperoxide (100 µM) decrease I_K and depolarize E_M in DASMC. This suggests that ROS could link the sensor with the effector in tissue specific means.

We recently evaluated the mechanism of O_2-constriction in 26 human DAs (12 female, age 9 ± 2 days) studied in their normal hypoxic state or following normoxic tissue culture. In fresh, hypoxic DAs, 4-aminopyridine (4-AP), a Kv inhibitor, and O_2 cause similar constriction and I_K.[7] Tissue culture for 72 h, particularly in normoxia, causes ionic remodeling, characterized by decreased O_2 and 4-AP constriction in DA rings and reduced O_2 and 4-AP sensitive I_K in DASMCs. Remodeled DAMSCs are depolarized and express less O_2-sensitive channels (including Kv2.1, Kv1.5, Kv9.3, Kv4.3, and BK_{Ca}). Kv2.1 adenoviral gene-transfer significantly reverses ionic remodeling, partially restoring both the electrophysiological and hemodynamic responses to 4-AP and O_2. In fresh DASMCs, ETC inhibitors (rotenone and antimycin) mimic hypoxia, increasing I_K and reversing constriction to O_2, but not phenylephrine. O_2 increases, whilst hypoxia and ETC inhibitors decrease, H_2O_2 production by altering mitochondrial membrane potential ($\Delta\Psi$m). H_2O_2, like O_2, inhibits I_K and depolarizes DASMCs.[7] We conclude that O_2 controls human DA tone by modulating the function of the mitochondrial ETC thereby varying $\Delta\Psi$m and the production of H_2O_2, which regulates DASMC Kv1.5 and 2.1 channel activity and DA tone.

Acknowledgments
Drs Michelakis and Archer are supported by the AHFMR, the Canadian Foundation for Innovation

and the Heart and Stroke Foundation of Canada and the CIHR.

References

1 Varvarigou A *et al.* Early ibuprofen administration to prevent patent ductus arteriosus in premature newborn infants. *JAMA* 1996; **275**: 539–44.

2 Thebaud B *et al.* Sildenafil reverses O_2 constriction of the rabbit ductus arteriosus by inhibiting type 5 phosphodiesterase and activating BK(Ca) channels. *Pediatr Res* 2002; **52**: 19–24.

3 Youngson C, Nurse C, Yeger H, Cutz E. Oxygen sensing in airway chemoreceptors. *Nature* 1993; **365**: 153–5.

4 Tristani-Firouzi M, Reeve HL, Tolarova S, Weir EK, Archer SL. Oxygen-induced constriction of the rabbit ductus arteriosus occurs via inhibition of a 4-aminopyridine-sensitive potassium channel. *J Clin Invest* 1996; **98**: 1959–65.

5 Fay FS, Nair P, Whalen WJ. Mechanism of oxygen induced contraction of ductus arteriosus. *Adv Exp Med Biol* 1977; **78**:123–34.

6 Michelakis E *et al.* Voltage-gated potassium channels in human ductus arteriosus. *Lancet* 2000; **356**: 134–7.

7 Michelakis ED. *et al.* O_2 sensing in the human ductus arteriosus: regulation of voltage-gated K^+ channels in smooth muscle cells by a mitochondrial redox sensor. *Circ Res* 2002; **91**: 478–86.

8 Coceani F, Kelsey L. Endothelin-1 release from lamb ductus arteriosus: relevance to postnatal closure of the vessel. *Can J Physiol Pharmacol* 1991; **69**: 218–21.

9 Coceani F, Kelsey L, Seidiltz E. Evidence of an effector role of endothelin in closure of the ductus arteriosus at birth. *Can J Physiol Pharmacol* 1992; **70**: 1061–4.

10 Fineman J, Takahashi Y, Roman C, Clyman R. Endothelin-receptor blockade does not alter closure of the ductus arteriosus. *Am J Physiol* 1998; **44**: H1620–6.

11 Coceani F *et al.* Endothelin A receptor is necessary for O2 constriction but not closure of ductus arteriosus. *Am J Physiol* 1999; **277**: H1521–31.

12 Archer S, Michelakis E. The mechanism(s) of hypoxic pulmonary vasoconstriction: potassium channels, redox O(2) sensors, and controversies. *News Physiol Sci* 2002; **17**: 131–7.

13 López-Barneo J, López-López JR, Ureña J, González C. Chemotransduction in the carotid body: K^+ current modulated by PO2 in type I chemoreceptor cells. *Science* 1988; **241**: 580–2.

14 Zhu WH, Conforti L, Czyzyk-Krzeska M F, Millhorn DE. Membrane depolarization in PC-12 cells during hypoxia is regulated by an O_2-sensitive K^+ current. *Am J Physiol* 1996; **271**: C658–65.

15 Roulet MJ, Coburn RF. Oxygen-induced contraction in guinea pig neonatal ductus arteriosus. *Circ Res* 1981; **4**: 997–1002.

16 Nakanishi T, Gu H, Hagiwara N, Momma K. Mechanisms of oxygen-induced contraction of ductus arteriosus isolated from the fetal rabbit. *Circ Res* 1993; **72**: 1218–28.

17 Archer SL *et al.* Molecular identification of the role of voltage-gated K^+ channels, Kv1.5 and Kv2.1, in hypoxic pulmonary vasoconstriction and control of resting membrane potential in rat pulmonary artery myocytes. *J Clin Invest* 1998; **101**: 2319–30.

18 Michelakis ED. *et al.* Diversity in mitochondrial function explains differences in vascular oxygen sensing. *Circ Res* 2002; **90**: 1307–15.

19 Duchen MR, Biscoe TJ. Relative mitochondrial membrane potential and $[Ca^{2+}]i$ in type I cells isolated from the rabbit carotid body. *J Physiol* 1992; **450**: 33–61.

20 Li Y, Stansbury KH, Zhu H, Trush MA. Biochemical characterization of lucigenin (bis-*N*-methylacridinium) as a chemiluminescent probe for detecting intramitochondrial superoxide anion radical production. *Biochem Biophys Res Commun* 1999; **262**: 80–7.

21 Archer SL, Huang J, Henry T, Peterson D, Weir EK. A redox based oxygen sensor in rat pulmonary vasculature. *Circ Res* 1993; **73**: 1100–12.

22 Herrero A, Barja G. Sites and mechanisms responsible for the low rate of free radical production of heart mitochondria in the long-lived pigeon. *Mech Ageing Dev* 1997; **98**: 95–111.

23 Duprat F *et al.* Susceptibility of cloned K^+ channels to reactive oxygen species. *Proc Natl Acad Sci USA* 1995; **92**: 11796–800.

24 Reeve HL, Weir EK, Nelson DP, Peterson DA, Archer SL. Opposing effects of oxidants and antioxidants on K^+ channel activity and tone in vascular tissue. *Exp Physiol* 1995; **80**: 825–34.

25 Lee S, Park M, So I, Earm Y. NADH and NAD modulates Ca^{2+}-activated K^+ channels in small pulmonary arterial smooth muscle cells of the rabbit. *Pflugers Arch* 1994; **427**: 378–80.

26 Archer S, Will J, Weir E. Redox status in the control of pulmonary vascular tone. *Herz* 1986; **11**: 127–41.

27 Reeve HL, Tolarova S, Nelson DP, Archer S, Weir EK. Redox control of oxygen sensing in the rabbit ductus arteriosus. *J Physiol* 2001; **533**: 253–61.

CHAPTER 52

Pharmacological manipulation of the fetal ductus arteriosus in the rat

Kazuo Momma, Toshio Nakanishi, Shinichiro Imamura, Katsuaki Toyoshima

Pharmacological animal studies of the fetal ductus arteriosus (DA) led to the current medical manipulation of patent ductus arteriosus (PDA) in prematures and in neonatal ductus-dependent congenital heart disease.[1,2] The following studies were done to develop new medical approaches to the neonatal PDA.

Pregnant Wistar rats (term = 21.5 days, weight = 420–530 g) were used as follows: the preterm fetus on the 19th day, and the near-term fetus on the 21st day.[3–6] Drugs were administered through orogastric tube, or injected intraperitoneally (i.p.) or subcutaneously (s.c., i.m.) in the back.[3–6] Doses were calculated assuming the weight of the mother rat as 0.5 kg. Fetal ductus was studied 2, 4, or 8 h after drug administration with delivery by cesarean section and rapid whole-body freezing method. The frozen fetal thorax was cut on a freezing microtome in frontal section, and inner diameters of the ductus, main pulmonary artery, and ascending aorta were measured with a microscope and micrometer.[3–6] In the control fetus with no treatment, the diameters of the ductus and main pulmonary artery (PA) are the same (0.80 mm), and DA/PA is 1.0.[3–6]

Ductus-dilating effects of prostaglandins (PG) (especially of PGE) and ductus-constricting effects of indomethacin have been well established,[1,2] and have been clinically applied.[1,2] We further studied cyclooxygenase (COX, prostaglandin (PG) synthase) inhibitors as follows. All conventional acidic nonsteroidal anti-inflammatory drugs (NSAIDs) such as indomethacin (Indo) constricted the fetal ductus arteriosus dose-dependently and severely in full dose in the near-term rat.[7,8] In rats, as well as in humans, fetal ductal constriction is very different at different gestational stages. Clinically, the human fetal ductus arteriosus does not constrict before 24 weeks of gestation. In the humans, fetal ductal constriction by maternally administered indomethacin begins to appear after 24 weeks, and increases as gestational age increases.[9] Even maximal doses of these drugs, including indomethacin, constricted the ductus only mildly in the preterm fetal rat on the 19th and 20th day of gestation 4. Recently-developed COX-2 inhibitors including celecoxib and rofecoxib in clinical dose constricted the fetal ductus to the same extent as mixed inhibitors including indomethacin10, as shown by Toyoshima et al. (see Chapter 53). Possibly, these COX-2 inhibitors can be used clinically to close the patent ductus arteriosus of the premature infant in place of indomethacin, with less gastrointestinal or other side-effects. COX-1 inhibitor (SC 560) constricted the ductus in the preterm fetus to the same extent as indomethacin and selective COX-2 inhibitors, but significantly less than in the near-term fetus.[11]

The physiological role of nitric oxide (NO) in dilating the fetal ductus arteriosus is not clear. We studied effects of nitric oxide synthase (NOs) inhibitor (L-NAME; N-nitro-L-arginine methyl ester, i.p., s.c.) as follows: in full dose, L-NAME constricted the ductus in the preterm fetus dose-dependently and severely, but only minimally in the near-term fetus.[6] These results combined with those with indomethacin indicate that nitric oxide and prostaglandins dilated the fetal ductus arteriosus, and the major physiologic role switches from NO to PG as the fetal stage advances from preterm to near-term. In addition, combined administration of indomethacin and L-NAME constricts the preterm and near-term fetal ductus synergistically[6,12] (Figs 52.1 & 52.2).

Steroid hormones constrict the ductus arteriosus of the fetal rat dose-dependently, and massive dose constricts the ductus severely.[3] We studied steroid hormones including dexamethasone and betamethasone. Steroid hormones in clinical doses constrict the fetal ductus moderately in the premature and near-term fetal rat.[3,5] Combined administration of dexamethasone and indomethacin constricted the ductus synergistically in the near-term and preterm fetus[5] (Figs 52.1 & 52.2), as shown by Takami and Momma (see Chapter 54). Although the precise mechanisms of ductus-constriction by corticosteroids are not clear, our results are compatible with the reported effect of steroid hormones on release of endothelin.

We have found that vitamin A and retinoic acid increase sensitivity of the fetal ductus to indomethacin and oxygen.[13,14] Our study showed that vitamin A (1 mg/kg, s.c.), administered 1 or 2 days before, potentiated drug-induced ductal constriction in the near-term and preterm fetus. Retinoic acid also potentiated drug-induced ductal constriction in the near-term fetus.[15]

We studied the role of endothelin (ET) in fetal ductal constriction as follows: used endothelin (ET) receptor inhibitors: bosentan (dual blocker) and CI-1020 (selective AT-A blocker).[16] Bosentan (i.p.) inhibited drug-induced ductal constriction in the near-term and preterm rat. In full dose, bosentan (30 mg/kg) and CI-1020 (10 mg/kg) reversed fetal drug-induced ductal constriction completely, indicating that pharmacological fetal ductal constriction depends on endothelin.

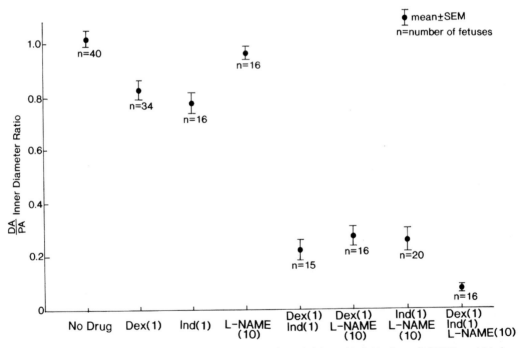

Fig. 52.1 Ductus-constricting effects of indomethacin (1 mg/kg, orogastric), dexamethasone (1 mg/kg, i.m.), and L-NAME (10 mg/kg, i.m.), 4 h after administration in the near-term rat (21st day of gestation). Indomethacin and dexamethasone constricted the fetal ductus only mildly when administered individually, and L-NAME constricted the ductus minimally. Combined administration of two of these three drugs constricted the ductus severely, and simultaneous administration of all three drugs constricted the ductus even more.

Combined Administration of Dex(1),Ind(1) & L-NAME(10) on FD 19

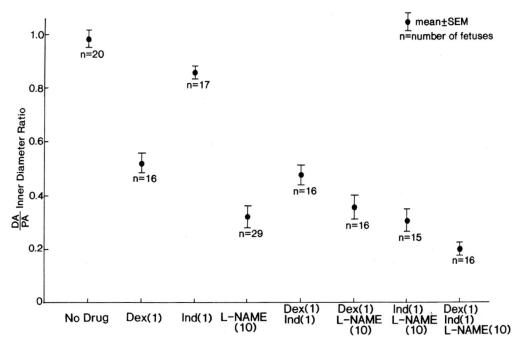

Fig. 52.2 Ductus-constricting effects of indomethacin (1 mg/kg, orogastric), dexamethasone (1 mg/kg, i.m.), and L-NAME (10 mg/kg, i.m.), 4 h after administration in the preterm rat (19th day of gestation). Compared to constriction at the near-term ductus, constriction of the fetal ductus was milder with indomethacin, more with dexamethasone, and severe with L-NAME. Combined administration of indomethacin and dexamethasone constricted the ductus synergistically. Because of severe constriction by L-NAME alone, the addition of indomethacin or dexamethasone to L-NAME did not further increase ductal constriction.

These studies lead to the following conclusions. Major physiological dilators of the fetal ductus are prostaglandins in the near-term fetus and nitric oxide in the preterm fetus. The major physiologic ductal constrictor is endothelin. Combined administration of indomethacin, L-NAME, and dexamethasone synergistically constrict the fetal ductus. Pretreatment with vitamin A potentiates ductal constriction. These experimental results provide a basis for better treatment for the patent ductus arteriosus in the premature infant.

References

1 Rudolph AM. *Congenital Diseases of the Heart.Clinical-Physiological Considerations*, 2nd edn. Armonk, NY: Futura, 2001: 155–96, 769–71.

2 Corbet AJ In: *The Science and Practice of Pediatric Cardiology*, 2nd edn. Garson A Jr, Bricker JT, Fisher DJ, Neish, SR eds. Baltimore, MD: Williams & Wilkins, 1998: 2489–514.

3 Momma K, Nishihara S, Ota Y. Constriction of the fetal ductus arteriosus by glucocorticoid hormones. *Pediatr Res* 1981; **15**: 19–21.

4 Momma K, Takao A. In vivo constriction of the ductus arteriosus by nonsteroidal antiinflammatory drugs in near-term and preterm fetal rats. *Pediatr Res* 1987; **22**: 567–72.

5 Momma K, Takao A. Increased constriction of the ductus arteriosus with combined administration of indomethacin and betamethasone in fetal rats. *Pediatr Res* 1989; **25**: 69–75.

6 Momma K, Toyono M. The role of nitric oxide in dilating the fetal ductus arteriosus in rats. *Pediatr Res* 1999; **46**: 311–15.

7 Momma K, Takeuchi H. Constriction of fetal ductus arteriosus by non-steroidal anti-inflammatory drugs. *Prostaglandins* 1983; **26**: 631–43.

8 Momma K, Takeuchi, H, Konishi T. Constriction of fetal ductus arteriosus by non-steroidal anti-inflammatory

drugs: study of additional 34 drugs. *Prostaglandins* 1984; **28**: 527–36.

9   Vermillion ST *et al.* The effect of indomethacin tocolysis on fetal ductus arteriosus with advancing gestational age. *Am J Obstet Gynecol* 1997; **177**: 256–61.

10 Toyoshima K, Takeda A, Momma K. Constriction of ductus arteriosus by selective cyclooxygenase (COX)-2 inhibitors in fetal rats. *Jap J Neonatol* 2001; **37**: 635–41 [in Japanese].

11 Takeda A. Constriction of ductus arteriosus by a selective cyclooxygenase (COX)-1 inhibitor in fetal rats. *Jap J Neonatol* 2002; **38** [in Japanese].

12 Seidner SR *et al.* Combined prostaglandin and nitric oxide inhibition produces anatomic remodeling and closure of the ductus arteriosus in the premature newborn baboon. *Pediatr Res* 2001; **50**: 365–73.

13 Momma K, Toyono M, Miyagawa-Tomita S. Accelerated maturation of fetal ductus arteriosus by maternally administered vitamin A in rat. *Pediatr Res* 1998; **43**: 629–32.

14 Wu GR, Jing S, Momma K, Nakanishi T. The effect of vitamin A on contraction of the ductus arteriosus in fetal rat. *Pediatr Res* 2001; 49: 747–54

15 Momma K. In: Clark EB, Nakazawa M, Takao A, eds. *Etiology and Morphogenesis of Congenital Heart Disease.* Armonk, NY: Futura, 2000: 261–264.

16 Momma K, Nakanishi T, Imamura S. Inhibition of *in vivo* constriction of fetal ductus arteriosus by endothelin receptor blockade in rats. *Pediatr Res* 2003; **53**: 479–85.

CHAPTER 53

Constriction of ductus arteriosus by selective inhibition of cyclooxygenase-1 and -2

Katsuaki Toyoshima, Atsuhito Takeda, Shinichiro Imamura, Kazuo Momma

A widely-patent ductus arteriosus is essential for fetal well-being because it allows 90% of the right ventricular output to bypass the high resistance pulmonary vascular bed *in utero*.[1]

Prostaglandin (PG)E plays an active role in dilating the ductus arteriosus (DA).[2,3] Cyclooxygenase (COX) is the central enzyme in the PG synthetic pathway. COX converts arachidonic acid to PGH_2, which is then further metabolized to various PGs. Since 1991, two COX isoforms have been identified, COX-1 and COX-2.[4] COX-1 is constitutively expressed by most tissues and seems to be responsible for homeostatic functions, while COX-2 is inducible and associated with inflammation.[4] Recently, selective COX-1 inhibitor and COX-2 inhibitor have been developed.[5,6] The selective COX-2 inhibitor is now being used as an anti-inflammatory agent with fewer side-effects owing to COX-1 inhibition.[5] The aim of this study was to examine the relative importance of COX-1 and COX-2 for dilating the DA in fetal rats. We studied the ductal constrictive effects of a selective COX-1 inhibitor and a selective COX-2 inhibitor, compared with a mixed COX inhibitor on the 19th day of pregnancy (preterm) and the 21st day of pregnancy (near-term) in rats. SC560 is a selec-tive COX-1 inhibitor (COX-1 $IC_{50} = 0.009\,\mu m$; COX-2 $IC_{50} = 6.3\,\mu m$).[5] Rofecoxib is a selective COX-2 inhibitor (COX-1 $IC_{50} = 63\,\mu m$; COX-2 $IC_{50} = 0.31\,\mu m$), which has been used as an anti-inflammatory drug in the USA. Indomethacin is a non-selective COX inhibitor (COX-1 $IC_{50} = $ 0.013 μm; COX-2 $IC_{50} = 0.13\,\mu m$), which has been used to close the patent ductus arteriosus in premature infants. The fetal ductus arteriosus was measured using the rapid whole-body freezing technique, as reported previously.[7,8] The inner diameters of the pulmonary artery (PA) and DA were measured under a binocular microscope with a micrometer. We calculated the ratio of DA/PA (1.0 in control) which was used to evaluate the constrictive effects of the drugs.

The results of the experiments are shown in Figs 53.1 and 53.2. The dose–response curves after administration of the three drugs show dose-dependent constriction of the DA. As shown in Fig. 53.1, on the 19th day there was no difference between the effects of SC560, rofecoxib, and indomethacin. As shown in Fig. 53.2, on the 21st day, the most prominent constriction of the fetal DA was caused by rofecoxib rather than SC560. As shown in Figs 53.1 and 53.2, fetal ductal constriction by rofecoxib and indomethacin was significantly stronger on the 21st day than on the 19th day. There was no statistical difference in the ductal constrictive effect of SC560 on the 19th day and the effect on the 21st day.

The present study demonstrates that COX-1 and COX-2 develop unevenly in the DA in fetal rat. Some reports have been published on the role of COX-2 in fetal lamb and pig DA.[9-12] Fetal lamb DA expressed both COX-1 and COX-2-immunoreactive protein by Western analysis. Although COX-1 was found in both endothelial and smooth muscle cells, COX-2

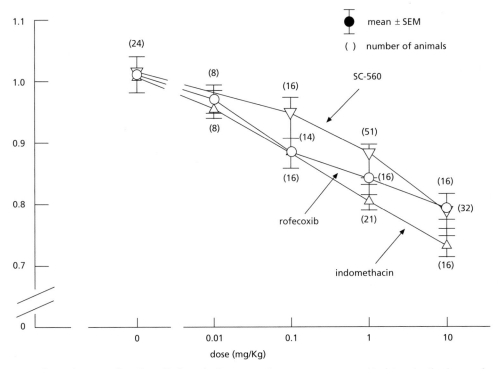

Fig. 53.1 Effects of SC-560, rofecoxib, and indomethacin on ductal constriction in 19-day gestation rat embryos. The ratio of the ductus arteriosus inner diameter to that of the pulmonary artery was used to determine the degree of ductal constriction (the ratio = 1 in controls) and is plotted on the y-axis.

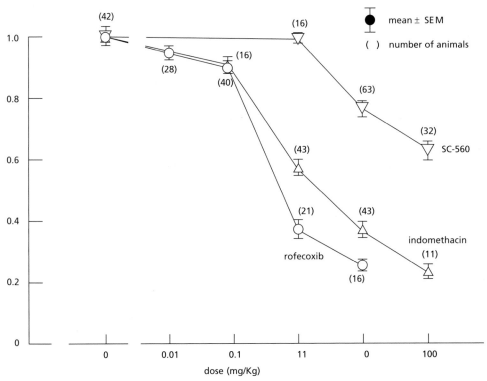

Fig. 53.2 Effects of SC-560, rofecoxib, and indomethacin on ductal constriction in 21-day gestation rat embryos. The ratio of the ductus arteriosus inner diameter to that of the pulmonary artery was used to determine the degree of ductal constriction (the ratio = 1 in controls) and is plotted on the y-axis.

was found only in the endothelial cells lining the ductus lumen by immunohistochemistry.[10] It was demonstrated that COX-1 and COX-2 develop unevenly in the DA. While the two enzymes sustain PGE formation at term gestation, COX-2 contributes little to this process in the preterm. COX-2 function, however, may increase upon exposure to a physiological stimulus such as oxygen, and during treatment with endotoxin.[12]

We found that both COX-1 and COX-2 play a minor role in dilating the DA in preterm fetal rats. PG induced by COX-2 assumes the major role in dilating the DA in the near-term. Both COX isoforms are found naturally in the amnion and chorion.[13] It has been shown that, at term, amnion COX-2 expression at the mRNA level exceeds that of COX-1 100-fold.[13,14] Sawdy *et al.* have found that fetal membranes contain both COX-1 and COX-2 at term, but only COX-2 contributes towards PG synthesis.[15] Previously, we showed that nitric oxide (NO) plays the major role and PG has a minor role in dilating the DA in preterm fetal rats. In contrast, PG plays the major role and NO plays a minor role in dilating the ductus in the near-term.[16] This changeover of the DA dilating mechanism resulting from a fetal environmental change, including that of the placenta, may have caused the increased COX-2 expression. It may lead to DA constriction immediately after birth when the supply of PGE from the placenta disappears.

Methods

Materials

Virgin Wistar rats were mated overnight from 17.00 to 09.00 hours, and the presence of sperm in vaginal smears was designated day 0 of gestation. Fetal rats from pregnant dams (term = 21.5 days) were used as follows: the preterm fetus on the 19th day, and the near-term fetus on the 21st day. SC560 (SC, Searle) is a COX-1 inhibitor.[5] Rofecoxib (Rof, Merk) is a COX-2 inhibitor.[6] Indomethacin (Indo, Banyu) is a mixed COX inhibitor.

Rapid whole-body freezing technique

Each drug was administered through an oro-gastric tube in a suspension of 2 mL water containing 5% arabic gum on the the 19th and 21st days of pregnancy. The fetal ductus arteriosus was measured

using the rapid whole-body freezing technique. The animals were killed 4 h later by cervical dislocation, and the fetuses were delivered quickly by cesarean section. The fetuses were fixed within 5 s by a rapid whole-body freezing technique using acetone cooled to –80°C by dry-ice. The frozen thorax was cut on a freezing microtome (Freezing Microtome; Komatsu Solidate Co., Tokyo, Japan) in the frontal plane. The frontal plane, defined as the plane perpendicular to the long axis of the DA was measured in the sections. The inner diameters of the pulmonary artery (PA) and DA were measured under a binocular microscope (Nikon Binocular Stereoscopic Microscope; Nihon Kogaku Co., Tokyo, Japan) with a micrometer (Nikon Ocular Micrometer, Nihon Kagaku Co., Tokyo, Japan). We calculated the ratio of DA/PA.

Statistics

The results are expressed as means ± SEM. Two- and three-way analysis of variance were used and the statistical significance of differences between group means was determined by the modified t statistics. The difference was considered to be significant if the p value was < 0.05.

Acknowledgment

The authors thank Ms Barbara Levene for editiorial help.

References

1 Heymann MA, Rudolph AM. Control of the ductus arteriosus. *Physiol Rev* 1975; **55**: 62–78.

2 Coceani F, Olley PM. The response of the ductus arteriosus to prostaglandins. *Can J Physiol Pharmacol* 1973; **51**: 220–5.

3 Momma K, Uemura S, Nishihara S et al. Dilatation of the ductus arteriosus by prostaglandins and prostaglandin's precursor. *Pediatr Res* 1980; **14**: 1074–7.

4 Vane JR, Botting RM. Mechanism of action of nonsteroidal anti-inflammatory drugs. *Am J Med* 1998; **104**: 2S-8S.

5 Warner TD, Giuliano F, Vane JR et al. Nonsteroid drug selectivities for cyclo-oxygenase-1 rather than cyclo-oxygenase-2 are associated with human gastrointestinal toxicity: A full *in vitro* analysis. *Proc Natl Acad Sci USA* 1999; **96**: 7563–8.

6 Smith CJ, Zhang Y, Koboldt CM et al. Pharmacological analysis of cyclooxygenase-1 in inflammation. *Proc Natl Acad Sci USA* 1998; **95**: 13313–18.

7 Momma K, Takeuchi H. Constriction of fetal ductus arteriosus by non-steroidal anti-inflammatory drug. *Prostaglandins* 1983; **26**: 631–43.

8 Momma K, Hagiwara H, Konishi T. Constriction of fetal ductus arteriosus by non-steroidal anti-inflammatory drug: study of additional 34 drugs. *Prostaglandins* 1984; **28**: 527–36.

9 Guerguerian AM, Hardy P, Clyman RI *et al*. Expression of cyclooxygenases in ductus arteriosus of fetal and newborn pigs. *Am J Obstet Gynecol* 1998; **179**: 1618–26.

10 Clyman RI, Hardy P, Waleh N *et al*. Cyclooxygenase-2 plays a significant role in regulating the tone of the fetal lamb ductus. *Am J Physiol* 1999; **276**: R913–21.

11 Takahashi Y, Roman C, Chomtob S *et al*. Cyclooxygenase-2 inhibitors constricts the fetal lamb ductus arteriosus both *in vitro* and *in vivo*. *Am J Physiol Regulatory Integrative Comp Physiol* 2000; **278**: R1496–505.

12 Coceani F, Ackerley C, Seidlitz E *et al*. Function of cyclo-oxygenase-1 and cyclooxygenase-2 in the ductus arteriosus from foetal lamb: differential development and change by oxygen and endotoxin. *Br J Pharmacol* 2001; **132**: 241–51.

13 Slater DM, Berger LC, Newton R *et al*. Expression of cyclooxygenase types 1 and 2 in human fetal membranes at term. *Am J Obstet Gynecol* 1995; **172**: 77–82.

14 Slater DM, Berger LC, Newton R *et al*. Expression of cyclooxygenase types 1 and 2 in human fetal membranes throughout pregnancy. *J Mol Endocrinol* 1999; **22**: 125–30.

15 Sawdy RJ, Slater DM, Dennes WJB *et al*. The roles of the cyclo-oxygenases types one and two in prostaglandin synthesis in human fetal membranes at term. *Placenta* 2000; **21**: 54–7.

16 Momma K, Toyono M. The role of nitric oxide in dilating the fetal ductus arteriosus in rats. *Pediatr Res* 1999; **46**: 311–15.

CHAPTER 54

Synergistic constriction of ductus arteriosus by indomethacin and dexamethasone in fetal rats

Takeshi Takami, Kazuo Momma

Indomethacin, one of the classical nonsteroidal anti-inflammatory drugs (NSAIDs), has been widely used to close the patent ductus arteriosus (PDA) in premature infants. However, it has some side-effects, such as renal failure, active bleeding, and thrombocytopenia, and may fail to close the PDA in some cases. Steroid hormone constricted the fetal ductus dose-dependently and moderately in premature and near-term fetal rats.[1] Dexamethasone is a pure glucocorticoid without mineralocorticoid activity and is approximately 30 times more potent than hydrocortisone. To find a better treatment for PDA in premature infants, we studied the synergism of regular doses of dexamethasone and indomethacin on the fetal ductus in rats.

Pregnant Wistar rats (term = 21.5 days) were used as follows: the preterm fetus on the 19th day and the near-term fetus on the 21st day. To study the *in situ* morphology of the fetal DA, a rapid whole-body freezing method was used as described in an earlier study.[1] Dexamethasone (0.3 mg/kg) or indomethacin (0.3 mg/kg) alone or in combination were administered either through an orogastric tube or injected intraperitoneally. From 2 to 8 h later, the fetuses were delivered by cesarean section with atlas dislocation of the mother, and frozen immediately in acetone cooled to −80°C by dry ice. The frozen thorax was cut on a freezing microtome in the frontal plane, and the inner diameters of the ascending aorta, the main pulmonary artery, and the DA were measured with a microscope and a micrometer. The narrowest diameter of the DA was used to get the ratio of the inner diameter of the DA to the main pulmonary artery (DA/PA). The DA/PA, which was 1.0 in controls, was studied at 2, 4, and 8 h after simultaneous administration of dexamethasone and/or indomethacin. Results are expressed as mean ± SEM. The statistical significance of differences between group means was determined separately by ANOVA and Fisher's PLSD methods.

In both the preterm (19th day) rats and near-term (21st day) rats, the fetal DA constricted more with combined administration of dexamethasone and indomethacin than with dexamethasone or indomethacin alone at 2, 4, and 8 h after administration (Figs 54.1 & 54.2). Especially in near-term rats, combined administration of dexamethasone and indomethacin caused severe ductal constriction, with a DA/PA of 0.56 ± 0.05 ($n = 16$) at 4 h and 0.52 ± 0.08 ($n = 16$) at 8 h, respectively.

Several mechanisms have been proposed in the literature for the reduction in the incidence of PDA associated with glucocorticoids. These include diuresis, interference with prostaglandin synthesis, and a reduced sensitivity of the ductal muscle to prostaglandin E_2.[2,3] Clinically, corticosteroid therapy has recently been widely used in the perinatal period. There is conclusive evidence that treatment of women with a course of corticosteroids before preterm delivery reduces the risk of respiratory distress syndrome (RDS), mortality, and intraventricular hemorrhage (IVH).[4] Meta-analyses showed that postnatal corticosteroids significantly reduced the risk of chronic lung disease (CLD) and death of

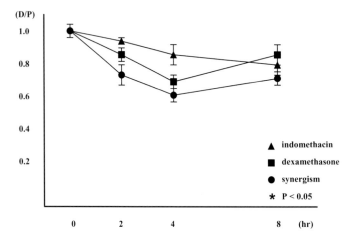

Fig. 54.1 Administration of dexamethasone and indomethacin in preterm (19th day) rats. The fetal DA constricted more with combined administration of dexamethasone and indomethacin than with dexamethasone or indomethacin alone at 2, 4, and 8 h after administration.

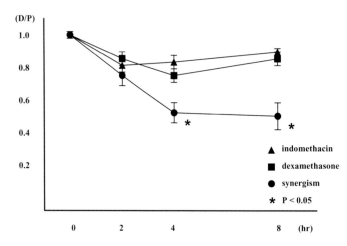

Fig. 54.2 Administration of dexamethasone and indomethacin in near-term (21st day) rats. The fetal DA also constricted more with combined administration of dexamethasone and indomethacin than with dexamethasone or indomethacin alone at 2, 4, and 8 h after administration.

infants at 28 postnatal days and 36 postmenstrual weeks, facilitated earlier extubation, and reduced the later use of corticosteroids.[5,6] Since respiratory distress syndrome (RDS) is associated with inflammation, it has been hypothesized that a long delay in anti-inflammatory therapy may lead to a critical degree of lung injury. The most common dosage regimen is 0.5 mg/kg/day divided into two daily doses and tapered over a period of 7–42 days. On the other hand, adverse effects of dexamethasone include poor growth and weight gain during treatment, hypertension, gastrointestinal hemorrhage and perforation, and hyperglycemia. Recently, there is increasing concern that postnatal corticosteroid treatment has adverse effects on neurodevelopment.[7]

In conclusion, we studied the time course of constriction of the fetal DA using regular doses of

dexamethasone and indomethacin. Ductal constriction was significantly increased by combined administration of dexametasone in near-term fetal rats. Clinically, further study is needed to evaluate the long-term risk and benefits of treating neonates with potent systemic steroids.

References

1 Momma K, Nishihara S, Ota Y. Constriction of the fetal ductus arteriosus by glucocorticoid hormones. *Pediatr Res* 1981; **15**: 19–21.
2 Heyman E, Ohlsson A, Shennan AT, Heilbut M, Coceani F. Closure of patent ductus arteriosus after treatment with dexamethasone. *Acta Paediatr Scand* 1990; **79**: 698–700.
3 Clyman RI, Mauray F, Roman C, Rudolph AM, Heymann MA. Glucocorticoids alter the sensitivity of the ductus arteriosus to prostaglandin E2. *J Pediatr* 1981; **98**: 126–8.

4 Crowley P. Prophylactic corticosteroids for preterm birth. *Cochrane Database Syst Rev* 2000; CD 000065.

5 Halliday HL, Ehrenkranz RA. Early postnatal (<96 hours) corticosteroids for preventing chronic lung disease in preterm infants. *Cochrane Database Syst Rev* 2000; CD 001146.

6 Halliday HL, Ehrenkranz RA. Moderately early (7–14 days) postnatal corticosteroids for preventing chronic lung disease in preterm infants. *Cochrane Database Syst Rev* 2000; CD 001144.

7 Whitelaw A, Thoresen M. Antenatal steroids and the developing brain. *Arch Dis Child Fetal Neonatal Ed* 2000; **83**: F154–7.

PART 13

Human clinical genetics and epidemiology

Editorial perspective

Deepak Srivastava

The epidemiology of congenital cardiovascular malformations has been studied for many decades, but only recently have genetic studies been possible. There are many genes, discussed throughout this book, that can cause congenital cardiovascular malformations (CCVMs) in an autosomal dominant fashion. In this section, examples are provided which show that mutations of genes responsible for familial CCVM can also cause sporadic disease but with incomplete penetrance and variable expressivity. The incidence of various genetic mutations in subsets of diseases is studied including those involving atrioventricular septation, the conotruncus, and valvular diseases. The combination of genetic factors and environmental agents is also explored in an attempt to link genetic risk factors to potential 'second hits'. An integrated approach combining human mutation screens of known candidate cardiac developmental genes along with epidemiologic and developmental studies will be instrumental in connecting the clinical genetics with cardiac developmental advances. The utility of this approach is highlighted in this section.

CHAPTER 55

Prevalence of congenital heart diseases in the Czech Republic

Milan Šamánek

Figures on the prevalence of congenital heart malformations (CHM) at birth range from 2.10[1] to 12.3[2] per 1000 live births. The oldest studies give a lower mean value of 5.2 per 1000 live births than the recent surveys which show the mean value of 7.7 per 1000 live births ranging from 4.23[3] to 12.23[4] per 1000 live births. In the countries neighboring the Czech Republic, a mean value of 8.07 was found. The lowest mean value of 7.1 per 1000 live births was found in German Bavaria and the highest of 10.60 in Szolnok Hungary in a study with small numbers. Much lower mean values of only 3.97 per 1000 live births were found in Canada, followed by the United States with 5.76 per 1000 live births. Having analyzed this data, we came to the conclusion that the majority were subject to some sources of error. Beside the inadequate size of some studies, those based on hospital statistics had the problem of selection bias, many were inaccurate because of diagnostic errors, or omission of clinically insignificant CHM, but a frequent source of error was incomplete validation of diagnoses by autopsy in those who died. This review outlines our own findings on the prevalence of CHM and on their severity.

The prevalence of CHM at birth was studied in all 816 569 children born live in Bohemia between the years 1980 and 1990.[5] All live-born children were examined by a pediatrician at birth, at 14 days and 6 weeks, and then 3 times in the first year and re-examined at the ages of 3, 7, and 15 years by a pediatrician. Children with suspected or confirmed CHM were referred to a pediatric cardiologist or directly to our Center for further investigation. This always included echocardiography and catheterization when necessary. Cardiac surgery was carried out only in

our Center. All children who died at home or in the hospital, not only those with heart disease, were autopsied.

In total, 5030 infants were born with CHM. This gives a CHM prevalence of 6.16 per 1000 live births. In addition to these congenital heart malformations, there were some other heart diseases such as 140 children with cardiomyopathy, 93 with a severe mitral valve prolapse, 44 with vascular ring, 9 with isolated aortic regurgitation, and 4 with isolated tricuspid regurgitation. The prevalence was higher to 1985 with a mean value of 6.68 per 1000 of live births than later on, when the figures of prevalence decreased to a mean value of 5.32 per 1000 of births. A reason for this difference is seen in the expansion of fetal diagnosis and the possibility of terminating cardiac-affected pregnancies. Of 561 CHM diagnosed prenatally, 61.5% of the parents opted to terminate the pregnancy and 15.3% of fetuses died spontaneously. There were a definite seasonal and regional differences in the prevalence of CHM and their individual types. The most frequent CHM was ventricular septal defect (41.59%), followed by atrial septal defect (8.67%) and aortic stenosis (7.77%) (Table 55.1).

Pulmonary stenosis, transposition of the great arteries, coarctation of the aorta, and patent ductus arteriosus occurred in a relative frequency from 5% to 6%. Atrioventricular septal defect (4%), hypoplastic left heart syndrome (3.42%), and tetralogy of Fallot (3.36%) were the next frequent malformations. Double outlet right ventricle, double inlet ventricle, common arterial trunk, and pulmonary atresia occurred in between 1.05% and 1.37% of all cases. The lowest prevalences were found for total anomalous

Table 55.1 Prevalence of congenital heart diseases at live birth

Heart malformation	No. of patients	Prevalence per 1000 live births	% of all heart malformations
Ventricular septal defect	2092	2.56	41.59
Atrial septal defect	436	0.53	8.67
Aortic stenosis	391	0.48	7.77
Pulmonary stenosis	292	0.36	5.81
Transposition of the great arteries	271	0.33	5.39
Coarctation of the aorta	266	0.33	5.29
Persistent ductus arteriosus	255	0.31	5.07
Atrioventricular septal defect	201	0.25	4.00
Hypoplastic left heart	172	0.21	3.42
Tetralogy of Fallot	169	0.21	3.36
Double-outlet right ventricle	69	0.08	1.37
Double inlet ventricle	67	0.08	1.33
Persistent truncus arteriosus	55	0.07	1.09
Pulmonary atresia with ventricular septal defect	55	0.07	1.09
Pulmonary atresia with intact ventricular septum	53	0.06	1.05
Total anomalous pulmonary venous drainage	40	0.05	0.80
Tricuspid atresia	39	0.05	0.78
Ebstein´s anomaly of the tricuspid valve	22	0.03	0.44
Interrupted aortic arch	19	0.02	0.38
Anomalous origin of the left coronary artery	11	0.01	0.22
Others	27	0.03	0.53
Total	5030	6.16	100.00

pulmonary venous connection (0.80%), tricuspid atresia (0.78), Ebstein's anomaly of the tricuspid valve (0.44%), interrupted aortic arch (0.38%), and anomalous origin of the coronary arteries (0.22%).

Within the category of critical CHM were placed children urgently admitted with deep cyanosis, severe congestive heart failure or both and those where CHM itself had terminated in death. In total, 35.3% of patients with CHM (2.36 per 1000 live births) suffered from a critical CHM, most frequently those with hypoplastic left heart (94%), transposition of the great arteries (84%), and double inlet ventricle and tricuspid atresia (77%). In total, 58% of neonates whose cause of death was identified as due to CHM died for other than cardiac reasons.

In conclusion, the prevalence of CHM in a 10-year study in which all children who died, not only those with CHM, were subjected to autopsy and those with suspected CHM were examined by echocardiography was 6.16 per 1000 live births. The prevalence before fetal detection and before possible termination of pregnancy was introduced 6.68 per 1000 live births and it decreased to 5.32 per 1000 after introducing fetal echocardiography and premature termination of pregnancy. The prevalence of critical CHM is 2.36 per 1000 live births. There are annual, seasonal, and regional variations in the total and individual prevalence. Ventricular and atrial septal defects are the most frequent CHM, followed by aortic and pulmonary stenoses and transposition of the great arteries.

References

1 Fyler DC. Report of the New England regional infant cardiac program. *Pediatrics* 1980; **65**(Suppl.): 376–461.

2 Manetti A, Pollini I, Cecchi F *et al.* Epidemiologia delle malformazion cardiovascollari III. Prevalenza e decorso in 46.895 nati vivi al Maternita di Carregi, Firenze, nel periodo 1975–1984. *G Ita Cardiol* 1993; **23**: 145–52.

3 Ferenz Ch, Loffredo Ch, Correa–Villaseñor A, Wilson PD. Genetic and environmental risk factors of major cardiovas-

cular malformations: The Baltimore–Washington Infant Study 1981–1989. In: *Perspectives in Pediatric Cardiology.* Armonk, NY: Futura, 1997: 337–58.

4 Robida A, Folger GM, Hajar HA. Incidence of congenital heart disease in Quatari children. *Int J Cardiol* 1997; **60**: 19–22.

5 Šamánek M, Vorísková M. Congenital heart disease among 818,569 children born between 1980 and 1990 and their 15-year survival: a prospective Bohemia survival study. *Pediatr Cardiol* 1999; **20**: 411–417.

CHAPTER 56

Gene–environment interactions in congenital heart disease: an epidemiological perspective

Christopher A. Loffredo

Epidemiologists study populations of affected and non-affected individuals to gain insights into the causes and prevention of diseases. In this context, the Baltimore–Washington Infant Study (BWIS) has advanced the understanding of congenital cardiovascular malformations (CCVM) by generating hypotheses about genetic and environmental risk factors.[1,2] At the present time of growing interest in using molecular tools to investigate basic mechanisms of normal and abnormal cardiogenesis, it is important to consider not only the separate roles of genetics and the environment, but also how they might interact to cause CCVM. For such studies to be successful, epidemiological science is needed to provide insights into how genes and environmental factors affect human populations, and basic science disciplines are needed to identify candidate genes and test possible teratogenic agents, and to develop experimental models to test hypotheses generated by population studies (Fig. 56.1). This report aims to summarize the findings of the BWIS in the context of gene–environment interactions, to stimulate productive future collaborations between the biological disciplines.

In a summary report on the prevention of birth defects and other adverse reproductive outcomes, the National Institute for Occupational Safety and Health identified major gaps in knowledge which have hindered the identification of risk factors and implementation of preventive strategies.[3] Among the identified research needs was a call to investigate the influence of genetic susceptibility, i.e. the genetic

basis for differential responses of individuals to exposures to developmental toxicants. A search for such gene–environment interactions in the etiology of CCVM represents an important, yet largely unexplored, research topic that may provide important clues for prevention of such malformations. Recent developments in molecular biology have identified genes that govern the metabolism of toxicants, and variants in these genes that result in altered metabolism. At the same time, epidemiological investigations have begun to describe associations of specific birth defects with maternal exposures to toxicants during pregnancy. These efforts have created a new research horizon by making it possible to examine the extent to which genotypic differences in key metabolic enzymes among individuals may mediate the developmental toxicity of prenatal environmental exposures. To move toward this new research goal, the identification of potential toxicants associated with specific types of CCVM is essential.

Materials and methods

The BWIS enrolled live-born infants during 1981–1989 in Maryland, the District of Columbia, and northern Virginia, USA. Methods of the study, its questionnaire, study forms, and major research findings have been published in two monographs[1,2] and in numerous manuscripts, as cited below. Cases ($n = 4,390$) were infants with structural CCVM diagnosed in the first year of life by pediatric cardiologists, and confirmed by echocardiography,

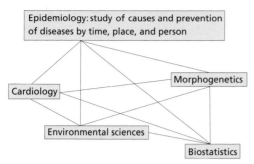

Fig. 56.1 A collaborative model for CCVM. Epidemiology as a biological discipline contributes to the study of congenital cardiovascular malformations (CCVM) by studying possible causes and preventive measures. Through collaborations of epidemiologists with experts in cardiology, environmental sciences, morphogenetics, and biostatistics, new progress may be achieved in defining the roles of genetics, environment, and gene–environment interactions in the etiology of CCVM.

cardiac catheterization, surgery, or autopsy. Subtypes of CCVM mentioned in the present report include the following numbers of enrolled cases: L-transposition of the great arteries ($n = 35$), D-transposition of the great arteries with intact ventricular septum ($n = 115$), atrioventricular septal defect ($n = 320$), hypoplastic left heart ($n = 162$), coarctation of the aorta ($n = 67$ with associated ventricular septal defect and $n = 126$ without), membranous ventricular septal defect ($n = 895$), total anomalous pulmonary venous return ($n = 60$), interrupted aortic arch ($n = 53$), and single ventricle ($n = 55$). Controls ($n = 3572$) were live-born infants free of CCVM, randomly sampled from the regional birth cohort by year and hospital of birth. Interviews were conducted with the parents, using a questionnaire about family history, medical and occupational history, use of medications, personal habits (use of alcohol, tobacco, and illicit drugs), and exposures to chemical and physical hazards at home and work. Case-control differences in these reported exposures during early pregnancy were assessed by logistic regression models, adjusting for known covariates of CCVM risk. Here we report the adjusted odds ratios (OR) for selected associations ($P<0.05$).

Results

Familial factors
Rates of CCVM among older siblings of the cases were highest for left-sided obstructive heart defects,[2,4] notably hypoplastic left heart in which 8% had affected older siblings. Coarctation of the aorta was similar with a 6% rate. In contrast, only 0.4% of control infants had an older sibling with CCVM.

In a successor, multicenter study (1990–1994) on familial aggregation of hypoplastic left heart and coarctation of the aorta, standardized echocardiography evaluations were performed on parents and siblings of affected probands. Familial CCVM were discovered in 19% of the families of hypoplastic left heart cases, and in 9% of the families of cases with coarctation of the aorta.[5] In most instances, the family members were concordant for the diagnosis of the case, or had previously undiagnosed aortic valve stenosis or bicuspid aortic valves, suggesting a strong role for genetic factors in left-sided obstructive types of CCVM.

Environmental factors
Maternal exposures to organic solvents at work and at home were associated in the BWIS with an increased risk of coarctation of the aorta (OR = 3.2), and hypoplastic left heart (OR = 3.4).[2,6] D-transposition of the great arteries (D-TGA) was also associated with maternal solvents exposures in the major analysis of the BWIS data, but later work on the expanded pesticides data collected in 1987–1989 revealed possible associations of D-TGA with rodenticidal chemicals (OR = 4.7) and with herbicides (OR = 2.8).[7] Membranous ventricular septal defects and total anomalous pulmonary venous return were also associated with maternal exposures to pesticides, and in the latter malformation group the association seemd to be much stronger in the presence of a reported family history of birth defects in older relatives.[2] Thus, the major classes of environmental exposures identified by the BWIS as possible hypotheses for future studies included organic solvent compounds, chemical rodenticides, and herbicides.

More recent analyses of the BWIS environmental and familial data focusing on diagnostic subtypes of CCVM have suggested that considerably more etiological heterogeneity may be present than has been appreciated in the past. For example, in cases with interrupted aortic arch compared to controls we found that type A interrupted aortic arch was associated with a family history of non-cardiac malformations and with maternal use of aspirin in the critical period, but the type B phenotype was associated with maternal reproductive factors (previous stillbirth, bleeding during the study pregnancy) and with use of arts and crafts paints.[8] Single ventricle with normal situs was associated with preconceptional paternal use of marijuana, while single ventricle in abnormal cardio-visceral situs was associated with maternal history of induced abortions and with preconceptional paternal alcohol consumption (>4 drinks per day).[9] Complete atrioventricular septal defect without trisomy was associated with maternal diabetes and use of antitussives, in contrast to partial forms of the heart defect which were associated with family history of CCVM.[10] In each of these examples, phenotypic heterogeneity correlated with differences in the patterns of possible risk factor associations.

Geographic information systems tools have been recently applied to the BWIS data on cases and controls. To date, these ongoing analyses suggested an increased risk for laterality and cardiac looping defects and other types of CCVM in areas where residential drinking water was supplied from wells, and where residences were close to hazardous waste disposal sites.[11] Common contaminants at these sites are chlorinated hydrocarbon compounds.

Gene–environment interactions

As mentioned above, the possible risk associated with pesticide exposures of mothers of infants with total anomalous pulmonary venous return was greater in the presence of a family history of CCVM than in the absence of such history. This may be an example of gene–environment interaction, whereby the risk from possible teratogens is modified by the genetic backgrounds of the mother and fetus. To further explore such interactions, neonatal blood spots were obtained from a subset of BWIS cases and controls, as a source of DNA for evaluating polymorphisms in candidate genes governing the metabolism of organic solvents.[12] Glutathione-S-transferase genes, GSTM1 and GSTT1, were selected on this basis. The results of this small pilot study (Fig. 56.2) showed an unmasking of solvent-associated increased risk of atrial septal defect, which had not been apparent before the GST genotypes were known.[13] Also, the results provided further refinement of the hypothesis of solvent-associated increased risk of pulmonic valve stenosis, in which the highest risk was observed for exposed infants carrying a specific genotype of GSTT1.[14]

Discussion

Although limited by self-report of environmental exposures and limited molecular genetic data, the BWIS data are a rich source for new studies testing hypotheses about the roles of genetics and environment in CCVM. Studies of developmental toxicity must now consider the role of the genetic

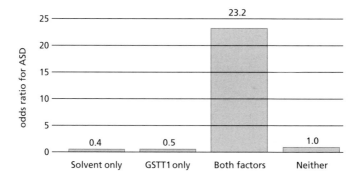

Loffredo et al. (1997) Am J Epidemiol 145:S30

Fig. 56.2 Possible genetic susceptibility to maternal solvent exposures. In this study, neonatal blood spots of cases and controls were retrieved from storage at the State of Maryland Newborn Screening Program, and genomic DNA was extracted. Genotypes at GSTM1 and GSTT1 were determined by standard polymerase chain reaction methods to identify homozygote deletion genotypes in comparison to non-homozygotes. For GSTT1 (glutathione-S-transferase theta type 1), cross-classification of subjects by maternal solvent exposures (paints and paint-cleaning chemicals) and GSTT1 non-deletion genotype in the infant suggested a large risk of atrial septal defect when both factors were present, relative to other combinations of genotype and exposure.

background in mediating effects of exposures. Such studies should assess the maternal genotype as well as the fetal genotype in mediating effects of exposures, since maternal, fetal, and placental metabolism can affect the concentration and types of metabolites reaching the fetus during development.

Summary

The BWIS established population-based data on the occurrence of CCVM in live-born infants, and generated novel hypotheses on possible etiologic risk factors. The results clearly suggest new avenues of experimental research into mechanisms of CCVM, especially: (1) organic solvents and pesticides as possible cardiac teratogens; (2) genetic factors responsible for the familial aggregation of left-sided obstructive heart defects; (3) models of gene–environment interactions.

Acknowledgments

The BWIS was funded by the NHLBI (R37HL25629) and was made possible only by the dedication and tireless efforts of the many pediatric cardiologists, research scientists, clinicians, and field and office staff who supported its work over nearly 2 decades. Special thanks go to Dr Charlotte Ferencz, MD, MPH, who founded and led the investigative team through all that time, and who continuously promoted the concept of interdisciplinary collaboration, including her enthusiastic participation in the original series of 'Takao' meetings.

References

1 Ferencz C, Loffredo CA, Correa-Villaseñor A, Wilson PD. *Genetic and Environmental Risk Factors of Major Cardiovascular Malformations*. Armonk, NY: Futura, 1997.

2 Ferencz C, Rubin JD, Loffredo CA, Magee CA. *Epidemiology of Congenital Heart Disease: the Baltimore–Washington Infant Study, 1981–1989*. Mt Kisco, NY: Futura, 1993.

3 National Institute for Occupational Safety and Health. *A Proposed National Strategy for the Prevention of Disorders of Reproduction*. Cincinnatio, OH: NIOSH, 1988.

4 Boughman JA, Berg KA, Astemborski JA *et al.* Familial risks of congenital heart defect assessed in a population-based epidemiological study. *Am J Med Genet* 1987; **26**: 839–49.

5 Loffredo CA, Chokkalingam A, Sill AM *et al.* Prevalence of congenital cardiovascular malformations among relatives of infants with hypoplastic left heart, coarctation of the aorta, and d-transposition of the great arteries. *Am J Med Genet* 2004; **124A**: 225–30.

6 Wollins DS, Ferencz C, Boughman JA, Loffredo CA. A population-based study of coarctation of the aorta: comparisons of infants with and without associated ventricular septal defect. *Teratology* 2001; **64**: 229–36.

7 Loffredo CA, Silbergeld EK, Ferencz C, Zhang J. Association of transposition of the great arteries in infants with maternal exposures to herbicides and rodenticides. *Am J Epidemiol* 2001; **153**: 529–36.

8 Loffredo CA, Ferencz C, Wilson PD, Lurie IW. Interrupted aortic arch: an epidemiologic study. *Teratology* 2000; **61**: 368–75.

9 Steinberger E, Ferencz C, Loffredo CA. Infants with single ventricle: a population-based epidemiological study. *Teratology* 2001; **65**: 106–15.

10 Loffredo CA, Hirata J, Wilson PD, Ferencz C, Lurie IW. Atrioventricular septal defects: possible etiologic differences between complete and partial defects. *Teratology* 2001; **63**: 87–93.

11 Kuehl KS, Loffredo CA. A population-based study of L-transposition of the great arteries: possible associations with environmental factors. *Birth Defects Res Part A Clin Mol Teratol* 2003; **67**: 162–7.

12 Loffredo CA, Ewing CK. Use of stored newborn blood spots in research on birth defects: variation in retrieval rates by type of defect and infant characteristics. *Am J Med Genet* 1997; **69**: 85–8.

13 Loffredo CA, Beaty TH, Silbergeld EK. Markers of polymorphic glutathione-S-transferase genes unmask an unsuspected risk factor for atrial septal defect in infants. *Am J Epidemiol* 1997; **145**(Suppl.): S30.

14 Loffredo CA, Beaty TH, Silbergeld EK. Solvent and paint exposures interact with polymorphisms in glutathione-S-transferase genes to increase the risk of congenital heart defects. *Teratology* 1997; **55**: 42.

CHAPTER 57

Familial recurrence risks of congenital heart defects

M. Cristina Digilio, Bruno Marino, Rossella Capolino, Anna Sarkozy, Bruno Dallapiccola

Nonsyndromic congenital heart defects (CHDs) are often a sporadic occurrence in the families, but multiple affected family members can also be found occasionally. In 1968, Nora introduced the multifactorial model for the etiology of nonsyndromic CHDs, suggesting that several genetic loci can interact together, in association with environmental factors.[1] However, familial recurrence of concordant CHDs within affected family members supports monogenic or oligogenic inheritance of CHD in selected pedigrees. In practical genetic counselling, the recurrence risk for CHD in sibs of patients with nonsyndromic CHD is considered as 1 to 3%.[2] In regard to the different types of CHD, it can be noted that ventricular and atrial septal defects, hypoplastic left heart, and atrioventricular canal defect (AVCD) are at greater risk of recurrence (3%), while for tricuspid atresia, Ebstein anomaly, and pulmonary atresia the risk is consistently lower (1%). A general concept in multifactorial inheritance is that if two first-degree relatives are affected, the recurrence risk for the next child becomes two to three times as great.

The experience of our group has focused on the evaluation of recurrence risk figures in sibs and the identification of families segregating specific CHDs in a possible Mendelian fashion. Particularly, we studied family history in patients with AVCD, tetralogy of Fallot (TF), and transposition of the great arteries (TGA).

Atrioventricular canal defect

AVCD is a genetically heterogeneous CHD. The recurrence risks for CHD among siblings of 103 patients with AVCD from our series corresponds to 3.6%[3] (Table 57.1). According to our experience and literature reports, large pedigrees with many affected members can be identified.[3–9] Most of these familial cases are compatible with an autosomal dominant mechanism of inheritance. The general concordance rate for CHD in familial cases from our series is 62%.[3] Interestingly, the concordance rate corresponds to 50% in sibs, but is much higher (100%) when one parent is affected. Information about cardiac abnormalities for the offspring of parents with complex CHDs is now becoming available because the first survivors of corrective surgical procedures are reaching adulthood. According to literature reports, recurrence risks for CHD in the offspring of parents affected by AVCD corresponds to 10%.[5,10] Nevertheless, it can be noted that affected mothers seem to have a higher risk to transmit the defect in comparison to affected fathers. In fact, the risk rate for offspring becomes 14% when the affected parent is the mother.[5] The detection of isolated cleft of the mitral valve or electrocardiographic left-axis deviation without cardiac malformation in families with autosomal dominant AVCD may indicate that these defects represent a mild expression of AVCD.[8]

AVCD in pedigrees with autosomal dominant inheritance probably results from a single gene defect. Up to now, two genes involved in nonsyndromic

Table 57.1 ••

Relationship	AVCD, risk (1)	TF, risk (2)	TGA, risk (3)
Siblings	3.6%	3.1%	1.8%
Parents	1.9%	0.5%	0.5%
Grandparents	0.0%	0.3%	0.06%
Uncles/aunts	0.8%	0.2%	0.2%
First cousins	0.3%	0.6%	0.5%

1: Digilio *et al.*, *Am J Dis Child*, 1993; 2: Digilio *et al.*, *J Med Genet*, 1997; 3: Digilio *et al.*, *Circulation*, 2001

AVCD have been identified,[11-13] but genetic heterogeneity with different genes causing AVCD in different families is suspected. A curious observation is the finding of rare families segregating AVCD in sibs with discordant karyotypes.[14,15] Of course, AVCD in Down and non-Down patients is genetically distinct, but the contemporary occurrence in the same family could imply that common predisposing genetic factors in parents could play a role in the etiology of both disorders.

Tetralogy of Fallot

Nonsyndromic TF has a frequency of CHD in sibs corresponding to 3.1% in our series of 102 patients, with a high concordance rate in affected sibs[16] (Table 57.1). An autosomal recessive mechanism of inheritance of nonsyndromic TF has been proposed by several authors, following the observation of TF recurrent in two or three sibs.[17,18] The absence of a detectable deletion 22q11.2 in patients included in our series supports the hypothesis that nonsyndromic TF, including familial and sporadic cases, is not the result of this chromosomal imbalance, and genes located on different chromosomes could be implicated.[16] The genetic basis of TF is probably complex. The results of the British collaborative study suggest a three-gene model for nonsyndromic TF as the best fitting model in their series of familial and sporadic cases.[10]

Transposition of the great arteries

TGA has been previously considered to be mostly a sporadic occurrence in families. Our clinical experience suggesting that familial TGA might be higher than thought[19] led us to design a study to investigate familial recurrence of CHD in 370 nonsyndromic patients enrolled inside an Italian multicentric study[20] (Table 57.1). Familial recurrence risk in sibs was 1.8%. TGA itself was the most common recurrent malformation, suggesting monogenic or oligogenic inheritance of TGA in selected pedigrees. Interestingly, complete TGA and congenitally corrected TGA have been found to segregate in the same family in several instances, indicating a pathogenetic link between some cases of TGA and the situs and looping abnormalities. Note that our observation disclosing a relationship between complete TGA and laterality defect is corroborated by molecular studies (the detection of complete TGA in mice heterozygous for both SMAD2 and Nodal mutations, the finding of complete TGA in humans with mutations of *CFC1* gene or *ZIC3* gene)[21-23] so as by pathogenetic evidences (the detection of complete TGA in animal models obtained by all-trans retinoic acid administration during pregnancy).[24,25]

Conclusions

The importance of the multifactorial polygenic model of inheritance for nonsyndromic CHDs is decreasing, owing to the increasing number of CHDs found to be related to a monogenic or oligogenic inheritance. Large families with multiple members affected by CHD are fundamental for the identification of the genes related to specific malformations using genetic techniques such as linkage analysis and positional cloning. The analysis of the anatomic types of CHD segregating in the same family is an important aid for the analysis of pathogenetic links between CHDs. The evaluation of risk figures in large series has practical implications in genetic counseling for families of probands with different types of CHD.

References

1 Nora JJ. Multifactorial inheritance hypothesis for the etiology of congenital heart diseases. The genetic-environmental interaction. *Circulation* 1968; **38**: 604–17.
2 Nora JJ, Berg K, Nora AH. *Cardiovascular Diseases: Genetics, Epidemiology and Prevention.* New York, NY: Oxford University Press, 1991: 53–80.

3 Digilio MC, Marino B, Cicini MP *et al.* Risk of congenital heart defects in relatives of patients with atrioventricular canal. *Am J Dis Child* 1993; **147**: 1295–7.

4 O'Nuallain S, Hall JG, Stamm SJ. Autosomal dominant inheritance of endocardial cushion defect. *Birth Defects: Original Article Series* 1977; **XIII**: 143–7.

5 Emanuel R, Somerville J, Inns A, Withers R. Evidence of congenital heart disease in the offspring of parents with atrioventricular defects. *Br Heart J* 1983; **49**: 144–7.

6 Wilson L, Curtis A, Korenberg JR *et al.* A large, dominant pedigree of atrioventricular septal defect (AVSD): exclusion from Down syndrome critical region on chromosome 21. *Am J Hum Genet* 1993; **53**: 1262–8.

7 Kumar A, Williams CA, Victorica BE. Familial atrioventricular septal defect: possible genetic mechanisms. *Br Heart J* 1994; **71**: 79–81.

8 Digilio MC, Marino B, Giannotti A, Dallapiccola B. Familial atrioventricular septal defects: possible genetic mechanism. *Br Heart J* 1994; **72**: 301.

9 Cousineau AJ, Lauer RM, Pierpont ME, Burns TL, Ardinger RH, Patil SR, Sheffield VC. Linkage analysis of autosomal dominant atrioventricular canal defects: exclusion of chromosome 21. *Hum Genet* 1994; **93**: 103–8.

10 Burn J, Brennan P, Little J *et al.* Recurrence risks in offspring of adults with major heart defects: results from first cohort of British collaborative study. *Lancet* 1998; **351**: 311–16.

11 Sheffield VC, Pierpont ME, Nishimura D *et al.* Identification of a complex congenital heart defect susceptibility locus using DNA pooling and shared segment analysis. *Hum Mol Genet* 1997; **6**: 117–21.

12 Zhao Y, Meng X, Cao H *et al.* Molecular cloning and characterization of a potential candidate gene for nonsyndromic atrioventricular septal defect on 1p31–1p21. *J Am Coll Cardiol* 2002; **39**: 408A.

13 Maslen CL, Robinson SW, Morris CD. Mutation of CRELD1 associated with an atrioventricular canal defect. *Am J Hum Genet* 2002; **71**: 209A.

14 Ferencz C, Boughman JA, Neill CA, Brenner JI, Perry LW. Congenital cardiovascular malformations: questions on inheritance. *J Am Coll Cardiol* 1989; **14**: 756–63.

15 Digilio MC, Marino B, Canepa SA *et al.* Congenital heart defect in sibs with discordant karyotypes. *Am J Med Genet* 1998; **80**: 169–72.

16 Digilio MC, Marino B, Giannotti A, Toscano A, Dallapiccola B. Recurrence risk figures for isolated tetralogy of Fallot after screening for 22q11 microdeletion. *J Med Genet* 1997; **34**: 188–90.

17 Miller ME, Smith DW. Conotruncal malformation complex: examples of possible monogenic inheritance. *Pediatrics* 1979; **63**: 890–893.

18 Wulfsberg EA, Zintz EJ, Moore JW. The inheritance of conotruncal malformations: a review and report of two siblings with tetralogy of Fallot and pulmonary atresia. *Clin Genet* 1991; **40**: 12–16.

19 Digilio MC, Marino B, Banaudi E, Marasini M, Dallapiccola B. Familial recurrence of transposition of the great arteries. *Lancet* 1998; **351**: 1661.

20 Digilio MC, Casey B, Toscano A *et al.*Complete transposition of the great arteries. Patterns of congenital heart disease in familial precurrence. *Circulation* 2001; **104**: 2809–14.

21 Nomura M, Li E. Smad2 role in mesoderm formation, left-right patterning and craniofacial development. *Nature* 1998; **393**: 786–90.

22 Goldmuntz E, Bamford R, Karkera JD *et al.* CFC1 mutations in patients with transposition of the great arteries and double-outlet right ventricle. *Am J Hum Genet* 2002; **70**: 776–80.

23 Mégarbané A, Salem N, Stephan E *et al.* X-linked transposition of the great arteries and incomplete penetrance among males with nonsense mutation in ZIC3. *Eur J Hum Genet* 2000; **8**: 704–8.

24 Pexieder T, Blanc O, Pelouch V, Ostadalova I, Milerova M, Ostadal B. Late fetal development of retinoic acid-induced transposition of great arteries: morphology, physiology, and biochemistry. In: Clark EB, Markwald RR, Takao A, eds. *Developmental Mechanisms of Heart Disease.* Armonk, NY: Futura, 1995: 297–307.

25 Nakajima Y, Morishima M, Yasui H, Nakazawa M, Momma K. Molecular mechanisms of complete transposition of the great arteries produced by all-trans retinoic acid in mouse embryo. In: Clark EB, Markwald RR, Takao A. eds. *Developmental Mechanisms of Heart Disease.* Armonk, NY: Futura 1995: 315–17.

CHAPTER 58

T-box gene family and congenital cardiovascular anomalies

Rumiko Matsuoka

Putative transcription factors of the *T-box* family genes[1-3] act to control early cell-fate decisions, and differentiation and morphogenesis/organogenesis. The spatial and temporal expression patterns of *T-box* genes[4] such as *Tbx1*, *Tbx2*, *Tbx3*, *Tbx4*, *Tbx5*, are unique although they overlap in their sites of expression. This overlapping indicates that T-box genes are differentially regulated during the developmental process, particularly in areas where inductive interactions are taking place. *Tbx1* shows very little overlap with the other two cognate gene sets, *Tbx2/Tbx3*, *Tbx4/Tbx5*, since the divergence of *Tbx1* occurred long before the relatively recent divergence of the other four genes from common ancestral genes, and recent studies of mouse genetics have suggested that *TBX1* is the major candidate gene for del22q11.2 syndrome.[5-7] Although the expression patterns of *Tbx2*[8] and *Tbx3* are similar to some temporal and spatial differences, *Tbx3*[9] is a disease gene for ulnar–mammary syndrome. *Tbx5* and *Tbx4* are exclusively expressed in the vertebrate forelimb and hind limb, respectively, and *Tbx5*[10,11] is a disease gene for Holt–Oram syndrome. When mutated, these genes may produce dramatic phenotypes in a number of human congenital malformations, including cardiovascular diseases, such as the key gene of del22q11.2 syndrome, Holt–Oram syndrome, ulnar-mammary syndrome, or similar syndromes. Del22q11.2 syndrome including conotruncal anomaly face syndrome (CAFS)/velo-cardio-facial syndrome (VCFS) and DiGeorge syndrome (DGS) with conotruncal anomaly face (CAF), is the most frequent known chromosomal microdeletion syndrome, with an incidence of 1 in 4000–5000 live births. This syndrome is characterized by a 3-Mb deletion on chromosome 22q11.2, cardiac abnormalities, anomaly face, T-cell deficits, cleft palate, and hypocalcemia. At least 30 genes have been mapped to the deleted region. However, the association of these genes with the cause of this syndrome is not clearly understood.[12-15] Therefore, in 1998 we established Holistic Molecular Genetic (HMG) medicine, which is a new system of molecular genetic medical care. The aim of HMG is to clarify the molecular genetic pathogenesis of congenital and hereditary heart disease throughout life. We have applied this system to test if *TBX1* is a candidate gene responsible for the CAFS and DGS with CAF in 22q11.2 deletion-minus patients, and analyzed the genotype/phenotype relationship of these *T-box* family genes in patients with Holt–Oram syndrome, with ulnar-mammary syndrome, and with other similar syndromes. To find the *TBX1* mutation, we focused on performing the precise diagnosis of CAFS or DGS with CAF based on a clear view of the phenotypes. In 96% (225/235) of the patients, there was a defined 1.5~3-Mb deletion at 22q11.2 which was not found in the remaining 10 patients (seven sporadic CAFS patients, one sporadic DGS with CAF patient and two patients from two CAFS families). We have identified three mutations of *TBX1* in two unrelated patients without the 22q11.2 deletion, one with sporadic CAFS/VCFS and one with sporadic DGS, and in three patients from a CAFS/VCFS family. Our results imply that the *TBX1* mutation is responsible for five major phenotypes in del22q11.2 syndrome, i.e. CAF, cardiovascular defects, thymic hypoplasia, velopharyngeal insufficiency with cleft palate, and parathyroid dysfunction with hypocalcemia. We conclude that *TBX1* is a major genetic determinant of the del22q11.2 syndrome in humans. Also, we found five mutations of *TBX5* in 50% (5/10) of unrelated patients with Holt–Oram syndrome. We did not find the mutations of *TBX3* in a patient with ulnar-mammary syndrome. It is important to emphasize that the correct diagnosis of a syndrome should be based on a clear view of the phenotypes to avoid confusion with other similar syndromes. HMG medicine will allow investigation of the prevention of crisis, based on a molecular genetic diagnosis, in the early-phase, and will aid precritical diagnosis and the choice of appropriate therapy. To try to understand their etiology, mutated genes are now being investigated further, including an expression study.[16]

Methods

Phenotypic evaluation

To investigate the molecular and clinical aspects of congenital heart disease, we constructed a system (HGM) for gene analysis. To investigate that *TBX1* is the major candidate gene for del22q11.2 syndrome, the genotype/phenotype relationship of the *T-box* family genes (*Tbx2*, *Tbx3*, *Tbx5*) in patients with Holt–Oram syndrome and patient with ulnar-mammary syndrome, we carefully evaluated each patient by history and physical examination and/or review of their medical records. The typical facial features of conotruncal anomaly face (CAF) are ocular hypertelorism, short palpebral fissures, "bloated" eyelids, a low nasal bridge, a small mouth, and the minor ear lobe anomalies.[17] Our findings indicated that CAF is always associated with deletion of 22q11.2.[18–20] An overlap of similar but varied phenotypes, including both the facial characteristics and structural anomalies, is seen in CAFS/VCFS and DGS with CAF. We found dysmorphism of the nose, which seems to be divided into two parts (upper part and lower part) at the joint of the wing and sides.[19,20] This makes physical diagnosis of del22q11.2 syndrome more certain and indicates that CAFS is the same pathologic entity as VCFS.[18–20] Facial features and anthropometric measurements were obtained from photographs.

Genetic analysis

Peripheral blood from the patients and their family members with congenital heart disease were used to prepare genomic DNA for mutation analysis or to perform chromosomal analysis, if needed, and the rest were used to construct an Epstein–Barr virus-transformed cell line (Plate 36). To test for the chromosomal deletion at 22q11.2, we carried out fluorescence *in situ* hybridization analysis using 10 probes on 22q11.2 in 235 unrelated patients with clinically evaluated CAFS or DGS with CAF. To investigate mutations in the coding sequence of *TBX1*, we also performed genetic analysis in 13 22q11.2 deletion-minus patients, (phenotypically, 8 sporadic CAFS or DGS, and 5 familial CAFS) from 10 families. Genetic analysis was also performed on the *T-box* family genes (*Tbx2*, *Tbx3*, *Tbx5*) in 10 patients with Holt–Oram syndrome and 1 patient with ulnar-mammary syndrome. Bidirectional direct sequencing of the purified PCR products (QIAGEN) was performed using a BigDye Terminator Sequencing Kit (Applied Biosystems) and a 3100 Genetic Analyzer (Applied Biosystems).

Acknowledgments

I thank H. Yagi MS, Y. Furutani PhD, K. Akimoto MD, PhD, M. Kimura MS, S. Imamura DVM, A. Takao MD, M. Nakazawa MD from Tokyo Women's Medical University, Tokyo, Japan, T. Sasaki MSD, S. Asakawa PhD, S. Minoshima PhD, N. Shimizu PhD from Department of Molecular Biology, Keio University School of Medicine, Tokyo, Japan, T. Tanaka from Japan Red Cross, Saitama Branch, Yono, Saitama, Japan, and Ms B. Levene for English correction of the manuscript.

References

1 Papaioannou VE, Silver LM. The T-box gene family. *BioEssays* 1998; **20**: 9–19.

2 Wilkinson DG, Bhatt S, Herrmann BG. Expression pattern of the mouse T gene and its role in mesoderm formation. *Nature* 1990; **343**: 657–9.

3 Peckam EA, Brook JD. T-box genes in human disorders. *Hum Mol Genet* 2003; **12**(Suppl. 1): R37–44.

4 Chapman DL, Garvey N, Hancock S *et al.* Expression of the T-box family genes, *Tbx1-Tbx5*, during early mouse development. *Dev Dyn* 1996; **206**: 381.

5 Jerome LA, Papaioannou VE. DiGeorge syndrome phenotype in mice mutant for the T-box gene, *Tbx1*. *Nature Genet* 2001; **27**: 286–91.

6 Lindsay EA, Vitelli F, Su H *et al. Tbx1* haploinsufficiency in the DiGeorge syndrome region causes aortic arch defects in mice. *Nature* 2001; **410**: 97–101.

7 Merscher S, Funke B, Epstein JB *et al. TBX1* is responsible for cardiovascular defects in velo-cardio-facial/DiGeorge syndrome. *Cell* 2001; **104**: 619–29.

8 Paxton C, Zhao H, Chin Y, Langner K, Reecy J. Murine Tbx2 contains domains that activate and repress gene transcription. *Gene* 2002; **283**: 117–24.

9 Bamshad M, Lin RC, Law DJ *et al.* Mutations in human *TBX3* alter limb, apocrine and genital development in ulnar-mammary syndrome. *Nature Genet* 1997; **16**: 311–5.

10 Li QY, Newbury-Ecob RA, Terrett JA *et al.* Holt–Oram syndrome is caused by mutations in *TBX5*, a member of the *Brachyury (T)* gene family. *Nature Genet* 1997; **15**: 21–9.

11 Basson CT, Bachinsky DR, Lin RC *et al.* Mutation in human cause limb and cardiac malformation in Holt–Oram syndrome. *Nature Genet* 1997; **15**: 30–5,.

12 MacQuade L, Christodoulou J, Budarf M *et al.* Patient with a 22q11.2 deletion with no overlap of the minimal DiGeorge syndrome critical region (MDGCR). *Am J Med Genet* 1999; **86**: 27–33.

13 Gong W, Gottelieb S, Collins *et al.* Mutation analysis of *TBX1* in non-deleted patients with features of DGS/VCFS or isolated cardiovascular defects. *J Med Genet* 2001; **38**: e45.

14 Conti E, Grifone N, Sarkozy A *et al.* DiGeorge subtypes of nonsyndromic conotruncal defects: evidence against a major role of TBX1 Gene. *Eur J Hum Genet* 2003; **11**: 349–51.

15 Stalmans I, Lambrechts D, De Smet F *et al.* VEGF: a modifier of the del22q11 (DiGeorge) syndrome? *Nat Med* 2003; **9**: 173–82.

16 Yamagishi H, Maeda J, Hu T *et al.* Tbx1 is regulated by tissue-specific forkhead proteins through a common Sonic hedgehog-responsive enhancer. *Genes Dev* 2003; **17**: 269–81.

17 Takao A, Ando M, Cho K, Kinouchi A, Murakami Y. Etiologic categorization of common congenital heart disease. In: Van Praagh R, Takao A, eds. *Etiology and Morphogenesis of Congenital Heart Disease.* New York: Futura, 1980: 253–69.

18 Matsuoka R, Takao A, Kimura M *et al.* Confirmation that the conotruncal anomaly face syndrome is associated with a deletion within chromosome 22q11. *Am J Med Genet* 1994; **53**: 285–9.

19 Matsuoka R, Kimura M, Scambler PJ *et al.* Molecular and clinical study of 183 patients with conotruncal anomaly face syndrome. *Hum Genet* 1998; **103**: 70–80.

20 Matsuoka R, Furutani M, Kimura M *et al.* Genotype–phenotype correlations in del22q11.2 syndrome. In: Clark EB, Nakazawa M, Takao A, eds. *Etiology and Morphogenesis of Congenital Heart Disease.* New York: Futura, 2000: 341–6.

CHAPTER 59

Deciphering the genetic etiology of conotruncal defects

Elizabeth Goldmuntz

Conotruncal defects are congenital malformations of the outflow tracts of the heart and historically include: tetralogy of Fallot (TOF), truncus arteriosus (TA), interrupted aortic arch (IAA), transposition of the great arteries (TGA), and double outlet right ventricle (DORV). They account for 16% of congenital heart disease presenting in the newborn period and are still associated with significant morbidity and mortality despite notable medical and surgical advances.[1] In the past decade, significant progress has been made in our understanding of the genetic contribution to the development of conotruncal defects. For our part, we have used a wide variety of molecular genetic approaches to begin to decipher the genetic basis of these important clinical problems, including the evaluation of genetic syndromes characterized in part by conotruncal defects and additional candidate genes identified from family studies or animal models. For these investigations, over the last decade, we have prospectively recruited a large cohort of patients with conotruncal defects ascertained solely on the basis of their cardiac anatomy.

Molecular analysis of genetic syndromes

Molecular genetic studies demonstrated that the vast majority of subjects with either DiGeorge, velo-cardio-facial or Conotruncal Anomaly Face syndromes shared a common genetic etiology, namely a chromosome 22q11 deletion (reviewed in ref. 2). Given that all of these syndromes are in part characterized by conotruncal cardiac defects, we and other investigators have evaluated the frequency

with which patients with a conotruncal defect have a 22q11 deletion. Over the past several years, we have prospectively studied a large cohort of patients with conotruncal defects by fluorescence *in situ* hybridization to detect a 22q11 deletion.[3] Our results are summarized in conjunction with those reported by other investigators in Table 59.1.[4–9] Of note, a substantial number of patients with either IAA, TA, or TOF but very few with DORV or TGA have a 22q11 deletion. These results indicate that a subset of IAA, TA, and TOF share a common genetic etiology, while DORV and TGA are not generally associated with this particular genetic alteration. We and others have also found that those subjects with either IAA, TA, or TOF and aortic arch anomalies have a higher deletion frequency than those with normal aortic arch anatomy.[3,10] Based on this finding, we studied subjects with aortic arch anomalies and normal intracardiac anatomy for 22q11 deletions and found a deletion in a substantial number of patients (24%) with a wide range of isolated aortic arch anomalies.[11]

Candidate genes identified from family studies

Conotruncal defects most commonly occur as a sporadic event within a family. While small families with a few affected members have been reported, large families with multiple members with conotruncal defects suitable for parametric linkage analyses have not been identified. Recently, Schott and colleagues[12] reported on four families with atrioventricular conduction block frequently accompanied by atrial septal defects whose affected members were found to have mutations of the homeobox gene, *NKX2.5*. We noted that two members of one family had TOF and hypothesized that additional subjects with TOF would have NKX2.5 mutations. We, therefore, evaluated a cohort of 114 subjects with TOF for mutations of NKX2.5 by Conformation-Sensitive Gel Electrophoresis and sequence analysis of PCR products demonstrating aberrant mobility.[13] We identified four heterozygous missense mutations in six subjects as summarized in Table 59.2. None of the mutation-positive subjects had atrioventricular conduction abnormalities. These mutations were not identified in 100 random normal control chromosomes.

In particular, two mutations (Arg216Cys, Ala219Val) map within a highly conserved domain, the NK2 specific domain. Mice carrying a homozygous mutation for the NK2 specific domain demonstrate congenital heart defects in the absence of atrioventricular conduction abnormalities.[14] The

Glu21Gln mutation is just 3' of another conserved domain, the TN domain, and changes a highly conserved amino acid. Thus, although further experiments are required, these mutations have a high likelihood of being disease-related. The Arg25Cys mutation deserves further mention since it was reported previously[15] and found in three subjects in this study. Because three of the four subjects identified with this alteration were African-American, we subsequently tested an African-American control population and identified that 2 of 43 (4.7%) African-American controls carried the Arg25Cys alteration.[13] Whether this mutation, which has been demonstrated to confer subtle functional alterations on protein function,[16] is a polymorphism or confers an increased susceptibility to congenital heart disease, remains to be determined. Nonetheless, mutations of NKX2.5 are associated with congenital heart defects, and in particular seem to play a role in the development of TOF. Further investigations to define the role of NKX2.5 in the development of other conotruncal and congenital cardiac defects are in progress.

Candidate genes identified by animal models

Multiple animal models where altered gene expression results in congenital cardiac defects have served to identify critical developmental pathways for conotruncal embryogenesis and candidate genes for similar human disorders. One such gene, *CFC1* (encoding cryptic) was found to participate in the

Table 59.1 Frequency of 22q11 deletions in conotruncal defects

Conotruncal defect	% Deleted[a]
Interrupted aortic arch	50–84%
Truncus arteriosus	34–41%
Tetralogy of Fallot	8–35%
Double outlet right ventricle	<5%
Transposition of the great arteries	<1%

[a] References 3–10.

Table 59.2 Summary of subjects with Tetralogy of Fallot and NKX2.5 mutations

Patient	Mutation	PV anatomy	Aortic arch anatomy	Other	Mutation positive relatives
229	G61C (Glu21Gln)	Stenosis	RAA, mirror	Retroaortic innominate vein	Mother, no reported phenotype
122	C73T (Arg25Cys)	Stenosis	LAA, normal	PFO or 2° ASD	
324	C73T (Arg25Cys)	Atresia	RAA, mirror	APC	
393	C73T (Arg25Cys)	Atresia	RAA, mirror	APC	Father, VSD
518	C646T (Arg216Cys)	Stenosis	RAA, unknown		
328	C656T (Ala219Val)	Atresia	RAA, mirror		Mother, no reported phenotype

PV, pulmonary valve; RAA, right-sided aortic arch; LAA, left-sided aortic arch; mirror, mirror image branching pattern; normal, normal branching pattern; APC, aortopulmonary collaterals; PFO, patent foramen ovale; 2° ASD, secundum atrial septal defect; VSD, ventricular septal defect.

establishment of left-right asymmetry when the mouse homozygous mutant for cryptic developed the equivalent of heterotaxy syndrome.[17,18] *CFC1* encodes an extracellular protein and is one of four family members characterized by an EGF-like domain and a cysteine rich, CFC domain which is highly conserved among the family members (reviewed in ref.19). Because of the homozygous mutant mouse phenotype, Bamford and colleagues[20] evaluated humans with heterotaxy syndrome and identified four mutations and one polymorphism in *CFC1*. Given that the cardiovascular abnormalities associated with heterotaxy syndrome include malposition of the great arteries, we hypothesized that human subjects with either TGA or DORV would also have mutations within CFC1. To that end, a cohort of subjects with either D-TGA ($n = 58$), L-TGA ($n = 6$), or DORV ($n = 22$) but without other signs of laterality abnormalities were evaluated for mutations in *CFC1* by single stranded conformation polymorphism and direct sequencing.[21] Two mutations predicted to alter protein function were identified. In particular, one subject with D-TGA exhibited a 20 base pair tandem duplication of the splice donor site at exon 4 that would introduce an alternative splice donor site. If the alternative site were used, then a frameshift would be introduced eliminating the CFC conserved domain and the hydrophobic domain. A second subject with DORV was found to have a one base pair deletion (G174del1) that would introduce a frameshift and interrupt the hydrophobic domain. Previous studies have demonstrated that the encoded mutant protein does not reach the cell surface.[20] Neither of these mutations were identified in 100 normal control subjects. A third mutation (R78W) was identified in one subject with DORV. The R78W mutation was also identified in multiple subjects with heterotaxy syndrome and found to confer subtle functional alterations in the mutant protein.[20] Though this mutation was not identified in 100 normal random controls, it was identified in 13.6% of African-American control subjects. Thus, this mutation is most likely a polymorphism, but may also increase susceptibility to disease. These findings represent the first report of a single gene defect in subjects with TGA or DORV. In addition, these data indicate that, in certain cases, subjects with heterotaxy syndrome and those with malposition of the great arteries in the absence of other laterality defects share a common genetic etiology.

Summary and conclusions

Multiple molecular genetic approaches have been used over the last decade to begin to decipher the genetic contribution to the development of conotruncal cardiac defects. Investigations into genetic syndromes, family studies, and animal models have all provided insight into genetic alterations associated with these defects. These investigations demonstrate that these malformations are genetically heterogeneous and extremely complex given that evidence of decreased penetrance is seen with each genetic alteration. Therefore, genetic and environmental modifiers must also be invoked as contributing to the risk of developing conotruncal defects. Future investigations will therefore include family-based association studies to identify genetic alterations that may increase or decrease the risk of developing this class of congenital heart defects.

References

1 Perry LW, Neill CA, Ferencz C, Rubin JD, Loffredo CA. Infants with congenital heart disease: the cases. In: Ferencz C, Rubin JD, Loffredo CA, Magee CA, eds. *Epidemiology of Congenital Heart Disease: The Baltimore-Washingtion Infant Study 1981–1989.* Mount Kisco: Futura, 1993; **4**: 33–62.

2 Emanuel BS, Budarf ML, Scambler PJ. The genetic basis of conotruncal cardiac defects: the chromosome 22q11.2 Deletion. In: Harvey RP, Rosenthal N, eds. *Heart Development.* Toronto: Academic Press, 1999: 463–78.

3 Goldmuntz E, Clark BJ, Mitchell LE *et al.* Frequency of 22q11 deletions in patients with conotruncal defects. *J Am Coll Cardiol* 1998; **32**: 492–8.

4 Fokstuen S, Arbenz U, Artan S *et al.* 22q11.2 deletions in a series of patients with non-selective congenital heart defects: incidence, type of defects and parental origin. *Clin Genet* 1998; **53**: 63–9.

5 Iserin L, de Lonlay P, Viot G *et al.* Prevalence of the microdeletion 22q11 in newborn infants with congenital conotruncal cardiac anomalies. *Eur J Pediatr* 1998; **157**: 881–4.

6 Mehraein Y, Wippermann CF, Michel-Behnke I *et al.* Microdeletion 22q11 in complex cardiovascular malformations. *Hum Genet* 1997; **99**: 433–42.

7 Momma K, Kondo C, Matsuoka R, Takao A. Cardiac anomalies associated with a chromosome 22q11 deletion

in patients with conotruncal anomaly face syndrome. *Am J Cardiol* 1996; **78**: 591–4.

8   Takahashi K, Kido S, Hoshino K *et al*. Frequency of a 22q11 deletion in patients with conotruncal cardiac malformations: a prospective study *Eur J Pediatr* 1995; **154**: 878–81.

9   Webber SA, Hatchwell E, Barber JC *et al*. Importance of microdeletions of chromosomal region 22q11 as a cause of selected malformations of the ventricular outflow tracts and aortic arch: a three-year prospective study. *J Pediatr* 1996; **129**: 26–32.

10 Momma K, Kondo C, Matsuoka R. Tetralogy of Fallot with pulmonary atresia associated with chromosome 22q11 deletion. *J Am Coll Cardiol* 1996; **27**: 198–202.

11 McElhinney DB, Clark BJ 3rd, Weinberg PM *et al*. Association of chromosome 22q11 deletion with isolated anomalies of aortic arch laterality and branching. *J Am Coll Cardiol* 2001; **37**: 2114–9.

12 Schott JJ, Benson DW, Basson CT *et al*. Congenital heart disease caused by mutations in the transcription factor NKX2-5 *Science* 1998; **281**: 108–11.

13 Goldmuntz E, Geiger E, Benson DW. NKX2.5 mutations in patients with tetralogy of Fallot. *Circulation* 2001; **104**: 2565–8.

14 Schinke M, Litovsky S, Usheva A *et al*. Lack of the conserved NK2-domain of the cardiac transcription factor

Nkx2.5 causes multiple heart defects. *Circulation* 2001; **104**: II-27.

15 Benson DW, Silberbach GM, Kavanaugh-McHugh A *et al*. Mutations in the cardiac transcription factor NKX2.5 affect diverse cardiac developmental pathways. *J Clin Invest* 1999; **104**: 1567–73.

16 Kasahara H, Lee B, Schott JJ *et al*. Loss of function and inhibitory effects of human CSX/NKX2.5 homeoprotein mutations associated with congenital heart disease. *J Clin Invest* 2000; **106**: 299–308.

17 Gaio U, Schweickert A, Fischer A *et al*. A role of the cryptic gene in the correct establishment of the left–right axis. *Curr Biol* 1999; **9**: 1339–42.

18 Yan YT, Gritsman K, Ding J *et al*. Conserved requirement for EGF-CFC genes in vertebrate left–right axis formation *Genes Dev* 1999; **13**: 2527–37.

19 Shen MM, Schier AF. The EGF-CFC gene family in vertebrate development. *Trends Genet* 2000; **16**: 303–9.

20 Bamford RN, Roessler E, Burdine RD *et al*. Loss-of-function mutations in the EGF-CFC gene CFC1 are associated with human left–right laterality defects. *Nat Genet* 2000; **26**: 365–9.

21 Goldmuntz E, Bamford R, Karkera JD *et al*. CFC1 mutations in patients with transposition of the great arteries and double-outlet right ventricle. *Am J Hum Genet* 2002; **70**: 776–80.

CHAPTER 60

Cardiovascular anomalies in patients with deletion 22q11.2: a multi-center study in Korea

In Sook Park, Young Hwue Kim, Jae Kon Ko, Jung Yun Choi, Soo Jin Kim, Hong Ryang Kil, June Huh, Heung Jae Lee, Jae Sook Ma, Sang Bum Lee, Eul Ju Seo, Han Wook Yoo

We reviewed clinical and laboratory data on 179 patients with deletion 22q11.2 by reviewing medical records from seven institutions in Korea. Genetic diagnosis was made by fluorescent *in situ* hybridization (FISH) method from peripheral lymphocyte using TUPLE 1 probe. Those patients whose clinical features were strongly suggestive of deletion but did not have genetic confirmation were not included in the study. There were 89 males and 90 females. Age distributions were: < 2 years, 32 patients; 2~6 years, 83 patients; 7~11 years, 28 patients; 12~16 years, 14 patients; >17 years, 22 patients. Congenital heart disease was seen in 156 patients (86%; Table 60.1): tetralogy of Fallot (TOF) in 98 [simple TOF, 48; TOF with absent pulmonary valve, 2; TOF with pulmonary atresia ± major aorto-pulmonary collateral arteries (a), 48], ventricular septal defect (VSD) 31; double outlet right ventricle (DORV) 7; interrupted aortic arch type B 7; ASD 7; truncus arteriosus 2; PDA 2; total anomalous pulmonary connection 1; and complete atrioventricular septal defect with DORV in 1 patient. Location of VSD were perimembranous 78%, subarterial 6%, total conal defect 12%, muscular 3% and mixed in 2%. The side of the aortic arch was right in 53%, left in 46%, and a double arch in one. Cervical arch was seen in 1 (Plate 37) and circumflex retroesophageal arch in 2 patients. Various anomalies in aortic arch branching were observed: retro-esophageal subclavian a ± Kom-

merell's diverticulum in 27 patients, origin of right subclavian artery from vertebral a in 1 patient, and isolation of subclavian artery in 2 patients. Anomalous origin of arch vessels was twice as common with the right arch (29%) than with the left arch (15%). Side of the aortic arch and branching pattern was not known in most patients with normal intracardiac structure. Other cardiovascular anomalies were bilateral SVCs in 14 patients, bicuspid aortic valve with aortic stenosis 3 patients, pericardial defect 3 patients, double chambered right ventricle 3 patients, aortopulmonary window 1 patients, juxtaposition of left atrial appendage 1 patient, partial anomalous pulmonary venous connection 1 patient, abnormal course of a pulmonary vein 1 patient, unroofed coronary sinus 1 patient, absent proximal left pulmonary a 1 patient, crossed pulmonary artery 1 patient, origin of right pulmonary artery from the ascending aorta 1 patient, and abnormal origin of left upper pulmonary artery from the right pulmonary artery in 1 patient (Fig. 60.1).

Study limitations

Since this is a retrospective study from many institutions, complete cardiovascular investigation is not available from all patients with "normal" heart. Therefore the incidence of various cardiovascular

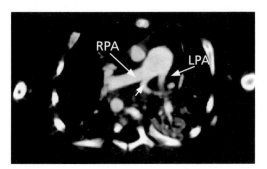

Fig. 60.1 CT image from a 1-month-old patient with huge PDA and mild isthmus hypoplasia, showing abnormal branch pulmonary artery to left upper lobe (short arrowhead) arising from the right pulmonary artery (RPA).

Table 60.1 Diagnosis of intra-cardiac lesions among 179 Korean patients (156 with congenital heart disease)

TOF	98 patients
"Simple"	48 patients
TOF with absent pulmonary valve	2 patients
TOF with pulmonary atresia	14 patients
TOF with pulmonary atresia and major aortopulmonary collateral arteries	34 patients
Ventricular septal defect	31 patients
Atrial septal defect	7 patients
Interrupted aortic arch with ventricular septal defect	7 patients
Double outlet right ventricle with pulmonary stenosis	7 patients
Persistent truncus arteriosus	2 patients
Patent ductus arteriosus	2 patients
Total anomalous pulmonary venous connection, supracardiac type	1 patients
Complete atrioventricular septal defect with double outlet right ventricle	1 patient

anomalies reported in this study probably represents a minimal estimate of the true incidence. Also, FISH study has been available for only 3–5 years in Korean hospitals and this syndrome is not well known to all medical specialists yet. As a result presumably only a small proportion of deletion patients are diagnosed and are included in this study.

Conclusion

A wide variety of cardiovascular anomalies, including some lesions not previously reported, were observed in our patients, expanding the spectrum of cardiovascular anomalies associated with this important genetic syndrome. A thorough cardiovascular investigation as well as noncardiac problems is essential in preoperative investigation and counseling.

Acknowledgments

This study was supported by a grant (no. 01-PJ10-PG6–01GN15–0001) from the Ministry of Health and Welfare, Republic of Korea.

CHAPTER 61

Atrioventricular canal defect: anatomical and genetic characteristics

Bruno Marino, Maria Cristina Digilio, Federica Mileto,
Emanuela Conti, Bruno Dallapiccola

The AVCD is a quite frequent CHD occurring in 3.5 per 10 000 live births, representing 7.3 of all CHD[1] and showing strong genetic impact and genetic heterogeneity.[2,3] There are essentially two main anatomic types of AVCD: a complete form, representing about the 70% of cases, and a partial form.

Our 15 years experience among > 600 patients shows that the DS represents 45% of cases and the heterotaxy 15% (Fig. 61.1). Moreover other genetic conditions, such as chromosomal or Mendelian syndromes or associations, are frequent, accounting for about 15% of cases. The nonsyndromic patients represent only 25% of all cases.

Down syndrome

Trisomy 21 is the classic genetic anomaly in children with AVCD. In this aneuploidy the complete form of AVCD is prevalent and additional cardiac defects (except TF) are rare.[4] In particular left-sided obstructive lesions are rare and anomalies of visceral situs, ventricular loop and TGA are virtually absent.[4,5] In the critical DS region of the chromosome 21 these are important candidate genes for the CHD including *DSCAM*,[6] *Collagen VI* and *XVIII*,[7] and *SH3BGR*.[8] All these genes could be involved in the mechanisms of cell adhesion and endocardial cushions fusion.

Heterotaxy

This complex syndrome may present with Mendelian, chromosomal or poligenic inheritance.

The two main groups of heterotaxy are asplenia and polysplenia presenting cardiac and extracardiac malformations different from each other. In particular, at cardiac level asplenia shows: complete AVCD with reduced number of leaflets and papillary muscle,[9] ventricular dominance, and transposition of the great arteries with pulmonary stenosis. In contrast, the cardiac defects of polysplenia are less complex including partial AVCD and normally related great arteries. Note that transposition of the great arteries is very rare in polysplenia. In these patients, in spite of ambiguity of the atrial situs, at ventricular and great arteries level, the following prevails: (1) the pattern of situs solitus with normal rightward spiraling of the ventricles (d-loop) and the great arteries (normally related) or (2) the pattern of situs inversus with leftward spiraling of the ventricles (l-loop) and of the great arteries (inversely normally related).[10] Studies on the genetics of heterotaxy show two contradictory aspects. Because familial recurrence includes the entire phenotypic spectrum and because the mutations of some human genes (such as *ZIC3*, *AVCR2*, and *CFC1*)[12] cause asplenia, polysplenia, and situs inversus, the first hypothesis suggests that a single genetic defect can cause multiple phenotypes. On the other hand, some recent studies suggest that there are different genetic pathways for asplenia and

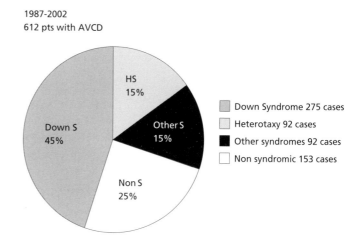

Fig. 61.1 Distribution of syndromes among patients with atrioventricular canal defects (AVCD).

polysplenia. In fact, target disruption in the mouse of some candidate genes results in more specific phenotypes. Animal knockout of PITX2 and SMAD2 cause right isomerism and TGA, and animal knockout of Sonic and Lefty 1 cause left isomerism with normally related great arteries. Moreover, human mutation of Lefty A and Lefty B is associated with left isomerism, complete AVCD, normally related great arteries, and left-sided obstructions.[11]

Other chromosomal syndromes

In our series of AVCD, the chromosomal defects represent 1.6% and the complete form is prevalent. The most frequent chromosomal anomaly after Trisomy 21 is deletion 8p consisting of growth and mental retardation and dysmorphic features. The AVCD is the most frequent CHD in this syndrome and the prevalent pattern includes the complete form of AVCD, cardiac malposition, and pulmonary valve stenosis recalling some cardiac features of heterotaxy. The critical region is a 5 cM area and *GATA4* is one of the candidate genes.[12] AVCD is also frequent in patients with deletion 3p. In this syndrome the critical region is at 3p25.3 and one of the candidate genes is *CRELD1*.[13]

Mendelian syndromes and associations

After the group of patients with Down syndrome and with heterotaxy, the group with Mendelian syn-

dromes and with associations is the most important.[2] In our experience these syndromes represent 9.3% of the entire series. The most frequent syndrome is the Noonan–Leopard syndrome. In this condition the common cardiovascular anomalies are pulmonary valve stenosis with dysplasia of the valve and hypertrophic cardiomyopathy, but also partial AVCD is quite frequent, with additional anomalies of the mitral valve causing subaortic stenosis.[14] PTPN11 is the causative gene, mapping to chromosome 12, showing different mutations in Noonan and in Leopard syndromes.[15]

A number of syndromes with polydactyly may be part of a common group of orofacioskeletal syndromes.[16] Ellis van Creveld syndrome, caused by a mutation of *EvC gene* to chromosome 4,[17] is the main syndrome of this group which presents polydactyly, short-limbed dwarphism, ectodermal anomalies and partial AVCD, common atrium, and persistent left superior vena cava.[16] Describing this cardiac phenotype, we indicated the anatomic similarities with some cardiac aspects of heterotaxy in particular with those of polysplenia.[16] Kaufman–McKusick syndrome, which has recently been grouped with the Bardet–Bield syndrome, is another example of these conditions characteristically associated with partial AVCD and common atrium. This syndrome is caused by a mutation of *BBS6* gene located on the short arm of chromosome 20. Smith–Lemli–Opitz syndrome is an autosomal recessive disorder of cholesterol metabolism also characterized by polydactyly and a complete AVCD,

Shh pathway in genetic syndromes with AVCD

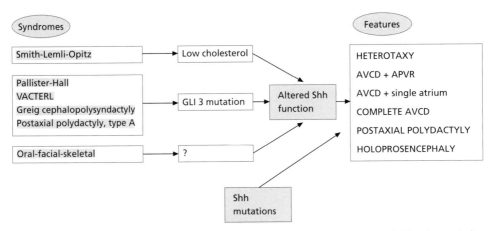

Fig. 61.2 Potential role of altered sonic hedgehog (shh) signaling in genetic syndromes associated with atrioventricular canal defects.

and a total anomalous pulmonary venous connection.[18] This pattern of cardiac defect also recalls some aspects of heterotaxy. The gene of this syndrome, *DHCR7*, maps to chromosome 11. A VACTERL association may also present the partial form of AVCD, perhaps in relation to a mutation of *Gli* genes and Sonic hedgehog signal transduction.

All these observations on OFS syndromes, SLO, VACTERL and other syndromes suggest the hypothesis that an altered function of Sonic pathways could lead to several different developmental errors presenting with partially overlapping manifestations including AVCD with or without heterotaxy, with or without polydactyly[19] (Fig. 61.2).

Nonsyndromic AVCD

The last group of AVCD consists of nonsyndromic patients and represents only 25% of the entire series. In this group, as we reported in 1986,[5] the partial form is prevalent and the left-sided obstructions are frequent. Moreover, familial recurrence is quite frequent, with autosomal dominant inheritance.[20] A linkage to chromosome 1p has been shown and a candidate gene is *p93*.[21]

Conclusions

It is evident that the AVCD shows a significant anatomic variability and genetic heterogeneity. The complete form of AVCD is prevalent in chromosomal imbalances and in patients with additional cardiac defects. Moreover additional heart malformations are prevalent also in children with Mendelian syndromes and associations. We even suggest that in many conditions it is possible to recognize a precise genotype–phenotype correlation.

Several mutations of different genes can activate a more limited number of pathogenetic mechanisms involved in the formation of AVC. These mechanisms lead to various phenotypes of AVCD with similar anatomic aspects. However, on some occasions the pathway is more specific and the phenotype is strictly correlated to the genetic cause: the anatomic form of AVCD and the type of additional cardiac defects can be characteristic of the syndrome.

An accurate phenotypic study and a description of cardiac anatomy is essential not only for surgical treatment but also to understand the cause and the pathogenesis of the cardiac malformations.

References

1 Loffredo CA, Hirata J, Wilson PD, Ferencz C, Lurie IW. Atrioventricular septal defects: possible etiologic differences between complete and partial defects. *Teratology* 2001; **63**: 87–93.

2 Digilio MC, Marino B, Toscano A, Giannoti A, Dallapiccola B. Atrioventricular canal defect without

Down syndrome: a heterogeneous malformation. *Am J Med Genet* 1999; **85**: 140–6.

3 Pierpont MEM, Markwald RR, Lin AE. Genetic aspects of atrioventricular septal defects. *Am J Med Genet* 2000; **97**: 289–96.

4 Marino B, Vairo U, Corno A *et al.* Atrioventricular canal in Down syndrome. Prevalence of associated cardiac malformations compared with patients without Down syndrome. *Am J Dis Child* 1990; **144**: 1120–2.

5 De Biase L, Di Ciommo V, Ballerini L *et al.* Prevalence of left-sided obstructive lesions in patients with atrioventricular canal without Down's syndrome. *J Thorac Cardiovasc Surg* 1986; **91**: 467–9.

6 Korenberg JR, Barlow GM, Chen XN *et al.* Down syndrome congenital heart disease: narrowed region and DSCAM as a candidate gene. In: Clark EB, Nakazawa M, Takao A, eds. *Etiology and Morphogenesis of Congenital Heart Disease: Twenty Years of Progress in Genetics and Developmental Biology.* Armonk, NY: Futura, 2000.

7 Jongewaard IN, Lauer RM, Behrendt DA, Patil S, Klewer SE. Beta 1 integrin activation mediates adhesive differences between trisomy 21 and non-trisomic fibroblasts on type VI collagen. *Am J Med Genet* 2002; **109**: 298–305.

8 Kerstann KF, Freeman SB, Feingolo E *et al.* Genetic variants associated with increased susceptibility for Down syndrome – associated atrioventricular septal defect. *Am J Hum Genet* (abstract) 2002; **71**: 445.

9 Francalanci P, Marino B, Boldrini R *et al.* Morphology of the atrioventricular valve in asplenia syndrome: a peculiar type of atrioventricular canal defect. *Cardiovasc Pathol* 1996; **5**: 145–51.

10 Marino B, Capolino R, Digilio MC, Di Donato R. Trasposition of the great arteries in asplenia and polysplenia phenotypes. *Am J Med Genet* 2002; **110**: 292–4.

11 Bamford RN, Roessler E, Burdine RD *et al.* Loss-of-function mutations in the EGF-CFC gene CFC1 are associated with human left-right laterality defects. *Nat Genet* 2000; **26**: 365–9.

12 Giglio S, Graw SL, Gimelli G *et al.* Deletion of a 5-cM region at chromosome 8p23 is assocaited with a spectrum of congenital heart defects. *Circulation* 2000; **102**: 432–7.

13 Maslen CL, Robinson SW, Morris CD. Mutation of CRELD1 associated with an atrioventricular canal defect. *Am J Hum Genet* (abstract) 2002; **71**: 209.

14 Marino B, Digilio MC, Toscano A, Gainnotti A, Dallapiccola B. Congenital heart diseases in children with Noonan syndrome: an expanded cardiac spectrum with high prevalence of atrioventricular canal. *J Pediatr* 1999; **135**: 703–6.

15 Digilio MC, Conti E, Sarkozy A *et al.* Grouping of multiple-lentigines/LEOPARD and Noonan syndromes on the PTPN11 gene. *Am J Hum Genet* 2002; **71**: 389–94.

16 Digilio MC, Marino B, Ammirati A *et al.* Cardiac malformations in patients with oral-facial-skeletal syndromes: clinical similarities with heterotaxia. *Am J Med Genet* 1999; **84**: 350–6.

17 Ruiz-Perez VL, Ide SE, Strom TM *et al.* Mutations in a new gene in Ellis-van Creveld syndrome and Weyers acrodental dysostosis. *Nat Genet* 2000; **24**: 283–6.

18 Lin AE, Ardinger HH, Ardinger RH, Cunniff C, Kelley RI. Cardiovascular malformations in Smith-Lemli-Opitz syndrome. *Am J Med Genet* 1997; **68**: 270–8.

19 Digilio MC, Marino B, Gainnotti A, Dallapiccola B, Opitz JM. Specific congenital heart defects in RSH/Smith-Lemli-Opitz syndrome: postulated involvement of the sonic hedgehog pathway in syndromes with postaxial polydactyly or heterotaxia. *Birth Defects Res Part A Clin Mol Teratol* 2003; **67**: 149–53.

20 Digilio MC, Marino B, Ciani MP *et al.* Risk of congenital heart defects in relatives of patients with atrioventricular canal. *Am J Dis Child* 1993; **147**: 1295–97.

21 Zhao Y, Meng X, Cao H *et al.* Molecular cloning and characterization of a potential candidate gene for nonsyndromic atrioventricular septal defect on 1p31–1p21. *J Am Coll Cardiol* 2002 (abstract); **39**: 408.

CHAPTER 62

A genetic approach to hypoplastic left heart syndrome

Paul Grossfeld

Introduction

Hypoplastic left heart syndrome (HLHS) comprises 2–3% of congenital heart defects, but accounts for 20–25% of mortality in all infants born with congenital heart disease. The first report of HLHS was described in 1851 by Dr Bardeleben, a German pathologist.[1] He described the constellation of findings in a newborn infant that died, which included a hypoplastic left ventricular cavity, atretic mitral and aortic valves, a hypoplastic aorta, an atrial septal communication, and a patent ductus arteriosus. Furthermore, he deduced that the systemic circulation depended upon the patency of the ductus arteriosus, and that closure of the ductus caused the infant's demise.

Two surgical options for HLHS currently exist.[2,3] The first, transplantation, is not a realistic option for the majority of HLHS infants, because of the shortage of available donor hearts. The other option, the three stage Norwood/Fontan procedure, ultimately converts the right ventricle to become the systemic ventricle. Both options have inherent limitations, and the 5-year survival of either is, at best, 70%. Furthermore, the long-term prognosis for either option is guarded. Hence, our current surgical modalities for HLHS can only be considered a palliation.

There is strong evidence for a genetic etiology for HLHS.[4]. For example, there are numerous reports of HLHS occurring in families. Recently, echocardiograms performed on siblings of infants with HLHS demonstrated a 30% occurrence of congenital heart defects, ranging in severity from a bicuspid aortic valve to HLHS.[5] HLHS has also been associated with multiple genetic loci and occurs in many dysmorphic syndromes, many of which are likely to be of a genetic etiology.

Three possible approaches can be used for identifying genes causing HLHS: linkage analysis, deletion disorders, and balanced translocations. Linkage analysis is a powerful tool for identifying candidate genes when large families are available, when there is high genetic penetrance, and when there are not multiple genetic loci involved. Thus, linkage analysis is unlikely to be useful for identifying genes that cause HLHS.

We have used a combined approach to identify a candidate gene for HLHS by studying a rare genetic deletion disorder, Jacobsen syndrome, in combination with the molecular cloning of a patient with a heart defect that carried a balanced translocation. Jacobsen syndrome (JS) was first reported in 1973 by the Danish geneticist, Dr Petrea Jacobsen.[6] Since her original publication, approximately 100 cases have been reported in the English literature.[7] We have subsequently studied prospectively over 100 cases of JS.[8]

JS is caused by the terminal deletion of the long (q) arm of chromosome 11 (Fig. 62.1), extending to the telomere. Previous studies have identified that the deletion breakpoints are variable, and that the breakpoints cluster around CCG trinucleotide repeat sequences.[9–11]

Our studies revealed that 57% of patients with Jacobsen syndrome have severe heart defects (Table 62.1).[12] We have divided these defects into two groups. The first, which includes about two-thirds of JS patients with heart defects, consists of left-sided obstructive lesions and ventricular septal defects, so-called flow lesions. HLHS occurs in about 5–10%

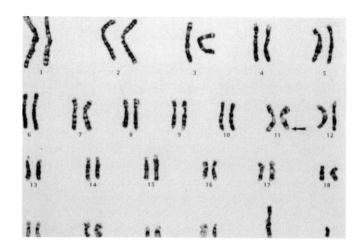

Fig. 62.1 Karyotype of a patient with Jacobsen syndrome. Arrow, deletion of 11q.

Table 62.1 Heart defects in Jacobsen syndrome

Flow lesions (common)	Miscellaneous lesions (uncommon)
Hypoplastic left heart syndrome	Secundum atrial septal defect
Shone's	Double outlet right ventricle
Coarctation of the aorta	Aberrant right subclavian artery
Bicuspid aortic valve	Atrioventricular canal defect
Aortic valve stenosis	d-Transposition of the great arteries
Mitral valve Stenosis	Dextrocardia
Membranous ventricular septal defect	Tricuspid atresia
	Type B interruption of the aortic arch/truncus arteriosus
	Left-sided superior vena cava

of all patients with JS, an unprecedented frequency of HLHS for any dysmorphic syndrome. This represents a frequency of 1000–2000 times that of the general population. The other third have a wide variety of heart defects, including atrioventricular canal defect, double outlet right ventricle, secundum atrial septal defects, and d-transposition of the great arteries. To summarize, HLHS occurs at an unprecedented frequency in JS, and many of the most common congenital heart defects occur in JS.

Experimental approach

Initially, we mapped the deletion breakpoints in 35 JS patients with heart defects by fluorescence *in situ* hybridization (FISH), There was no apparent correlation between the deletion breakpoints and the type of heart defect. Thus, the patient with the smallest deletion with a heart defect (in this case, HLHS), defined a cardiac 'minimal' region in 11q. Analysis of

this region using the human genome database revealed the presence of about 20 known genes in this minimal region. At least two of these genes, *KCNJ5* and *JAM3*, are expressed in the heart. *KCNJ5* encodes a cardiac potassium channel. A mouse knockout model of this gene caused sinus arrhythmias, a nonlethal phenotype, and there was no evidence of structural heart defects in these knockout mice.[13] Patients with isolated HLHS were analyzed for mutations in *JAM3*, but none were found.[14]

To identify an individual candidate gene(s) in the Jacobsen syndrome cardiac minimal region, we mapped and cloned the molecular breakpoint of a patient with a balanced translocation whose breakpoint is in 11q. This patient had a severely dysplastic pulmonary valve that required surgical valvotomy. In addition, she had a submucosal cleft palate, developmental delay, and craniofacial defects. All of these disorders occur in Jacobsen syndrome. Although still possible, the association of the balanced translocation in this patient with the clinical phenotype described (i.e., a 'partial JS phenotype') seemed unlikely to be coincidental.

The karyotype of this patient (t:11;17:25;21) suggested that the breakpoint in 11q could be in the JS cardiac minimal region. We hypothesized that interruption of a gene in the cardiac minimal region would define that gene as a candidate gene for causing at least a subset of the heart defects in JS. Towards that end, we mapped the breakpoint of the translocation. Initially, we used overlapping BAC clones and identified the molecular breakpoint to be within the JS cardiac minimal region. Next, we performed genomic southern hybridization and subsequently cloned the chromosome 11 and 17 translocation breakpoints.[12] No genes or expressed sequence tags seemed to be interrupted by the chromosome 17 breakpoints. The chromosome 11 breakpoint, however, was found to be between exons 1 and 2 of a known gene in the 11q cardiac minimal region: *OBCAM* (opiate binding cell adhesion molecule).

OBCAM is a member of the immunoglobulin superfamily of genes. The protein is 345 amino acids long and contains three immunoglobulin binding domains, as well as a carboxyl-terminus glycosylphophatidyl (GPI) binding domain that is required for attachment of protein to the cell surface.[15] OBCAM is a member of the IgLON subfamily of proteins, consisting of three other closely related genes: Neurotrimin, LAMP (limbic-associated membrane protein), and Kilon (kindred of IgLONs).[16–20] The IgLONs are highly conserved genes across human, mouse, rat, chick, and bovine genomes; they are located at 11q25, 3q13.2-q21, and 1p31. Interestingly, Neurotrimin is located next to OBCAM at 11q25, in a tail to tail configuration. The sequence of exon 1 of OBCAM and Neurotrimin is identical.

Previous studies of the IgLONs have been on their function in the brain, where they are most abundantly expressed, and in a unique pattern.[17–19,21–24]

These studies have implicated a putative role for the IgLONs as a cell adhesion molecule that mediates essential cell–cell interactions during axon formation. Prior studies have not detected expression of any of the IgLONs in the heart.[19–23]

All patients with Jacobsen syndrome and heart defects have both Neurotrimin and OBCAM deleted.[12] To determine if the IgLONs are expressed in human heart, we performed Northern blot analysis to mRNA from fetal and adult human heart. Interestingly, all four genes were found to be expressed in the heart, in a chamber-specific pattern (Table 62.2). Furthermore, multiple isoforms were detected whose expression pattern is regulated during development. Recent studies in chick heart have identified both a cell membrane-bound and a cytosolic form of OBCAM, suggesting multiple functions for OBCAM in the heart [unpubl. data]. Thus, the region-specific expression pattern of the IgLONs in the heart is reminiscent of that in the brain. Taken together, the IgLONs seem to have an important function in cardiac development and function.

To determine whether mutations in OBCAM might occur in patients with isolated heart defects that occur in Jacobsen syndrome, we performed DNA sequencing analysis on 35 patients with flow lesions. No mutations were detected. We are currently analyzing patients for possible microdeletions spanning OBCAM and Neurotrimin, using quantitative real time polymerase chain reaction[25] (Fig. 62.2).

Future studies

To date, the function of the IgLONs in the heart is unknown. No functional or genetic knockouts have been reported. Based on our current data, it seems that interruption of OBCAM (i.e. by the balanced translocation), causes defective pulmonary valve development (dsyplasia), whereas deletion of both OBCAM and Neurotrimin causes more severe heart

Table 62.2 Human cardiac expression pattern of IgLONs

	Fetal	Adult	Aorta	Apex	RA	LA	RV	LV	Dev
OB	+	++	++	++	+	+	++	++	Yes
NT	+++	+	+	++++	+	+	+	+	Yes
KILON	+	+	ND	+	+	+	+	+	No
LAMP	ND	+	ND	++	ND	ND	++	++++	Yes

OBCAM EXON 2 COPY NUMBER

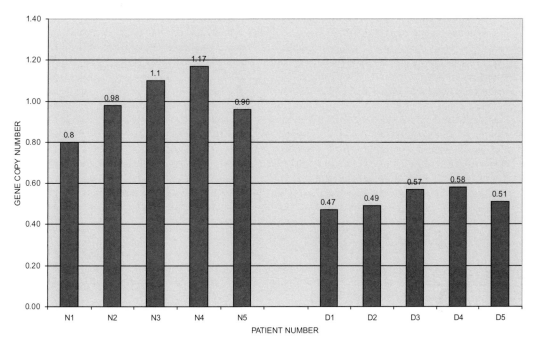

Fig. 62.2 Relative copy number of OBCAM in five normal (N1–N5), and five Jacobsen syndrome patients (D1–D5) that are hemizygous for OBCAM (mapped previously by FISH), using quantitative real time polymerase chain reaction. The probe to OBCAM was to exon 2. Control probe was to RNAseP.

defects, including HLHS. The molecular basis of the incomplete penetrance and variable cardiac phenotype is unknown. We are currently generating knockouts of the IgLONs in order to elucidate the function of these genes in cardiac development and in causing congenital heart defects.

Recently, we obtained cardiac tissue from a newborn infant with Jacobsen syndrome and HLHS. This tissue may prove valuable for studying the effect of hemizygosity of OBCAM and Neurotrimin on IgLON gene expression, as well as on other genes involved in cardiac development.

Summary

Jacobsen syndrome is a rare chromosomal disorder caused by terminal deletions of 11q. Using a combination of deletion mapping and the cloning of a patient with a balanced translocation, we have implicated a role for the IgLONs in cardiac development and congenital heart defects. Clearly, the combined approach of the human, chick, and mouse systems will help elucidate the exact functions of this interesting subfamily of genes in cardiac development and congenital heart disease.

Acknowledgments
The author would like to thank Drs Ju Chen and Abraham Rothman for their critical review of this manuscript, and to all of the 11q families for their unrelenting support and participation in this research.

References

1 Josef Gehrmann, MD; Thomas Krasemann, MD; Hans Gerd Kehl, MD and Johannes Vogt, MD, PhD. Hypoplastic left-heart syndrome: the first description of the pathophysiology in 1851; translation of a publication by Dr Bardeleben From Giessen, Germany. *Chest* 2001; **120**: 1368–71.

2 Razzouk AJ, Chinnock RE, Gundry ST *et al.* Transplantation as a primary treatment for hypoplastic left heart syndrome: Intermediate term results. *Ann Thorac Surg* 1996; **62**: 1–8.

3 Norwood WI. Hypoplastic left heart syndrome. *Ann Thorac Surg* 1991; **52**: 688–95.

4 Grossfeld PD. The molecular genetics of hypoplastic left heart syndrome. *Cardiol Young* 1999; **9**: 627–32.

5 Loffredo C *et al*. Prevalence of congenital cardiovascular malformations among relatives of infants with hypoplastic left heart, coarctation of the aorta, and d-transposition of the great arteries. *Am J Med Genet* 2004; **124A**: 225–30.

6 Jacobsen P, Hauge M, Henningsen K *et al*. An (11; 21) translocation in four generations with chromosome 11 abnormalities in the offspring. *Hum Hered* 1973; **23**: 568–85.

7 Leegte B, Kerstjens-Frederikse WS, Deelstra K, Begeer JH, van Essen AJ. 11q-syndrome: three cases and a review of the literature. *Genet Couns* 1999; **10**: 305–13.

8 Grossfeld PD *et al*. The terminal 11q deletion disorder: a prospective study of 109 cases. *Am J Med Genet* 2004; **129A**: 51–61.

9 Penny LA, Dell'Aquila M, Jones MC *et al*. Cliniical and molecular characterization of patients with distal 11q deletions. *Am J Hum Genet* 1995; **56**: 676–83.

10 Tunnacliffe A, Jones C, Le Paslier D *et al*. Localization of Jacobsen syndrome breakpoints on a 40-Mb physical map of distal chromosome 11q. *Genome Res* 1999; **9**: 44–52.

11 Jones C, Mullenbach R, Grossfeld P *et al*. Co-localization of CCG repeats and chromosome deletion breakpoints in Jacobean syndrome: evidence for a common mechanism of chromosome breakage. *Hum Mol Genet* 2000; **9**: 1201–8.

12 Grossfeld PD *et al*. The 11q deletion disorder: Identification of a candidate gene for heart defects. In press.

13 Wickman K, Nemec J, Gendler SJ, Clapham DE. Abnormal heart rate regulation in GIRK4 knockout mice. *Neuron* 1998; **20**: 103–14.

14 Phillips HM, Renforth GL, Spalluto C *et al*. Narrowing the critical region within 11q24-qter for hypoplastic left heart and identification of a candidate gene, *JAM3*, expressed during cardiogenesis. *Genomics* 2002; **79**: 475–8.

15 Shark KB, Lee NM. Cloning, sequencing and localization

16 Lippman DA, Lee NM, Loh HH. Opioid-binding cell adhesion molecule (OBCAM)-related clones from a rat brain cDNA library. *Gene* 1992; **177**: 249–54.

17 Wilson DJA, Kim DS, Clark GA, Marshall-Clarke S, Moss DJ. A family of glycoproteins (gp55), which inhibit neurite outgrowth, are members of the Ig superfamily and are related to OBCAM, neurotrimin, LAMP and CEPU-1. *J Cell Sci* 1996; **109**: 3129–38.

18 Lodge AP, Howard MR, McNamee CJ, Moss DJ. Co-localization, heterophilic interactions and regulated expression of IgLON family proteins in the chick nervous system. *Mol Brain Res* 2000; **82**: 84–94.

19 Struyk AF *et al*. Cloning of Neurotrimin defines a new subfamily of differentially expressed neural cell adhesion molecules. *J Neurosci* 1995; **15**: 2141–56.

20 Funatsu N *et al*. Characterization of a novel rat brain GPI-anchored protein (kilon), a member of the IgLON cell adhesion molecule family. *J Biol Chem* 1999; **274**: 8224–30.

21 Hachisuka A, Yamazaki T, Sawada J, Terao T. Characterization and tissue distribution of opioid-binding cell adhesion molecule (OBCAM) using monoclonal antibodies. *Neurochem Int* 1996; 28: 373–9.

22 Hachisuka A *et al*. Localization of opioid-binding cell adhesion molecule (OBCAM) in adult rat brain. *Brain Res* 1999; **842**: 482–6.

23 Hachisuka A, Nakajima O, Yamazaki T, Sawada J. Development expression of opioid-binding cell adhesion molecule (OBCAM) in rat brain. *Dev Brain Res* 2000; **122**: 183–91.

24 Lodge AP, McNamee CJ, Howard MR, Reed JE, Moss DJ. Identification and characterization of CEPU-Se- A secreted isoform of the IgLON family protein, CEPU-1. *Mol Cell Neurosci* 2001; **17**: 746–60 .

25 Kariyazono H, Ohno T, Ihara K *et al*. Rapid detection of the 22q11.2 deletion with quantitative real-time PCR. *Mol Cell Probes* 2001; **15**: 71–3.

16 ... to chromosome 11 of a cDNA encoding a human opioid-binding cell adhesion molecule (OBCAM). *Gene* 1995; **155**: 213–17.

CHAPTER 63

Char syndrome and *TFAP2B* mutations

Bruce D. Gelb

Clinical description of Char syndrome

Florence Char, an American geneticist, described a novel syndrome in 1978, based on her observations with a four-generation Arkansas family.[1] The principal features that she noted were facial dysmorphia consisting of a short philtrum, patulous lips, ptosis, and low-set ears (Fig. 63.1a), aplasia of a phalanx in the 5th fingers (Fig. 63.1b), and patent ductus arteriosus. Dr Char noted that the mode of inheritance of this disorder was autosomal dominant and that expression of the trait was variable.

Since that description of the trait, which is now referred to eponymously, a limited number of additional publications have described additional families inheriting Char syndrome.[2–8] In addition, the original kindred described by Dr Char was re-evaluated 30 years later, by which time a number of additional affected individuals were available.[9] Clinical descriptions of the affected individuals in those families expanded the range of abnormalities associated with Char syndrome (Table 63.1). Most of these features have varied significantly between and within families inheriting Char syndrome. The exception is the dysmorphia, which has been present in all patients although less marked among affected individuals in one family.[4] Disease penetrance seems to be complete. The variability of the expression of the Char syndrome phenotype was compared between two large kindreds with 19 and 14 affected individuals (the original Char and Sletten kindreds, respectively).[9] Patent ductus arteriosus prevalence was 21% in the former and 71% in the latter, while the prevalence of 5th finger abnormalities was 89%

and 0%, respectively. In all families with several affected individuals, the pattern of inheritance is autosomal dominant with complete penetrance.

There are no data about the anatomy or histology of the ductus arteriosus or other affected structures in Char syndrome.

Genetic mapping and disease gene discovery

Satoda and co-workers identified *TFAP2B* as the Char syndrome disease gene using a positional candidacy approach.[10] Initially, two multigenerational kindred, the original family discovered by Florence Char[1] and a second kindred identified by Sletten and Pierpont,[4] were used to perform linkage analysis.[9] Significant linkage was found with several polymorphic DNA markers mapping to chromosome 6p12-p21. The maximal two-point LOD score was 8.39, achieved with marker *D6S1638*. Both families contributed positively to the LOD scores obtained with markers from that region and independently provided evidence for linkage. Haplotype analysis identified recombinant events that defined the Char syndrome locus with high probability to a 3.1-cM region between *D6S459/D6S1632/D6S1541* and *D6S1024*. While genetic heterogeneity is suspected for Char syndrome (discussed below), no proof of that has been reported using linkage exclusion mapping.

Next, Satoda and co-workers discovered that missense mutations in *TFAP2B* cause Char syndrome.[10] They physically mapped *TFAP2B*, which had been assigned to chromosomal band 6p21 with FISH, into the critical region for Char syndrome and then

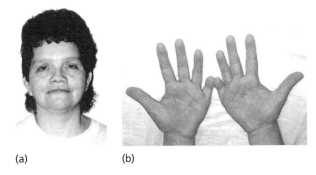

(a)   (b)

Fig. 63.1 (a) Typical facial features of Char syndrome in an affected 46-year-old woman from the Arkansas family. The short philtrum, prominent lips, flat nasal bridge with upturned nares, midface hypoplasia, and ptosis are evident. (b) Hands of the same individual with Char syndrome. The 5th middle phalanges are absent, and the 5th proximal and distal phalanges are hypoplastic.

Table 63.1 Clinical features of Char syndrome

Dysmorphia	Broad forehead
	Hypertelorism
	Ptosis
	Flat nasal bridge
	Flat nasal tip
	Short philtrum
	Patulous lips
	Low set pinnae
Cardiovascular	Patent ductus arteriosus
	Muscular ventricular septal defect
	Complex defects
Skeletal	Clinodactyly of 5th fingers
	Hypoplasia or aplasia of middle phalanx of the 5th fingers
	Polydactyly of the toes
	Partial syndactyly of the toes
	Abnormal 5th toes (broad, externally rotated)
Ophthalmalogic	Strabismus
	Myopia
Polythelia Dental/Oral	Hypodontia of permanent teeth
	High arched palate
Developmental delay, mild	

performed mutation analysis with the original Char kindred and a modest Scottish family.[3] Both families were inheriting exon 5 missense mutations, which were, respectively, a C-to-A transversion at nucleotide 791 that predicted the substitution of an alanine by an aspartic acid residue at codon 264

(A264D) and a C-to-T transition at nt 865 that predicted the substitution of an arginine by a cysteine at codon 289 (R289C). Subsequently, this research group genotyped an additional eight unrelated patients and families with Char syndrome.[11] They identified four additional missense mutations (Table 63.2). No mutation was found in four individuals with Char syndrome. While the mutation analysis scanned only the coding exons and their intron boundaries, the dominant negative effects of the mutations that were identified suggested that changes in regulatory regions of the *TFAP2B* gene would be unlikely to cause Char syndrome. Thus, Char syndrome may prove to be genetically heterogeneous.

Tfap2b and its protein product

Moser and co-workers cloned the mouse *Tfap2b* cDNA using its homology to *Tfap2a*.[12] First, a human genomic bacteriophage library was screened with a portion of the human *TFAP2A* cDNA. This resulted in the isolation of two weakly hybridizing phage clones that contained sequences homologous to exons 2–6. This, in turn, led to a screening of a mouse fetal cDNA phage library and the isolation of cDNAs with the entire coding region. Williamson and co-workers isolated the orthologous human cDNA from a breast cancer-derived cell line.[13] The 1391-bp human cDNA has 5′ and 3′ untranslated regions of 32 and 9 bp, respectively. The open reading frame of 1350 bp encodes a 450-residue polypeptide with a predicted unglycosylated $M_r = 49\ 266$. The predicted protein sequence has the typical organization of AP-2 transcription factors: an N-terminal transactivation domain, a basic domain, and a

Table 63.2 TFAP2B Mutations causing Char syndrome

Family	Nucleotide substitution	Exon	Amino acid substitution	Functional domain
Minnesota	C185>G	2	P62R	Transact.
Palestine	C673>T	4	R225C	Basic
England	C673>A	4	R225S	Basic
Arkansas	C791>A	5	A264D	Basic
Australia	G821>A	5	R274Q	Basic
Scotland	C865>T	5	R289C	HSH

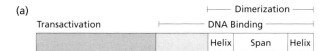

(a)

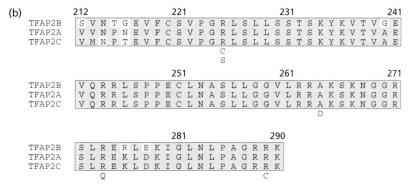

(b)

Fig. 63.2 (a) Cartoon showing the domain arrangement of a prototypical AP-2 protein. (b) Clustal W alignment of the basic and helix-span-helix (HSH) regions of the human TFAP2 protein sequences with five Char syndrome mutations. Identical amino acid residues are shaded in gray. The basic region of TFAP2B extends from residue 212–287 and the first helix of the HSH motif extends from residue 288–315.[30]

C-terminal helix-span-helix (HSH) domain (Fig. 63.2a). The sequence of the basic and HSH domain are highly conserved with the other three human AP-2 proteins (Fig. 63.2b) as well as those in other organisms such as mouse, chicken, frog, and fly (e.g., *Drosophila* AP-2 and human TFAP2A are 68% identical). The transactivation domains are far more divergent among the AP-2 proteins (e.g. Drosophila AP-2 and human TFAP2A are only 28% identical). The TFAP2B transactivation domain, like those of most of the AP-2 proteins, contains a PY motif (XPPXY) and certain other conserved residues, which are critical for transactivating gene expression.[14]

The expression pattern of *Tfap2b* has been studied during mouse embryogenesis.[15] At the earliest stage examined, day 8 post coitum (p.c.), *Tfap2b* expression is observed in the lateral head mesenchyme, neural fold, and the extraembryonic trophoblast. At day 10 p.c., *Tfap2b* is expressed in the mid- and hindbrain, the spinal cord, dorsal root ganglia, and the facial mesenchyme, the first branchial arch, and the surface ectoderm. Later, during organogenesis, *Tfap2b* continues to be expressed in the midbrain and facial mesenchyme and is expressed in the kidney and corneal epithelium. This tissue-specific expression pattern has overlap with other AP-2 genes in some structures at certain time points, but is unique overall.

Moser and co-workers generated a mouse model with complete deficiency of Tfap2b using targeted gene disruption in embryonic stem cells.[16] Mice that were heterozygous for the *Tfap2b* allele were phenotypically normal, while homozygotes died in the newborn period. It was shown that *Tfap2b-/-* mice have polycystic kidneys with cysts in the collecting ducts and distal tubules. These renal changes occurred relatively late in kidney development and were due to excessive apoptosis in the affected regions that was accompanied by downregulation of anti-apoptotic genes. These investigators did not note any malformations in structures comparable to those affected in Char syndrome.

The genome of the fruit fly *Drosophila melanogaster* contains a single AP-2 gene (*dAP-2*). The gene has been cloned[17,18] and several mutant alleles have been generated.[19,20] Flies with null mutations die as adults or late pupae. They have an abnormal phenotype that includes severely shortened legs with absent tarsal joints as well as reduced proboscis. While embryonic brain development is normal, defects do exist in the central complex of the protocerebrum. Hypomorphic *dAP-2* alleles have less severe effects on leg shortening. Interestingly, these mutations result in ectopic growth in the eye territory including supernumerary antennae, potentially through a developmental mechanism that might be relevant for the polythelia observed in some individuals with Char syndrome.

One particularly interesting *Drosophila dAP-2* mutation is R243C,[20] which alters the arginine residue corresponding to the one mutated in the Char syndrome allele, R225C. In flies, R243C is a null mutant associated with a severe phenotype comparable to that observed with CRIM-negative mutants. When paired with hypomorphic mutations, the R243C allele caused a more severe phenotype, evidence of a dominant negative effect. These results provided confirmation *in vivo* of the dominant negative effects that were documented *in vitro* and in cell culture with the TFAP2B R225C mutant protein.

Molecular pathology of Char syndrome

As noted above, six *TFAP2B* mutations associated with Char syndrome have been identified to date. Several features are noteworthy. First, they are all missense mutations. This makes it less likely that they cause haplo-insufficiency, a notion bolstered by the mutant protein characterization studies described below. Second, five of the six *TFAP2B* gene defects affect residues in the basic or HSH domain (Fig. 63.2b). Since those domains are critical for DNA binding, it seems that the pathogenic mechanism underlying Char syndrome relates to perturbed binding of AP-2 dimers containing mutant TFAP2B to their target gene regulatory sites. Third, four of the six Char syndrome mutations alter arginine residues. As discussed by Zhao *et al.*,[11] the disproportion of arginine missense mutations observed in *TFAP2B* and other transcription factors[21,22] can be attributed to synergism between fundamental genetic and structural mechanisms. A genetic mechanism is invoked because four of the six codons coding for arginine contain CpG dinucleotides, which are susceptible to mutagenesis.[23] In fact, all four *TFAP2B* arginine residues that are mutated are encoded by CGX codons. The structural mechanism relates to that fact that arginine residues are known to play critical functions in the binding of transcription factors to their target sequences.[24] Specifically, they can form hydrogen bonds with bases as well as with phosphate groups in the DNA backbone.

The effects of the six TFAP2B mutant proteins have been characterized *in vitro* and in cell culture.[10,11] Electromobility shift assays (EMSAs) were used to assess the ability of mutant TFAP2B proteins to bind TFAP2 target DNA sequence. Wild type and mutant proteins were translated *in vitro* and incubated with the palindromic TFAP2 recognition sequence from position −180 of the human metallothionein-2A gene (*MT2A* -180). The P62R protein, which has normal basic and HSH sequence, engendered a normal shift (Fig. 63.3). Among the mutants affecting the basic or HSH domains, the R274Q protein weakly bound sequence while the other four mutants did not. When these mutants were co-expressed with a truncated TFAP2A protein

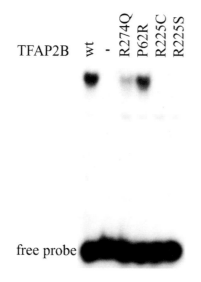

Fig. 63.3 Autoradiograms of electromobility shift assays (EMSAs) performed using recombinant TFAP2B proteins. EMSAs performed with singly translated recombinant TFAP2B proteins that had been incubated with [^{32}P]-labeled DNA with the consensus TFAP2 binding sequence. Free probe is indicated below. EMSA performed with co-translated TFAP2B and truncated TFAP2A proteins. Truncated TFAP2A (ΔN165), which retains dimerization and DNA-binding properties, was co-translated with wild type and mutant TFAP2B. TFAP2 protein were incubated with [^{32}P]-labeled DNA with the consensus TFAP2 binding sequence and electrophoresed. The two homodimer species (upper and lower shifted complexes) and the heterodimer (intermediate shifted complex) are indicated.

that retains its dimerization and DNA binding functions, it was observed that heterodimers containing R225S, R274Q, and R289C did bind target sequence while R225C heterodimers were not able to do so (Fig. 63.3). Protein cross-linking documented that R225C protein dimerizes, establishing its deficit as a failure of DNA binding per se.

The six TFAP2B mutants have been expressed transiently in NIH3T3 cells, either alone or with wild type TFAP2B, and their ability to transactivate a chloramphenicol acetyl transferase (CAT) reporter gene assessed.[10,11] When expressed singly, all mutants engendered significantly less CAT expression than wild type (Fig. 63.4a). When co-expressed with wild type TFAP2B, all mutants significantly reduced the CAT expression expected from the wild type protein (Fig. 63.4b). This documented that the mutant-wild type heterodimers were not trans-

activating efficiently, clear evidence that the mutants have dominant negative effects. There were some significant differences among the mutants with the R225C and A264D proteins having the most negative effects.

Genotype/phenotype correlation

As documented above, five of the six *TFAP2B* mutations have affected DNA binding, while one mutation, P62R, affected the transactivation domain. While the functional profile of P62R was similar to that of R274Q and R289C, the phenotype associated with P62R was strikingly different.[4,9] The facial dysmorphism originally described by Florence Char has been consistent among affected individuals with relatively little intra- or interfamilial variation. The affected members in the family bearing the P62R mutation consistently had a much milder facial dysmorphism, such that the original assignment of affectation status for some individuals in that kindred without PDA was in error. In addition, other families with multiple affected individuals have revealed some persons with abnormalities of the hands, ranging from aplasia of the middle phalanx of the fifth digit to clinodactyly. None of the 14 affected members of the family inheriting the P62R mutation had such hand defects.

Despite the mild facial and hand phenotype, the prevalence of PDA and other cardiovascular defects in the family inheriting P62R was high. This discrepancy between the effects of P62R on cardiac development versus those on craniofacial and hand development requires explanation, particularly since two other mutants with comparable dominant negative effects are associated with the typical Char syndrome phenotype. One potential basis for this phenomenon would depend on the expression patterns of TFAP2 coactivators. The PY motif has been shown to mediate interactions between transcription factors and coactivators.[25] Thus, adverse effects of P62R could be more marked in certain tissues, in which coactivators interacting with the PY motif play a greater role in modulating transcriptional activation. Testing of this hypothesis, particularly with respect to cardiovascular development, must await identification of the relevant TFAP2B coactivators.

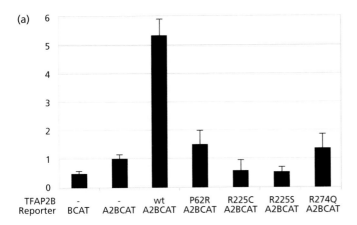

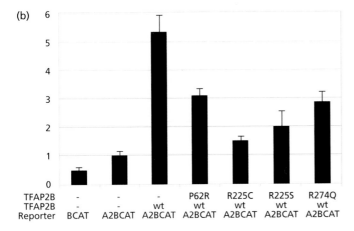

Fig. 63.4 Transactivation assays with wild type and mutant TFAP2B in NIH3T3 cells. (a) Cells were transfected transiently with 1.5 µg of the CAT reporter construct (A2BCAT) with three copies of TFAP2 binding sequence or an equivalent amount of the CAT-only construct (BCAT). To test for transactivation, 0.3 µg wild type (wt) or mutant *TFAP2B* construct was co-transfected with A2BCAT. After 48 h, cells were lysed and the CAT concentrations in the lysates determined. To normalize for transfection efficiency, 0.5 µg of pQB125 was co-transfected, and GFP fluorescence measured. The bars indicate the mean and standard errors from three independent transfections. Units are arbitrary and the mean from the condition with only A2BCAT was set at 1.0. (b) Transient co-expression of wild and mutant *TFAP2B* genes in NIH3T3 cells. Co-transfections and analysis were performed as described in Fig. 63.4(a). Total DNA used during the transfection was made equivalent for all conditions with an unrelated plasmid.

Acknowledgments

This work was supported in part from awards from the National Institutes of Health (HD38018) and the March of Dimes (FY00–246).

References

1 Char F. Peculiar facies with short philtrum, duck-bill lips, ptosis and low-set ears – a new syndrome? *Birth Defects Orig Artic Ser* 1978; **14**: 303–5.

2 Temple IK. Char syndrome (unusual mouth, patent ductus arteriosus, phalangeal anomalies). *Clin Dysmorphol* 1992; **1**: 17–21.

3 Davidson HR. A large family with patent ductus arteriosus and unusual face. *J Med Genet* 1993; **30**: 503–5.

4 Sletten LJ, Pierpont ME. Familial occurrence of patent ductus arteriosus. *Am J Med Genet* 1995; **57**: 27–30.

5 Slavotinek A, Clayton-Smith J, Super M. Familial patent ductus arteriosus: a further case of CHAR syndrome. *Am J Med Genet* 1997; **71**: 229–32.

6 Sweeney E, Fryer A, Walters M. Char syndrome: a new family and review of the literature emphasising the presence of symphalangism and the variable phenotype. *Clin Dysmorphol* 2000; **9**: 177–82.

7 Bertola DR, Kim CA, Sugayama SM *et al.* Further delineation of Char syndrome. *Pediatr Int* 2000; **42**: 85–8.

8 Zannolli R, Mostardini R, Matera M *et al.* Char syndrome: an additional family with polythelia, a new finding. *Am J Med Genet* 2000; **95**: 201–3.

9 Satoda M, Pierpont ME, Diaz GA, Bornemeier RA, Gelb BD. Char syndrome, an inherited disorder with patent ductus arteriosus, maps to chromosome 6p12-p21. *Circulation* 1999; **99**: 3036–42.

10 Satoda M, Zhao F, Diaz GA *et al.* Mutations in TFAP2B cause Char syndrome, a familial form of patent ductus arteriosus. *Nat Genet* 2000; **25**: 42–46.

11 Zhao F, Weismann CG, Satoda M *et al.* Novel TFAP2B mutations that cause Char syndrome provide a genotype-phenotype correlation. *Am J Hum Genet* 2001; **69**: 695–703.

12 Moser M, Imhof A, Pscherer A *et al.* Cloning and characterization of a second AP-2 transcription factor: AP-2 beta. *Development* 1995; **121**: 2779–88.

13 Williamson JA, Bosher JM, Skinner A *et al.* Chromosomal mapping of the human and mouse homologues of two new members of the AP-2 family of transcription factors. *Genomics* 1996; **35**: 262–4.

14 Wankhade S, Yu Y, Weinberg J, Tainsky MA, Kannan P. Characterization of the activation domains of AP-2 family transcription factors. *J Biol Chem* 2000; **275**: 29701–8.

15 Moser M, Ruschoff J, Buettner R. Comparative analysis of AP-2 alpha and AP-2 beta gene expression during murine embryogenesis. *Dev Dyn* 1997; **208**: 115–24.

16 Moser M, Pscherer A, Roth C *et al.* Enhanced apoptotic cell death of renal epithelial cells in mice lacking transcription factor AP-2beta. *Genes Dev* 1997; **11**: 1938–48.

17 Monge I, Mitchell PJ. DAP-2, the Drosophila homolog of transcription factor AP-2. *Mech Dev* 1998; **76**: 191–5.

18 Bauer R, McGuffin ME, Mattox W, Tainsky MA. Cloning and characterization of the Drosophila homologue of the AP-2 transcription factor. *Oncogene* 1998; **17**: 1911–22.

19 Kerber B, Monge I, Mueller M, Mitchell PJ, Cohen SM. The AP-2 transcription factor is required for joint formation and cell survival in Drosophila leg development. *Development* 2001; **128**: 1231–8.

20 Monge I, Krishnamurthy R, Sims D, Hirth F *et al.* *Drosophila* transcription factor AP-2 in proboscis, leg and brain central complex development. *Development* 2001; **128**: 1239–52.

21 Basson CT, Huang T, Lin RC *et al.* Different TBX5 interactions in heart and limb defined by Holt-Oram syndrome mutations. *Proc Natl Acad Sci USA* 1999; **96**: 2919–24.

22 International Agency for Research on-Cancer. IACR PT53 Mutation Database: 2001.

23 Holliday R, Grigg GW. DNA methylation and mutation. *Mutat Res* 1993; **285**: 61–7.

24 Pabo CO, Sauer RT. Transcription factors: structural families and principles of DNA recognition. *Annu Rev Biochem* 1992; **61**: 1053–95.

25 Yagi R, Chen LF, Shigesada K, Murakami Y, Ito Y. A WW domain-containing yes-associated protein (YAP) is a novel transcriptional co-activator. *Embo J* 1999; **18**: 2551–62.

CHAPTER 64

The genetic origin of atrioventricular conduction disturbance in humans

D. Woodrow Benson

The atrioventricular (AV) conduction system is comprised of specialized cells that permit synchronized cardiac excitation resulting in contraction of the atria during ventricular filling and rapid depolarization of the ventricles. Anatomic components of the AV conduction system can be identified in the postnatal heart: the sinoatrial node, the AV node, His bundle, left and right bundle branches, and Purkinje ramifications. These elements are distinguished from the ordinary working myocardium by developmental, anatomic, electrophysiologic, and gene expression characteristics (reviewed in refs 1, 2).

AV block refers to any abnormality in which conduction of sinus or atrial impulses to the ventricle is delayed or interrupted. AV block taxonomy has been based on extent (degree) of block and site of block (Plate 38). First degree AV block manifests as prolongation of the PR interval (mild conduction delay) while in third degree or complete AV block, no atrial impulse conducts to the ventricle. Second degree AV block is intermediate, and some atrial impulses conduct to the ventricle.[3] AV block is termed 'progressive' if the electrocardiographic features worsen over time, e.g. block progresses from second to third degree.

The classification can be extended by subdividing the PR interval into three subintervals related to conduction in specific anatomic sites: PA interval (intra-atrial conduction), AH interval (AV node conduction), and HV interval (distal His–Purkinje conduction) (Plate 38). This electroanatomical classification (extent, progression, and site of AV block)

has been useful in guiding indications for pacing therapy, but the genetic significance of this scheme is not known.

Several causes of AV block have been identified in the pediatric patient. AV block as a surgical complication has diminished to ~1% as a result of improved understanding of conduction system anatomy.[4] Maternal antibody-associated AV block is usually detected between 16 and 24 weeks of gestation in an otherwise normally developing heart and is irreversible; over 60% of affected children require lifelong pacemakers.[5] The target antigens have been extensively characterized, but pathogenicity remains to be clarified. AV block may also be the major cardiac manifestation of neuromuscular disease (Table 64.1).

Despite an increasing number of entries in Online Mendelian Inheritance in Man (OMIM), in some cases an obvious cause of AV block is not identifiable. Familial clustering of AV block of unknown or idiopathic cause has been recognized, and published pedigrees show autosomal dominant inheritance.[11] Some individuals with AV block have a health history or family history of other forms of cardiovascular disease in the young including cardiomyopathy or congenital cardiac anomaly. This is not surprising given the common origin of the specialized conduction system elements and the working myocardium.[12,13]

To identify the genetic basis of AV block, models using reduced penetrance (presence of disease genotype in absence of phenotype) and variable expressivity (presence of a disease genotype with variable

Table 64.1 Genetic causes of neuromuscular disease in which AV block is the principal cardiac manifestation

Neuromuscular disorder	Inheritance	Gene	OMIM	Reference
Emery Dreifus muscular dystrophy	X-linked	emerin	310300	17
Emery Dreifus muscular dystrophy	AD	Lamin A/C	181350	5, 9
Kearns-Sayre syndrome	AD	MtDNA deletion	530000	1
Myotonic dystrophy	AD	DMPK	160900	7

phenotypes) have been employed. An association between AV conduction abnormalities and congenital cardiac abnormalities has long been observed. Using genetic linkage and candidate gene analysis, heterozygous mutations in the transcription factor, NKX2.5, were identified as a cause of both AV block and varied congenital heart defects.[14,15] The AV block phenotype develops even in the absence of associated malformation.[14,16] Mutations exhibiting reduced DNA binding and transcriptional activation are most likely to result in the AV block phenotype.[17] NKX2.5-associated AV block is characterized by conduction delay in the AV node that progresses during postnatal life such that most individuals have advanced second or third degree AV block by the third decade of life.[14] The developmental basis for progressive AV nodal block, which is similar to that observed in association with heterozygous TBX5 (a T-box transcription factor) mutation has not been elucidated.[18]

Mutations in PRKAG2, the gene for the γ2 regulatory subunit of AMP-activated protein kinase also result in AV block.[19] Affected individuals also manifest Wolff–Parkinson–White syndrome and cardiac hypertrophy. The cardiac pathology demonstrates that, rather than the characteristic features of hypertrophic cardiomyopathy, hypertrophy results from myocardial storage disease characterized by vacuoles filled with glycogen-associated granules. Detailed clinical electrophysiology studies of this phenotype have shown that accessory AV connections are responsible for pre-excitation.[20] The AV block is progressive, with a site of block in the distal His-Purkinje system (below the His bundle recording site). Accumulation of glycogen-associated granules in conductive tissue may lead to AV block, but how such accumulation accounts for the presence of accessory AV connections remains an open question.

Two distinct inherited syndromes of cardiac arrhythmia, the congenital long QT syndrome and Brugada syndrome, have been previously associated with mutations in the cardiac sodium channel α-subunit gene (SCN5A). Recently, heterozygous SCN5A mutations were detected in individuals with AV block thus identifying a third cardiac sodium channelopathy.[21]

Biophysical characterization of AV block-causing SCN5A mutation has revealed distinct patterns of abnormalities not previously observed for other SCN5A alleles.[22–24] In vitro studies of single, AV block-causing SCN5A mutations demonstrate competing shifts in activation and inactivation gating, with the net effect being reduced levels of sodium current density, which in turn slows the rise time of the cardiac action potential and slows conduction velocity, resulting in conduction delay rather than another arrhythmia phenotype. Based on the limited studies performed to date, when AV block is due to SCN5A mutation the extent, progression, and site of block is variable.

Considerable progress has been made in the diagnosis and treatment of AV block, and recently identified genetic causes are providing insight into the molecular pathogenesis of this important clinical problem. These findings are significant, since they provide insight into the molecular basis of a clinical condition previously defined only by biophysical characteristics. AV block-causing mutations identified to date have not conformed precisely to the electromechanical classification scheme. Models of AV block pathophysiology, based on electrocardiographic and electrophysiologic characteristics, have been useful for diagnosis and treatment of affected individuals, but identification of genetic causes promises to lead to improved understanding of pathogenesis and natural history. For the electrophysiologist, understanding the mode of inheritance is essential for identifying individuals at risk of developing AV block. For the molecular geneticist, patterns of transmission can direct strategies for identification of the disease-causing gene mutations. For the developmental biologist, disease-causing mutations become reagents for dissecting the processes whereby cells from common ancestry are recruited into the atrium, ventricle, or conduction system and the tubular embryonic heart is transformed into the four-chambered adult heart. These insights promise to lead to alternative diagnostic methods and new therapeutic strategies for this challenging clinical problem.

References

1 Moorman AFM, Lamers WH. Development of the conduction system in the vertebrate heart. In: Harvey RP, Rosenthal N, eds. *Heart Development*. San Diego, CA: Academic Press, 1999: 195–208.

2 Thomas PS, Kasahara H, Edmonson AM *et al*. Elevated expression of Nkx-2.5 in developing myocardial conduction cells. *Anat Rec* 2001; **263**: 307–13.

3 Fish, FA, Benson, DW. Disorders of cardiac rhythm and conduction. In: Allen HD, Gutgesell HP, Clark EB, Driscoll DJ, eds. *Heart Disease in Infants, Children, and Adolescents*. Philadelphia: Lippincott, Williams and Wilkins, 2001: 462–533.

4 Ho SY, Rossi MB, Mehta AV *et al*. Heart block and atrioventricular septal defect. *Thorac Cardiovasc Surg* 1985; **33**: 362–5.

5 Buyon JP, Hiebert R, Copel J *et al*. Autoimmune-associated congenital heart block: Demographics, mortality, morbidity and recurrence rates obtained from a national neonatal lupus registry. *J Am Coll Cardiol* 1998; **31**: 1658–66.

6 Nagano A, Koga R, Ogawa M *et al*. Emerin deficiency at the nuclear membrane in patients with Emery-Dreifuss muscular dystrophy. *Nat Genet* 1996; **12**: 254–9.

7 Bonne G, Di Barletta MR, Vanous S *et al*. Mutations in the gene encoding lamin A/C cause autosomal dominant Emery-Dreifuss muscular dystrophy. *Nat Genet* 1999; **21**: 285–8.

8 Fatkin, D, MacRae C, Sasaki T *et al*. Missense mutations in the rod domain of the lamin A/C gene as causes of dilated cardiomyopathy and conduction-system disease. *N Eng J Med* 1999; **341**: 1715–24.

9 Anan R, Nakagawa M, Miyatta M *et al*. Cardiac involvement in mitochondrial diseases. A study on 17 patients with documented mitochondrial DNA defects. *Circulation* 1995; **91**: 955–61.

10 Brook JD, McCurrach ME, Harley HG *et al*. Molecular basis of myotonic dystrophy: expansion of a trinucleotide (CTG) repeat at the 3' end of a transcript encoding a protein kinase family member. Cell 1992; **68**: 799–808.

11 Brink PA, Ferreira A, Moolman JC *et al*. Gene for progressive familial heart block type I maps to chromosome 19q13. *Circulation* 1995; **91**: 1631–40.

12 Gourdie RG, Kubalak S, Mikawa T. Conducting the embryonic heart: orchestrating development of specialized cardiac tissues. *Trends Cardiovasc Med* 1999; **9**: 18–26.

13 Takebayashi-Suzuki K, Pauliks LB, Eltsefon Y, Mikawa T. Purkinje fibers of the avian heart express a myogenic transcription factor program distinct from cardiac and skeletal muscle. *Dev Biol* 2001; **234**: 390–401.

14 Benson DW, Silberbach GM, Kavanaugh-McHugh A *et al*. Mutations in *NKX2.5*, a cardiac transcription factor, affect diverse cardiac developmental pathways. *J Clin Invest* 1999; **104**: 1567–73.

15 Schott J-J, Benson DW, Basson CT *et al*. Congenital heart disease caused by mutations in the transcription factor *NKX2.5*. *Science* 1998; **281**: 108–11.

16 Goldmuntz E, Geiger E, Benson DW. NKX2.5 mutations in patients with tetralogy of Fallot. *Circulation* 2001; **104**: 2565–8.

17 Kasahara H, Lee B, Schott J-J *et al*. Loss of function and inhibitory effects of human CSX/NKX2.5 homeoprotein mutations associated with congenital heart disease. *J Clin Invest* 2000; **106**: 299–308.

18 Basson CT, Bachinsky DR, Lin RC *et al*. Mutations in human *TBX5* cause limb and cardiac malformation in Holt-Oram syndrome. *Nat Genet* 1997; **15**: 30–5.

19 Arad M, Benson DW, Perez-Atayde AR *et al*. Constitutively active AMP kinase mutations cause glycogen storage disease mimicking hypertrophic cardiomyopathy. *J Clin Invest* 2002; **109**: 357–62.

20 Mehdirad AA, Fatkin D, DiMarco JP *et al*. Electrophysiologic characteristics of accessory atrioventricular connections in an inherited form of Wolff–Parkinson–White syndrome. *J Cardiovasc Electrophysiol* 1999; **10**: 629–35.

21 Schott JJ, Alshinawi C, Kyndt F *et al*. Cardiac conduction defects associate with mutations in SCN5A. *Nat Genet* 1999; **23**: 20–21.

22 Tan HL, Bink-Boelkens MT, Bezzina CR *et al*. A sodium-channel mutation causes isolated cardiac conduction disease. *Nature* 2001; **409**: 1043–7.

23 Viswanathan PC, Benson DW, Balser JR. A common SCN5A polymorphism modulates the biophysical effects of an SCN5A mutation in a patient with cardiac conduction disease. *J Clin Invest* 2003; **111**: 341–6.

24 Wang DW, Viswanathan PC, Balser JR, George AL Jr, Benson DW Clinical, genetic, and biophysical characterization of SCN5A mutations associated with atrioventricular conduction block. *Circulation* 2002; **105**: 341–6.

CHAPTER 65

Noonan syndrome and *PTPN11* mutations

Marco Tartaglia, Bruce D. Gelb

Noonan syndrome is the eponymous name for the disorder that Jacqueline Noonan, a pediatric cardiologist, described in an oral presentation in 1963 and published in 1968.[1,2] Her description of this syndrome was based on observations made in nine patients with valvar pulmonic stenosis, a distinctive dysmorphic facial appearance with hypertelorism, ptosis, and low-set ears, webbed neck, and chest deformities (Fig. 65.1). Several male patients also had cryptorchidism. John Opitz suggested that this disorder be called Noonan syndrome,[3] which was subsequently adopted. The clinical features observed in Noonan syndrome are summarized in Table 65.1.

Noonan syndrome is inherited in an autosomal dominant manner, although rare apparently autosomal recessive cases have been described. Like many autosomal dominant disorders, a substantial proportion of cases seem to be sporadic. The prevalence of Noonan syndrome is not known precisely, but the best estimate is between 1:1000 and 1:2500 live births. Disease incidence is higher since loss of affected fetuses occurs.

Genetic mapping and disease gene discovery

The first genetic mapping studies for Noonan syndrome were performed with small kindreds, with the first report appearing in 1992. Since Noonan syndrome shares some features in common with neurofibromatosis (particularly in certain individuals), markers flanking *NF1* on chromosome 17q and *NF2* on chromosome 22q were used to exclude allelism of Noonan syndrome to those traits.[4,5] Jamieson and co-workers used a large Dutch kindred inheriting the disorder to perform a genome-wide scan and observed linkage with several markers at chromosome 12q22-qter, which they named *NS1*.[6] They also documented that Noonan syndrome was genetically heterogeneous, based on linkage exclusion for the *NS1* locus with some other smaller kindreds. The *NS1* locus was refined to a region of approximately 7.5 cM using novel STRs. Legius and co-workers studied a four-generation Belgian family in which some affected individuals had findings consistent with Noonan syndrome while others had a phenotype more consistent with cardiofaciocutaneous syndrome.[7] They achieved independent linkage to *NS1*, and refined the critical interval further to approximately 5 cM. A positional candidacy approach was taken to identify the Noonan syndrome disease gene residing at *NS1*.

Tartaglia and co-workers discovered that missense mutations in *PTPN11* cause Noonan syndrome.[8] They studied two medium-sized kindreds inheriting the disorder, documenting probable linkage to *NS1* but failing to reduce the critical region further. *PTPN11* was considered a candidate gene because it mapped to the proper genetic interval at chromosomal band 12q24.1 and because its protein product, SHP-2, occupied a critical role in several intracellular signal transduction pathways controlling diverse developmental processes, including cardiac semilunar valvulogenesis.[9] Bi-directional sequencing of the fifteen *PTPN11* coding region exons and their intron boundaries for one family revealed a G-to-T transversion at position 214 in exon 3, predicting the substitution of Ala[72] by a Ser residue (A72S) in the N-SH2 domain. This sequence change was confirmed with a PCR-based RFLP assay that docu-

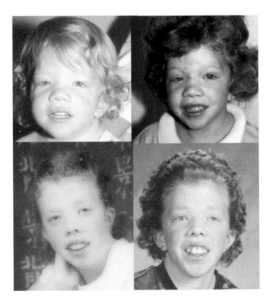

Fig. 65.1 Dysmorphic facial features in Noonan syndrome. Series of one affected girl from age 2 to 17 years, showing the evolution of the facial features. (Kindly provided by J. Allanson.)

mented its presence in all affected family members and its absence among unaffected ones. This change was not observed in more than 200 control individuals. Sequence comparison of SHP-2 with its orthologues and other closely related PTPases revealed complete conservation of Ala[72]. Analysis of the second family revealed an A-to-G transition at position 236 in exon 3. This change predicted the substitution of Gln[79] by an Arg (Q79R), affecting another highly conserved residue in the N-SH2 domain. This sequence change was confirmed in all affected individuals in this family, but was absent in unaffected family members and controls. Taken together, these findings established *PTPN11* as the *NS1* disease gene.

PTPN11 and IT protein product, SHP-2

Ahmad and co-workers cloned the human *PTPN11* cDNA from an umbilical cord library based on its homology to other protein tyrosine phosphatases in the catalytic domain.[10] The predominant cDNA contained an open reading frame of 1,799 nucleotides, resulting in a predicted protein of 593 amino acid residues that is named SHP-2. SHP-2 has

Table 65.1 Clinical features of Noonan syndrome

Dysmorphia	Epicanthal folds
	Ptosis
	Downslanting palpebral fissures
	Triangular facies
	Low set, thickened pinnae
	Light colored irises
	Curly, coarse hair
Cardiovascular	Congenital heart defects (pulmonic stenosis > atrioventricular septal defects > aortic coarctation > secundum atrial septal defects > mitral valve defects > tetralogy of Fallot > ventricular septal defects > patent ductus arteriosis)
	Hypertrophic cardiomyopathy
Short stature	
Webbed neck with low posterior hairline	
Skeletal	Pectus excavatum and/or carinatum
	Cubitus valgus
	Scoliosis
	Vertebral anomalies
Cryptorchidism	
Feeding difficulties	
Developmental	Delay
	Attention deficit/hyperactivity disorder
Hematologic	Bleeding diathesis (von Willebrand disease, factors XI and XII deficiency)
	Thrombocytopenia
	Leukemia
Ophthalmologic	Strabismus
	Myopia
Hearing Loss	
Dental/Oral	Malocclusion
	High arched palate
Lymphatic	Lymphedema
	Lymphangiectasia

a domain arrangement identical to another non-membranous protein tyrosine phosphatase, SHP-1, with two tandemly arranged src-homology 2 (SH2) domains at the N-terminus followed by the catalytic, or protein tyrosine phosphatase (PTP), domain. There is 60% identity between the PTP domains of SHP-1 and SHP-2 but slightly lower homology across the SH2 domains. Ahmad and co-worker also identified a second *PTPN11* transcript that contains 12 additional base pairs within the catalytic domain. Little additional information is available about this alternative transcript.

The expression pattern of *PTPN11* has been explored in humans and mice. In humans, a 7.0-kb transcript is detected in several tissues (heart, brain, lung, liver, skeletal muscle, kidney, and pancreas) with highest steady-state levels in heart and skeletal muscle.[10] The age of the subjects from whom the RNAs were derived was not specified. The expression pattern of SHP-2 was assessed in adult human brain using immunoblot and immunohisto-chemistry.[11] While SHP-2 was detected diffusely in the brain, immunohistochemical analysis revealed signal from neurons but not glial or endothelial cells. In the developing mouse, a 7.0-kb *Ptpn11* transcript was detected at all time points examined (E7.5–E18.5) with northern analysis.[12] *Ptpn11* was detected using *in situ* hybridization in embryonic and extra-embryonic tissues at E7.5. At later time points, signal was present in all tissues with highest levels in heart and neural ectoderm.

A mouse model of Shp-2 deficiency was generated using targeted disruption in embryonic stem cells.[13,14] The allele, which deleted several residues of the N-SH2 domain and obliterated activation of the MAPK pathway, was a recessive embryonic lethal. Developing embryos nullizygous for Shp-2 had defects in gastrulation and patterning, resulting in severe abnormalities in axial mesoderm development.

Chimeric mice were generated by associating *Ptpn11*-nullizygous embryonic stem cells with wild type morulas.[15,16] Among phenotypically normal chimeric embryos, mutant cells were absent in the heart, somites, limb buds, and nasal placode, all regions that require Fgf signaling. There was also absence of a contribution of *Ptpn11*-mutant cells to hematopoietic progenitors in fetal liver and bone marrow. Extensive characterization of limb development in chimeras demonstrated that the absence of *Ptpn11*-mutant cells in the developing progress zone resulted from abnormal chemokinesis or cell adhesion, but not from inadequate proliferation.[16] When *Ptpn11*-mutant cells were present in the progress zone, limb development was abnormal, evidence that Shp-2-related signaling is required for limb development.

Of particular relevance to the potential pathogenesis of Noonan syndrome, Shp-2 has a role in semilunar valvulogenesis. Chen and co-workers studied the effects of a hypomorphic allele of *Egfr* (called *Egfr^{wa2}*), which produces a protein with 10–20% residual kinase activity.[9] Mice with combined homozygosity for *Egfr^{wa2}* and heterozygosity for a null *Ptpn11* allele had aortic and pulmonic stenosis due to thickening of the valve leaflets with excessive numbers of mesenchymal cells. Embryos with only *Egfr^{wa2}* homozygosity also had abnormal semilunar valves, but to a significantly lesser extent. While the nature of the *PTPN11* alleles differs between these mice and patients with Noonan syndrome (haploinsufficiency vs. gain-of-function), these data suggest that the pulmonic stenosis associated with Noonan syndrome results from abnormal SHP-2 activity in the EGFR pathway.

The *Drosophila* homologue of *PTPN11* is *corkscrew* (*csw*), which was cloned by Perrimon's group in 1992.[17] This X-linked gene is named for the shape of misshapen fly embryos that result from deficiency of this protein tyrosine phosphatase. Corkscrew is maternally required for determination of cell fates for terminal structures. Corkscrew acts downstream of torso, which is a receptor tyrosine kinase that is homologous to fibroblast growth factor receptor 3.[18–22] After binding its ligand, torso autophosphorylates and initiates a signal cascade that results in activation of mitogen-activated protein kinase (MAPK, Fig. 65.2). Activated MAPK dimerizes and translocates into the nucleus where it induces expression of two transcription factors, *tailless* and *huckebein* at the anterior and posterior embryonic poles.

As shown in Fig. 65.2, the interactions between torso and corkscrew are complex. Using an SH2 domain, corkscrew binds to torso at the phosphorylated residue Y630(20). This binding activates corkscrew, which then dephosphorylates torso at Y918. This dephosphorylation prevents GAP1, a negative regulator of the MAPK cascade, from bind-

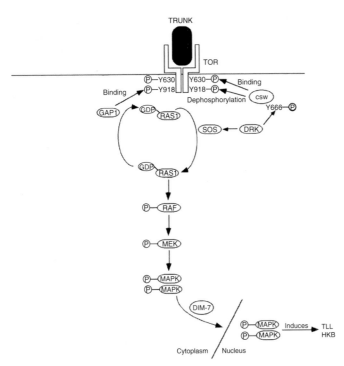

Fig. 65.2 Torso (TOR) signal transduction pathway. The signaling pathway from the receptor tyrosine kinase, TOR, to stimulation of gene transcription by mitogen activated protein kinase (MAPK) in *Drosophila* embryos. Corkscrew (CSW) binds phosphorylated Y630 residue and dephosphorylates Y918. The latter prevents the binding of GTPase activating protein 1 (GAP1), which negatively regulates the MAPK pathway. Activated TOR also phosphorylates CSW at Y666, potentiating the binding of DRK. This activates the MAPK cascade, resulting in increased expression of TLL and HKB. Abbreviations: Downstream-of-receptor-kinases, DRK; Son-of-sevenless (SOS); MAP kinase kinase, MEK; Tailless, TLL; Huckebein, HKB.

ing to torso. Activated torso also phophorylates corkscrew at Y666, facilitating docking of the protein, downstream-of-receptor-kinases (the *Drosophila* homologue of the mammalian adapter protein GRB-2). Downstream-of-receptor-kinases, in turn, binds son-of-sevenless, activating it and stimulating the MAPK cascade. Epistatic analyses have also documented that corkscrew interacts with additional members of the MAPK cascade, although its specific targets remain to be determined. Recently, it was shown that corkscrew binds with *Drosophila* importin-7, which binds to dimerized MAPK and translocates it across the nuclear membrane.[23]

In addition to its role in the development of terminal structures through the torso signal cascade, corkscrew also is important for several other receptor tyrosine kinase pathways that result in MAPK activation.[22] Among these, the best characterized is the sevenless pathway in the developing *Drosophila* eye.[24] The *Drosophila* eye is comprised of 800 units, called ommatidia, that contain eight photo-receptor cells (R1–R8), as well as lens and accessory cells. While the development of all photoreceptor cells is dependent on the *Drosophila* epidermal growth factor (EGF) receptor, only R7 development also re-

quires signaling from sevenless. Mutant corkscrew alleles perturb R7 development, producing the rough eye phenotype.[25] While the sevenless pathway to MAPK is quite similar to that used by torso, the interactions of corkscrew within the cascades are not identical. In particular, corkscrew binds sevenless independent of the phosphorylation state of sevenless (whereas it binds torso only after ligand binding and autophosphorylation). In addition, activated corkscrew binds and dephosphorylates the Gab2 homologue, daughter-of-sevenless, which is phosphorylated by activated sevenless.[26,27] Daughter-of-sevenless then acts as a multisite adapter in promoting signaling to MAPK in a RAS-dependent or RAS-independent fashion.

Phenotypic characterization of several *corkscrew* alleles has documented that corkscrew participates in signal cascades for several other receptor tyrosine kinases.[22,28] EGF (a.k.a. DER) is important for the development of ventral ectoderm (including the central nervous system), eyes, antennae, legs, and wings. All of these structures develop abnormally when corkscrew is deficient. Similarly, the fibroblast growth factor receptor 1, breathless, is a receptor tyrosine kinase that is critical for tracheal development. When corkscrew is deficient, tracheal cell precursors are produced normally but fail to migrate properly. Finally, another fibroblast growth factor receptor, heartless, is critical for specification of pericardial cells. Deficiency of corkscrew disrupts or deletes their development.

Molecular pathology of Noonan syndrome

In the original gene discovery paper as well as in a subsequent publication, Tartaglia and co-workers investigated the relative importance of *PTPN11* defects in the epidemiology of NS as well as the spectrum of molecular defects observed in the disorder.[8,29] Mutation screening was performed with 141 apparently unrelated individuals affected with NS, either sporadic ($n = 81$) or familial ($n = 60$) cases. Among the familial cases, the trait was linked to *NS1* in 11 of the kindreds and excluded in four. For the remaining 45 families, their small size pre-

cluded genetic linkage analysis. Missense mutations were identified in 66 cases or 47% (Table 65.2). A total of 22 different molecular defects were observed in this cohort and one mutation, the 922A-to-G transition that predicted an N308D substitution constituted nearly one-third of the defects. Several sporadic N308D cases, for whom the parents did not carry that allele, were observed, indicating a mutational hotspot.

Two lines of evidence suggest that Noonan syndrome caused by *PTPN11* mutations is almost completely penetrant. First, *PTPN11* mutation analysis with 11 families for which there was significant or suggestive linkage to the NS1 locus revealed mutations in all affected individuals but none of the unaffected ones. Second, genotyping of a number of unaffected parents for defects discovered in their offspring with apparently sporadic Noonan syndrome provided only a single instance of a genotypically affected, phenotypically normal parent. While it is possible that similar analysis for 'milder' cases of

Table 65.2 *PTPN11* Mutations in Noonan syndrome

No. of cases	Nucleotide substitution	Exon	Amino acid substitution	Domain
2	A124>G	2	T42A	N-SH2
2	G179>C	3	G60A	N-SH2
1	G181>A	3	D61N	N-SH2
2	A182>G	3	D61G	N-SH2
2	T184>G	3	Y62D	N-SH2
4	A188>G	3	Y63C	N-SH2
1	G214>T	3	A72S	N-SH2
2	C215>G	3	A72G	N-SH2
2	C218>T	3	T73I	N-SH2
1	G228>C	3	E76D	N-SH2
6	A236>G	3	Q79R	N-SH2
3	A317>C	3	D106A	N-SH2/C-SH2 linker
1	G417>C	4	E139D	C-SH2
1	G417>T	4	E139D	C-SH2
1	A836>G	7	Y279C	PTP
2	A844>G	7	I282V	PTP
1	T853>C	7	F285L	PTP
1	T854>C	8	F285S	PTP
20	A922>G	8	N308D	PTP
2[a]	A923>G	8	N308S	PTP
1	A925>G	8	I309V	PTP
1	G1502>A	13	R501K	PTP
4	A1510>G	13	M504V	PTP

[a]Affected members of one family exhibited the Noonan-like/multiple giant cell lesion condition.

NS might uncover some instances of incomplete penetrance, the strict criteria for Noonan syndrome employed clinically identifies a cohort with almost 100% penetrance.

The 68 Noonan syndrome mutations identified to date are not randomly distributed in the *PTPN11* gene (Fig. 65.3). Sixty-five of the mutations (96%) affect residues residing at or adjacent to the interface between the N-SH2 and PTP domains. The N-SH2 domain interacts with the PTP domain and binds to phosphotyrosyl-containing targets on activated receptors or docking proteins using two separate sites. These sites show negative cooperativity so that N-SH2 can work as intramolecular switch to control SHP-2 catalytic activity. In the inactive state, the N-SH2 and PTP domains share a broad interaction surface. More precisely, the N-SH2 D'E loop and flanking βD' and βE strands closely interact with the catalytic cleft, blocking the PTP active site. Crystallographic data on SHP-2 in the inactive conformation revealed a complex interdomain hydrogen bonding network involving Asn58, Gly60, Asp61, Cys459, and Gln506, which stabilizes the protein.[30] Numerous polar interactions between N-SH2 residues located in strands βF and βA, helix αB and residues of the PTP domain further stabilize the inactive conformation. Significantly, most of the residues mutated in Noonan syndrome are either

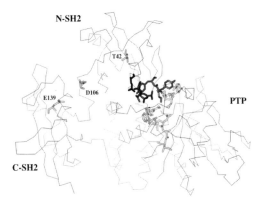

Fig. 65.3 Location of mutated residues in SHP-2 in the inactive conformation. Cα trace of N-SH2, C-SH2 and PTP domains according to Hof et al. (1998). Mutated residues are indicated with their side chains as thick lines (N-SH2 residues located in or close to the N-SH2/PTP interaction surface, black; linker, C-SH2 and N-SH2-phosphopeptide binding residues, gray; PTP residues located in or close to the N-SH2/PTP interaction surface, gray).

directly involved in these interdomain interactions (Gly60, Asp61, Ala72, Glu76, and Gln79) or are in close spatial proximity to them (Tyr62, Tyr63, Thr73, Tyr279, Ile282, Phe285, Asn308, Ile309, Arg501, and Met504). This distribution of molecular lesions suggests that the pathogenetic mechanism in Noonan syndrome involves altered N-SH2/PTP interactions that destabilize the inactive conformation without altering SHP-2's catalytic capability. Consistent with this view, no mutation altered Cys459 (the residue essential for nucleophilic attack), the PTP signature motif (positions 457–467), or the TrpProAsp loop (positions 423–425), which are all essential for phosphatase activity.

Three of the Noonan syndrome mutations affected residues outside of the interacting regions of the N-SH2 and PTP domains (Fig. 65.3). One recurrent mutation affected Asp106, which is located in the linker stretch connecting the N-SH2 and C-SH2 domains. Although functional studies are required to understand the functional significance of the Asp→Ala substitution, Tartaglia and co-workers hypothesized that this mutation might alter the flexibility of the N-SH2 domain, thus inhibiting the N-SH2/PTP interaction.[29] Two mutated residues, Thr42 (N-SH2 domain) and Glu139 (C-SH2 domain), are spatially far from the N-SH2/PTP interaction surfaces. In contrast to the other mutated residues, Thr42 and Glu139 are implicated in the intermolecular interactions of the SH2 domains with phosphotyrosyl-containing peptides.[31,32] Specifically, Thr42 directly interacts with the tyrosine phosphate and Glu139 is adjacent to Arg138 and Ser140, which form hydrogen bonds to that phosphate. Since the phenotype of the subjects bearing these mutations was typical for Noonan syndrome, molecular characterization is needed in order to understand how defects in phosphotyrosine binding result in similar developmental perturbations to those affecting SHP-2 inactivation.

The mechanism of action of the mutant SHP-2 proteins appears to be a gain of function. Tartaglia and co-workers used thermodynamic analysis to explore the molecular consequences of two Noonan syndrome mutants, A72S and A72G.[8] The technique of Monte Carlo[33] with scaled collective variables[34] (MC-SCV) was used to determine the energetically accessible conformations of the segment Gly[68]-Glu[76] in the context of N-SH2 in the activated (A) conformation. From this procedure, more than 30 structures were analyzed to relate their structure and energy. For the wild type (Fig. 65.4a), only three low-energy structures had Cα-root mean square distance (rmsd) ″ 2Å. The lowest energy structure (rmsd = 0.86Å) was ~8 kcal/mol below the other two states with small rmsd, supporting the observed stability of the active conformation of isolated N-SH2(32). In addition to the two low-rmsd states around 8 kcal/mol above the lowest energy conformation, several conformations were found at this energy with considerably larger rmsd values. Therefore, shuttling of wild-type SHP-2 between the A and inactivated (I) conformations becomes energetically plausible if, upon interacting with the PTP domain, the energy gap between the lowest energy conformation and the nearby states decreases. This would make those conformations accessible and confer the requisite flexibility to this segment of N-SH2. In contrast, both A72G and A72S had large populations with small rmsd and low energies (Fig. 65.4b,c). Even if the energies of these states shifted relative to each other upon binding of the PTP domain, there would still be several low-energy conformations available that were close to the A conformation, but none that would confer the flexibility required for transition to the I state. Consequently, the ability of these two mutants to shuttle between the A and I states is predicted to be impaired, implying that the equilibrium is shifted toward the A state relative to the wild-type protein.

There are functional data supporting the conclusions of the foregoing energetics-based structural analyses. O'Reilly and co-workers created and char-acterized two SHP-2 mutants, D61A and E76A, which they postulated would be gain-of-function changes since both are N-SH2 residues that interact directly with the PTP domain.[35] Both mutants showed increased basal phosphatase activity (E76A>>D61A>WT) and retained normal phosphopeptide binding properties. When expressed in *Xenopus* ectodermal explants, both mutants induced changes mimicking some aspects of development that are fibroblast growth factor-inducible, documenting basal stimulation of some signaling cascades *in vivo*. D61G, found in a case of Noonan syndrome, was extremely similar to D61A, providing strong evidence that this mutation has gain-of-function effects. E76D, observed in another case, affected the same residue as the E76A, but was more a more conservative change. Glu[76], however, is invariant among the SHP-2 orthologues and homologues. The similarity in function of Asp[61], Ala[72] and Glu[76] in stabilizing the I state[30] provides further evidence that NS is caused by increased activity of SHP-2.

Genotype/phenotype correlation

Because of the clinical heterogeneity observed in Noonan syndrome, Tartaglia and co-workers investigated possible associations between genotype and phenotype.[29] The distribution of several major clinical features of Noonan syndrome in subjects with and without mutations in *PTPN11* is shown in Table 65.3. A statistically significant association with pulmonary valve stenosis was found among the group with *PTPN11* mutations (70.6% vs. 46.2%, $P=$

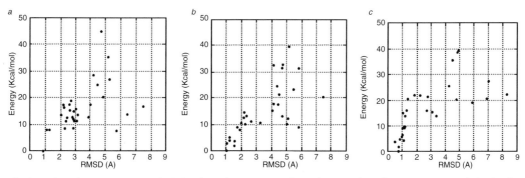

Fig. 65.4 Plots of root mean-square deviation (RMSD) against energy for the wild type and two mutant N-SH2 segments of SHP-2. For each case, the lowest energy conformation was arbitrarily set to an energy of 0 kcal mol-1. (a) Wild type; (b) Ala72Gly; (c) Ala72Ser.

Table 65.3 Clinical features in Noonan patients with and without *PTPN11* mutations

Clinical feature	Proportion (%) of patients with PTPN11 mutation	Proportion (%) of patients without PTPN11 mutation	P[1]
Cardiac defects:			
HCM	3/51 (5.9)	17/65 (26.1)	0.004
Pulmonic stenosis	36/51 (70.6)	30/65 (46.2)	0.008
Septal defects	6/50 (12.0)	11/63 (17.5)	NS
Short stature	39/51 (76.5)	45/64 (70.3)	NS
Special education	11/46 (23.9)	21/59 (35.6)	NS
Pectus deformities	39/50 (78.0)	46/61 (75.4)	NS
Cryptorchidism	26/31 (83.9)	25/35 (71.4)	NS

[1] NS indicates a statistically not significant difference

0.008). In contrast, a statistically significant lower incidence of HCM was observed in this group (5.9% vs. 26.2%, *P* = 0.004). There was no significant difference in the prevalence of atrial and/or ventricular septal defects or other congenital heart malformations between the *PTPN11* mutation and non-mutation groups. Similarly, there was no difference in the rates of short stature, pectus deformities, cryptorchidism, or enrollment in special education (as a marker of developmental delay).

The cohorts with N-SH2 and PTP mutations, respectively, were compared for the same clinical manifestations of NS. While this analysis had less statistical power due to sample size, no significant differences were identified. The phenotype observed in subjects with the common Asn308Asp substitution (*n* = 17) was not qualitatively different from those with other mutations, except none carrying the Asn308Asp change was enrolled in special education.

PTPN11 mutations have now been identified in two phenotypes related to classic Noonan syndrome. Tartaglia and co-workers identified an A-to-G transition at position 923 (Asn308Ser) in a previously described family with Noonan-like syndrome with multiple giant cell lesions in bone (MIM no. 163955).[29] In this family, two siblings had lesions in the mandible while their mother only had typical features of Noonan syndrome.[36] The same Asn308Ser mutation was observed in another family with Noonan syndrome that had no known bony involvement.

Digilio and co-workers screened eight independent individuals with LEOPARD syndrome (MIM no. 151100) for *PTPN11* defects and identified missense mutations in seven.[37] They also found mutations in two individuals with Noonan syndrome with café-au-lait spots. Among these nine apparently independent mutations, three were A-to-G transitions at position 386 (Tyr279Cys) and six were C-to-T transitions at position 1403 (Thr468Met). The Tyr279Cys mutation had been found previously in an infant diagnosed with Noonan syndrome; re-examination later in life revealed the presence of multiple café-au-lait spots [S. Jeffery, pers. comm.]. These results suggest specificity for these mutations for the development of these dermatological abnormalities.

Two other genetic disorders that share some features with Noonan syndrome are cardiofaciocutaneous and Costello syndrome. Geneticists had also proposed that one or both might be allelic with Noonan syndrome. Two independent studies excluded *PTPN11* mutations in medium-sized cohorts of individuals with cardiofaciocutaneous syndrome[38,39] and one achieved the same for Costello syndrome.[40] Thus, it can be concluded that neither of these two disorders is allelic with the genetic form of Noonan syndrome caused by *PTPN11* mutations.

Acknowledgments

This work was supported in part from awards from the National Institutes of Health (HD01294 and HL71207) and March of Dimes (FY03–52) to BDG and Progetto di ricerca finalizzata 1% FSN 2002 'Valutazione molecolare e funzionale delle malformazioni e disfunzioni cardiache su base genetica' to MT.

References

1 Noonan J, Ehmke D. Associated non cardiac malformations in children with congenital heart disease. *J Pediatr* 1963; **63**: 468–70.

2 Noonan JA. Hypertelorism with Turner phenotype. A new syndrome with associated congenital heart disease. *Am J Dis Child* 1968; **116**: 373–80.

3 Opitz JM. The Noonan syndrome. *Am J Med Genet* 1985; **21**: 515–18.

4 Sharland M, Taylor R, Patton MA, Jeffery S. Absence of linkage of Noonan syndrome to the neurofibromatosis type 1 locus. *J Med Genet* 1992; **29**: 188–90.

5 Flintoff WF, Bahuau M, Lyonnet S *et al.* No evidence for linkage to the type 1 or type 2 neurofibromatosis loci in Noonan syndrome families. *Am J Med Genet* 1993; **46**: 700–5.

6 Jamieson CR, van der Burgt I, Brady AF *et al.* Mapping a gene for Noonan syndrome to the long arm of chromosome 12. *Nat Genet* 1994; **8**: 357–60.

7 Legius E, Schollen E, Matthijs G, Fryns JP. Fine mapping of Noonan/cardio-facio cutaneous syndrome in a large family. *Eur J Hum Genet* 1998; **6**: 32–7.

8 Tartaglia M, Mehler EL, Goldberg R *et al.* Mutations in PTPN11, encoding the protein tyrosine phosphatase SHP-2, cause Noonan syndrome. *Nat Genet* 2001; **29**: 465–8.

9 Chen B, Bronson RT, Klaman LD *et al.* Mice mutant for Egfr and Shp2 have defective cardiac semilunar valvulogenesis. *Nat Genet* 2000; **24**: 296–9.

10 Ahmad S, Banville D, Zhao Z, Fischer EH, Shen SH. A widely expressed human protein-tyrosine phosphatase containing src homology 2 domains. *Proc Natl Acad Sci USA* 1993; **90**: 2197–201.

11 Reeves SA, Ueki K, Sinha B, Difiglia M, Louis DN. Regional expression and subcellular localization of the tyrosine-specific phosphatase SH-PTP2 in the adult human nervous system. *Neuroscience* 1996; **71**: 1037–42.

12 Feng GS, Hui CC, Pawson T. SH2-containing phosphotyrosine phosphatase as a target of protein-tyrosine kinases. *Science* 1993; **259**: 1607–11.

13 Arrandale JM, Gore-Willse A, Rocks S *et al.* Insulin signaling in mice expressing reduced levels of Syp. *J Biol Chem* 1996; **271**: 21353–8.

14 Saxton TM, Henkemeyer M, Gasca S *et al.* Abnormal mesoderm patterning in mouse embryos mutant for the SH2 tyrosine phosphatase Shp-2. *Embo J* 1997; **16**: 2352–64.

15 Qu CK, Yu WM, Azzarelli B *et al.* Biased suppression of hematopoiesis and multiple developmental defects in chimeric mice containing Shp-2 mutant cells. *Mol Cell Biol* 1998; **18**: 6075–82.

16 Saxton TM, Ciruna BG, Holmyard D *et al.* The SH2 tyrosine phosphatase shp2 is required for mammalian limb development. *Nat Genet* 2000; **24**: 420–3.

17 Perkins LA, Larsen I, Perrimon N. Corkscrew encodes a putative protein tyrosine phosphatase that functions to transduce the terminal signal from the receptor tyrosine kinase torso. *Cell* 1992; **70**: 225–36.

18 Lu X, Perkins LA, Perrimon N. The torso pathway in Drosophila: a model system to study receptor tyrosine kinase signal transduction. *Development* 1993; Suppl.: 47–56.

19 Perrimon N, Lu X, Hou XS *et al.* Dissection of the Torso signal transduction pathway in Drosophila. *Mol Reprod Dev* 1995; **42**: 515–22.

20 Cleghon V, Feldmann P, Ghiglione C *et al.* Opposing actions of CSW and RasGAP modulate the strength of Torso RTK signaling in the *Drosophila* terminal pathway. *Mol Cell* 1998; **2**: 719–27.

21 Ghiglione C, Perrimon N, Perkins LA. Quantitative variations in the level of MAPK activity control patterning of the embryonic termini in Drosophila. *Dev Biol* 1999; **205**: 181–93.

22 Perkins LA, Johnson MR, Melnick MB, Perrimon N. The nonreceptor protein tyrosine phosphatase corkscrew functions in multiple receptor tyrosine kinase pathways in Drosophila. *Dev Biol* 1996; **180**: 63–81.

23 Lorenzen JA, Baker SE, Denhez F *et al.* Nuclear import of activated D-ERK by DIM-7, an importin family member encoded by the gene moleskin. *Development* 2001; **128**: 1403–14.

24 Raabe T. The sevenless signaling pathway: variations of a common theme. *Biochim Biophys Acta* 2000; **1496**: 151–63.

25 Allard JD, Chang HC, Herbst R, McNeill H, Simon MA. The SH2-containing tyrosine phosphatase corkscrew is required during signaling by sevenless, Ras1 and Raf. *Development* 1996; **122**: 1137–46.

26 Herbst R, Carroll PM, Allard JD, Schilling J, Raabe T, Simon MA. Daughter of sevenless is a substrate of the phosphotyrosine phosphatase Corkscrew and functions during sevenless signaling. *Cell* 1996; **85**: 899–909.

27 Herbst R, Zhang X, Qin J, Simon MA. Recruitment of the protein tyrosine phosphatase CSW by DOS is an essential step during signaling by the sevenless receptor tyrosine kinase. *Embo J* 1999; **18**: 6950–61.

28 Firth L, Manchester J, Lorenzen JA, Baron M, Perkins LA. Identification of genomic regions that interact with a viable allele of the Drosophila protein tyrosine phosphatase corkscrew. *Genetics* 2000; **156**: 733–48.

29 Tartaglia M, Kalidas K, Shaw A *et al.* PTPN11 mutations in Noonan syndrome: molecular spectrum, genotype-phenotype correlation, and phenotypic heterogeneity. *Am J Hum Genet* 2002; **70**: 1555–63.

30 Hof P, Pluskey S, Dhe-Paganon S, Eck MJ, Shoelson SE. Crystal structure of the tyrosine phosphatase SHP-2. *Cell* 1998; **92**: 441–50.

31 Huyer G, Ramachandran C. The specificity of the N-terminal SH2 domain of SHP-2 is modified by a single point mutation. *Biochemistry* 1998; **37**: 2741–7.

32 Lee CH, Kominos D, Jacques S *et al.* Crystal structures of peptide complexes of the amino-terminal SH2 domain of the Syp tyrosine phosphatase. *Structure* 1994; **2**: 423–38.

33 Allen M. Tildesley. *Computer Simulation of Liquids.* Oxford: Clarendon, 1987.

34 Noguti T, Go N. Efficient Monte Carlo method for simulation of fluctuating conformations of native proteins. *Biopolymers* 1985; **24**: 527–46.

35 O'Reilly AM, Pluskey S, Shoelson SE, Neel BG. Activated mutants of SHP-2 preferentially induce elongation of Xenopus animal caps. *Mol Cell Biol* 2000; **20**: 299–311.

36 Bertola DR, Kim CA, Pereira AC *et al.* Are Noonan syndrome and Noonan-like/multiple giant cell lesion syndrome distinct entities? *Am J Med Genet* 2001; **98**: 230–4.

37 Digilio MC, Conti E, Sarkozy A *et al.* Grouping of Multiple-Lentigines/LEOPARD and Noonan Syndromes on the PTPN11 Gene. *Am J Hum Genet* 2002; **71**: 389–94.

38 Kavamura MI, Pomponi MG, Zollino M *et al.* PTPN11 mutations are not responsible for the Cardiofaciocutaneous (CFC) syndrome. *Eur J Hum Genet* 2003; **11**: 64–8.

39 Ion A, Tartaglia M, Song X *et al.* Absence of PTPN11 mutations in 28 cases of cardiofaciocutaneous (CFC) syndrome. *Hum Genet* 2002; **111**: 421–7.

40 Tartaglia M, Cotter PD, Zampino G, Gelb BD, Rauen KA. Exclusion of *PTPN11* mutations in Costello syndrome: further evidence for distinct genetic etiologies of Noonan, cardio-facio-cutaneous, and Costello syndromes. *Clin Genet* 2003; **63**: 423–6.

CHAPTER 66

Missense mutations in the *PTPN11* as a cause of cardiac defects associated with Noonan syndrome

Mitsuhiro Kamisago, Kayoko Hirayama-Yamada,
Taichi Kato, Shinichiro Imamura, Kunitaka Joo,
Masahiko Ando, Atsuyoshi Takao, Kazuo Momma,
Makoto Nakazawa, Rumiko Matsuoka

Noonan syndrome (NS) is characterized by dysmorphic face, short stature, chest deformity, and congenital heart disease (CHD).[1] More than 50% of the patients with NS have some cardiac defects, most commonly pulmonary stenosis (PS), atrial septum defect (ASD), and hypertrophic cardiomyopathy (HCM).[2–4] The estimated incidence of this syndrome is between one per 1000 and one per 2500 live births.[5] In 1994, a candidate gene for Noonan syndrome was mapped to chromosome 12q24.1 and genetic heterogeneity was also noted.[6] In 2001, mutations in *PTPN11*, encoding the protein-tyrosine phosphatase SHP-2, were reported to cause NS.[7,8] To further characterize the genotype/cardiac-phenotype correlation, we reviewed the clinical data and genotyped NS patients.

We evaluated 34 probands of Japanese NS with cardiac defects, among whom there was only one familial case (Table 66.1). Their age ranged from 2 months to 37 years. There were 23 males and 11 females. In the screening of the 34 patients, 10 different *PTPN11* missense mutations were identified in 15 probands, including two novel ones (Glu69Gln, Ser502Ala) (Table 66.2). Two pairs of three unrelated subjects shared the same missense mutation Tyr63Cys in exon 3 and Asn308Ser in exon 8, respectively. Two unrelated subjects carried the same de novo missense mutation Tyr62Asp in exon 3. Eleven of these mutations were located in or around inter-acting portion of N-terminal SH2 domain and protein tyrosine phosphatase (PTP) domain[9] (Fig. 66.1). The rest, three Asn308Ser and one Asn308Asp, resided in the PTP domain of exon 8. These mutations are thought to be in a hot spot. There were eight cases of valvular pulmonary stenosis, including five cases of dysplastic valve. There were seven cases of atrial septal defects, six of which were secundum defect type and one multiple fenestrated type. Only one case of the secundum type was isolated and the rest were accompanied by PS. There was one case each of HCM, infundibular PS with VSD, and ASD, and supravalvular PS. A novel mutation, Ser502Ala, was identified in exon13. It was located at the site of the PTP domain interacting with the N-SH2 domain.[9] The Ser502Ala mutation resulted in valvular PS accompanied by ASD, peripheral PS and supravalvular AS. One missense mutation, Asn308Ser, was identified in a NS proband with HCM. It is interesting that the Asn308Ser mutation has been seen by us and others to be associated with PS without HCM.

These findings strongly suggest that PTPN11 plays an important role in valvulogenesis and cardiac septum formation, and that additional genetic and/or environmental factors must be involved in bringing about the observed variation in cardiac phenotypes resulting from a single *PTPN11* mutation.

Methods

Clinical evaluation

Informed consent was obtained from all participants in accordance with the Ethics Committee of Tokyo Women's Medical University. Noonan syndrome was diagnosed on the basis of the presence of the following major characteristics: typical facial features (ocular hypertelorism, ptosis, epicanthic folds, anti-mongoloid slant of palpebral fissures), cardiac defects (PS, ASD, and HCM), short stature, and chest deformity. Cardiac defects were evaluated by history, physical examination, 12-lead electrocardiography and transthoracic echocardiography, cardiac catheterization, and angiography without knowledge of the genotype status.

Genetic studies

Genomic DNA was extracted from peripheral blood lymphocytes or Epstein–Barr virus-transformed lymphocytes. By comparing the cDNA sequence of the Human PTPN11 gene (GenBank accession number NM002834) and BAC clone RP3–329E11 (GenBank accession number AC004086) which were used in a previous study,[7] we determined the genomic structure and made adequate primers to amplify each exon (2–15)(Table 66.3). (We used the sequence of primer pairs for exon 1, which was suggested by Tartaglia.[7])

The coding region (exons 1–15) with flanking introns of PTPN11 were amplified from genomic DNA by PCR using 15 sets of primers (Table 66.3). For exons 2–15, PCRs were performed in a 50 μL reaction volume containing 50–100 ng genomic DNA, 1U AmpliTaq, 25 pmol of each primer, 200 μM of each dNTP and 1xPCR buffer (Applied Biosystems), through the use of Gene Amp PCR System 2400 (Applied Biosystems). For exon1, we used GC buffer I or II (TaKaRa) instead of 1xPCR buffer. Cycling parameters were as follows: 95°C for 4 min (first

Table 66.1 Subjects classified by cardiac defects

Cardiac defects	Total: 34
PS without ASD	10
PS with ASD	7
HCM	7
PS with VSD	3
PS with HCM	2
ASD with HCM	2
ASD	2
Tetralogy of Fallot with ASD	1

PS, pulmonary stenosis; ASD, atrial septal defect; VSD, ventricular septal defect; HCM, hypertrophic cardiomyopathy

Table 66.2 *PTPN11* Mutations in Noonan syndrome

No.	Nucleotide change	EXON	Amino acid change	Heart disease
1	GGT-GCT	3	Gly60Ala	PS, ASD
2	GAT-GGT	3	Asp61Gly	ASD
3	TAC-GAC	3	Tyr62Asp	PS(valv.), ASD
4	TAC-GAC	3	Tyr62Asp	PS(infund.), VSD,ASD
5	TAT-TGT	3	Tyr63Cys	PS(valv.), ASD
6	TAT-TGT	3	Tyr63Cys	PS(mild,valv.)
7	TAT-TGT	3	Tyr63Cys	PS, small VSD
8	GAG-CAG	3	* Glu69Gln	PS(mild,valv.)
9	CAG-CGG	3	Gln79Arg	ASD, PS(valv.)
10	TTT-TCT	8	Phe285Ser	PS(dysplstic, infund.)
11	AAT-AGT	8	Asn308Ser	HCM
12	AAT-AGT	8	Asn308Ser	VSD, PS(valv.)
13	AAT-AGT	8	Asn308Ser	PS(supra valv.)
14	AAT-GAT	8	Asn308Asp	PS(mild,valv.)
15	TCA-GCA	13	* Ser502Ala	PS(dysplastic), ASD

valv., valvular; infund., infundibular; *, novel mutation

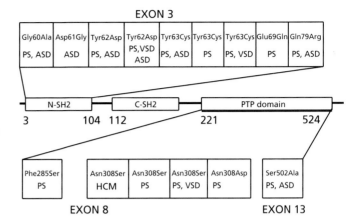

Fig. 66.1 Distribution of *PTPN11* missense mutations in Noonan syndrome with cardiac defect. The functional domains of the SHP-2 protein are composed of two tandemly arranged SH2 domains and a protein tyrosine phosphatase (PTP) domain. Numbers below the domain structure indicate the amino acid boundaries of those domains.

Table 66.3 Primer pairs for amplifying the *PTPN11* coding sequence

PTPN 1F	GCTGACGGGAAGCAGGAAGTGG	PTPN 1R	CTGGCACCCGTGGTTCCCTC
PTPN 2F	GCCCAGGGCTCAGATAAGG	PTPN 2R	GCAGGGAGGAGGCATTGAC
PTPN 3F	AAAATCCGACGTGGAAGATGAGAT	PTPN 3R	GTCACAAGCCTTTGGAGTCAGAGA
PTPN 4F	TGAAACCCCATCTGTAGGTGATAG	PTPN 4R	ATCCCTTGGAGGAATGTGTCTACT
PTPN 5F	TGGAGGCTGATGATACTATTCTGT	PTPN 5R	CACCCAGCCTATTATCTGTCTTT
PTPN 6F	CAACTTGCTCCGTGTCAATCAAT	PTPN 6R	AACCCTCTGTCCGTGCCTTTAT
PTPN 7F	CTAAGGCCTCCGATGTGCTAAC	PTPN 7R	CACGCCTGACCCAGATGAAC
PTPN 8F	TTCAGGCTAGAAATTTAGGAAGAA	PTPN 8R	TAGGCTGGGGAGTAACTGATTTG
PTPN 9F	TCCTAAACATGGCCAATCTGACA	PTPN 9R	AATGCAAATATCATCATGGTAAGC
PTPN 10F	TGAGTAACGGCAAGACCCTGAAT	PTPN 10R	AGGCCATTTTCCATGTTGGTG
PTPN 11F	TGTCCCTCAATGCAGTTGCTCTAT	PTPN 11R	AACCTGGGGAGATTCTCTTCCTCT
PTPN 12F	GAAGTCTTCAGCCCAGATTTTT	PTPN 12R	TTGCCAACATATTTTCAAACATAA
PTPN 13F	TTCCCATTCCGAAATCAAACAGT	PTPN 13R	TAGCCATTGCAACATGCTCAGTTA
PTPN 14F	ACTAACAGTAGGGCAACAGGAACG	PTPN 14R	TCAGTATTCTCAACCCGTCTATCA
PTPN 15F	TTGCTTGCCTGCTTAAAAATACT	PTPN 15R	TATCTGGTGCCCAAAGAATGTAGT

denaturing step); 35 cycles of 95°C for 20 s, 60°C for 30 s, and 72°C for 1 min; and 72°C for 5 min (last extension step). The PCR products were purified using PCR purification kits (QIAGEN, Santa Clarita, CA) and sequenced directly with a ABI BigDyeterminator cycle-sequencing Kit (Perkin Elmer) and an ABI 3100 Capillary Array Sequencer (Perkin Elmer). Sequences were analyzed using SeqMan II software (DNASTAR).

References

1 Noonan J, O'Connor W. Noonan syndrome: a clinical description emphasizing the cardiac findings. *Acta Paediatr Jpn* 1996; **38**: 76–83.

2 Sharland M, Burch M, McKenna WM, Paton MA. A clinical study of Noonan syndrome. *Arch Dis Child* 1992; **67**: 178–83.

3 Ishizawa A, Oho S, Dodo H, Katori T, Homma SI. Cardiovascular abnormalities in Noonan syndrome: the clinical findings and treatments. *Acta Paediatr Jpn* 1996; **38**: 84–90.

4 Marino B, Digilio MC, Toscano A, Giannotti A, Dallapiccola B. Congenital heart diseases in children with Noonan syndrome: An expanded cardiac spectrum with high prevalence of atrioventricular canal. *J Pediatr* 1999; **135**: 703–6.

5 Noonan JA. Noonan syndrome. An update and review for the primary pediatrician. *Clin Pediatr (Phila)* 1994; **33**: 548–55.

6 Jamieson CR, van der Burgt I, Brady AF *et al*. Mapping a gene for Noonan syndrome to the long arm of chromosome 12. *Nat Genet* 1994; **8**: 357–60.

7. Tartaglia M, Mehler EL, Goldberg R *et al.* Mutations in PTPN11, encoding the protein tyrosine phosphatase SHP-2, cause Noonan syndrome. *Nat Genet* 2001; **29**: 465–8.

8. Tartaglia M, Kalidas K, Shaw A *et al.* PTPN11 mutations in Noonan syndrome: molecular spectrum, genotype-phenotype correlation, and phenotypic heterogeneity. *Am J Hum Genet* 2002; **70**: 1555–63.

9. Hof P, Pluskey S, Dhe-Paganon S, Eck MJ, Shoelson SE. Crystal structure of the tyrosine phosphatase SHP-2. *Cell* 1998; **92**: 441–50.

CHAPTER 67

Novel gene mutations in patients with left ventricular noncompaction and evidence for genetic heterogeneity

Fukiko Ichida, Chen Rui, Tohru Tsuji, Noriyuki Haneda, Karla R. Bowles, Shinichi Tsubata, Keiichiro Uese, Keiichi Hirono, Sayaka Watanabe, Yuji Hamamichi, Ikuo Hashimoto, Toshio Miyawaki, Neil E. Bowles, Jeffrey A. Towbin

Left ventricular noncompaction (LVNC), a form of cardiomyopathy, presents in infancy with a hypertrophic and dilated left ventricle with deep trabeculations and commonly with reduced systolic function. Deletion of the FK Binding protein 12 (FKBP12) gene result in nonisolated LVNC associated with congenital heart disease in mice.[1] Mutations in the gene *G4.5*, which maps to chromosome Xq28, have been described in patients with isolated LVNC, suggesting that LVNC and Barth syndrome (X-linked disorder associated with dilated cardiomyopathy, skeletal myopathy, neutropenia, and abnormal mitochondria) are allelic.[2,3] Female patients with LVNC, however, have been also reported suggesting non-X-linked inheritance in some instances.[4,5]

The purpose of this study was to investigate patients with LVNC for disease-causing mutations in a series of candidate genes selected using the "final common pathway hypothesis"[6] including α-dystrobrevin.

DNA was isolated from 27 patients including six families with isolated LVNC and from 10 patients with nonisolated LVNC including two families after informed consent. Patient samples were screened for mutations in FKBP and G4.5, as well as cytoskeletal protein-encoding gene α-dystrobrevin, using single-strand DNA conformation polymorphism (SSCP) analysis and DNA sequencing.

A C>T mutation was identified at nucleotide 362 of α-dystrobrevin, resulting in a change from proline to leucine (P121L) in all six affected individual from one family with LVNC, including five with nonisolated LVNC and one with isolated LVNC (Plate 39). The pattern of transmission is most consistent with an autosomal dominant trait over four generations. All patients with the nonisolated form had one or more VSDs. Computer modeling predicted this mutation to result in a change in the secondary structure of this protein. No mutations were identified in FKBP12 and G4.5 in these patients.

A novel splice-site mutation of intron 8 in *G4.5* gene was found in the proband and four female carriers from one family with isolated LVNC, being consistent with X-linked transmission over four generations (Plate 40). This mutation results in deletion of exon 9 from the mRNA, and is predicted to significantly disrupt the protein product. Neither of the affected individuals nor any other family members presented with signs or symptoms of BTHS.

Genotype–phenotype correlation were analyzed in all of 38 cases with G4.5 mutation reported up to the present time.[7–11] The individual G4.5 mutations in 38 patients are heterogeneous, and there are no obvious genotype–phenotype correlations that allow the systemic manifestations of BTHS and the differentiation of clinical course to be predicted. In patients with X-linked LVNC, associated findings of BTHS are either absent or inconsistent. Additional factors to G4.5 mutations influence the clinical phenotype, which may also account for the large phenotypic heterogeneity of the symptoms within families.

These data suggest that there is genetic heterogeneity in LVNC, which like dilated cardiomyopathy, is a disease of the cytoskeleton. This mutation in the α-dystrobrevin represents the first mutation identified in patients with LVNC. In addition, we believe that G4.5 mutations should be considered as a possible cause of infantile cardiomyopathy affecting males, even in the absence of signs of BTHS.

References

1 Shou W *et al.* Cardiac defects and altered ryanodine receptor function in mice lacking FKBP12. *Nature* 1998; **391**: 489–92.

2 Bleyl SB *et al.* Neonatal, lethal noncompaction of the ventricular myocardium is allelic with Barth syndrome. *Am J Hum Genet* 1997; **61**: 868–72.

3 Bione S *et al.* A novel X-linked gene, G4.5 is responsible for Barth syndrome. *Nat Genet* 1996; **12**: 385–9.

4 Ichida F *et al.* Clinical features of isolated noncompaction of the ventricular myocardium. Long-term clinical course, hemodynamic properties, and genetic background. *J Am Coll Cardiol* 1999; **34**: 233–40.

5 Ichida F *et al.* Novel gene mutations in patients with left ventricular noncompaction or Barth syndrome. *Circulation* 2001; **10**: 1256–63.

6. Towbin JA *et al.* Etiologies of cardiomyopathy and heart failure. *Nat Med.* 1999; **5**: 266–7.

7 Johnston J *et al.* Mutation characterization and genotype-phenotype correlation in Barth syndrome. *Am J Hum Genet* 1997; **61**: 1053–8.

8 Cantlay AM *et al.* Genetic analysis of the G4.5 gene in families with suspected Barth syndrome. *J Pediatr* 1999; **135**: 311–5.

9 Barth PG *et al.* An X-linked mitochondrial disease affecting cardiac muscle, skeletal muscle and neutrophil leucocytes. *J Neurol Sci* 1983; **62**: 327–55.

10 Gedeon AK *et al.* X-linked fatal infantile cardiomyopathy maps to Xq28 and is possibly allelic to Barth syndrome. *J Med Genet* 1995; **32**: 383–8.

11 D'Adamo P *et al.* The X-linked gene G4.5 is responsible for different infantile dilated cardiomyopathies. *Am J Hum Genet* 1997; **61**: 862–7.

CHAPTER 68

Mitochondrial 16189 DNA variant and left ventricular hypertrophy in diabetes mellitus

Yukihiko Momiyama, Michiko Furutani, Yoshihiko Suzuki,
Shinichiro Imamura, Kazuhiro Hosokawa, Yoshihito Atsumi,
Kempei Matsuoka, Mitsuru Kimura, Hiroshi Kasanuki,
Fumitaka Ohsuzu, Rumiko Matsuoka

About 1% of type 2 diabetes mellitus (DM) is known to be associated with a mitochondrial (mt) DNA mutation at nucleotide position (np) 3243.[1] Recently, common mtDNA variants at 1310, 1438, 3290, 3316, 3394, 12026, 15927, and 16189 have been suggested to be associated with DM.[2–7] Among these mtDNA abnormalities, the 3243 mutation and the variants at 3316, 15927, and 16189 have also been reported to be associated with cardiomyopathies.[7–10] Left ventricular hypertrophy (LVH) is common in DM. DM was reported to be associated with LVH independent of hypertension and obesity.[11] However, the mechanism of LVH in DM remains unclear. Some mtDNA abnormalities may play a role in the development of LVH in patients with type 2 DM.

We investigated the prevalence of a mtDNA mutation at 3243 and variants at 1310, 1438, 3290, 3316, 3394, 12026, 15927, and 16189 in 33 diabetic patients with echocardiographically detected LVH (wall thickness >12 mm), 79 diabetic patients without LVH, and 100 non-DM controls. Patients with valvular heart disease or any wall motion abnormalities on echocardiograms were excluded. Controls were healthy blood donors.

After informed consent was obtained, peripheral blood samples were taken, and lymphoblastoid cell lines were established by Epstein-Barr virus transformation. To detect a heteroplasmic mutation at np

3243, DNA extracted from blood was used. The mtDNA fragments encompassing the mutation site were amplified by PCR.[1] The PCR products were digested with Apa I and then analyzed by polyacrylamide gel electrophoresis. To detect homoplasmic variants at 1310, 1438 (12SrRNA), 3290 (tRNA^{Leu}), 3316, 3394 (ND1), 12026 (ND4), 15927 (tRNA^{Thr}), and 16189 (Control), DNA extracted from cell lines was used, and the mtDNA fragments encompassing the polymorphic sites were amplified by PCR. Using an ABI Prism sequencer, we sequenced the six regions, where the eight variants described above are present, and adjacent three regions: tRNA^{Phe} (np 577–647), 12SrRNA (648–1601), tRNA^{Leu} (3230–3304), ND1 (3307–4262), ND4L (10470–10766), ND4 (10760–12137), tRNA^{Thr} (15888–15953), tRNA^{Pro} (15955–16023), and Control (16024–16576) regions. A total of 9 mtDNA regions (4982 bp) were sequenced, and the results were compared with the MITOMAP human mtDNA revised Cambridge sequence.

Among the three groups, age and gender were not different (Table 68.1). Compared with diabetic patients without LVH, those with LVH had higher rates of obesity (body mass index >26 kg/m^2) and hypertension (blood pressures ≥160/95 mgHg or on drugs). DM duration and HbA1c level were not different. In mtDNA analysis, none had the mutation at

Table 68.1 Clinical characteristics in the three groups

	Patients with LVH	P value	Patients without LVH	P value	Non-DM controls
Age (years)	62 ± 9	NS	63 ± 7	NS[a]	62 ± 10
Gender (male)	23 (70%)	NS	46 (58%)	NS[b]	65 (65%)
Body mass index	25 ± 3	<0.001	22 ± 3		
Obesity	12 (36%)	<0.05	12 (15%)		
Duration of DM (years)	14 ± 9	NS	13 ± 9		
Family history of DM in mothers	13 (39%)	NS	15 (19%)		
Insulin therapy	5 (15%)	NS	30 (38%)		
HbA1c (%)	7.8 ± 1.5	NS	8.3 ± 1.8		
Systolic blood pressure (mmHg)	144 ± 18	NS	137 ± 15		
Hypertension Echocardiograms	23 (70%)	<0.01	32 (41%		
LV internal dimension	44.4 ± 4.3	NS	43.2 ± 3.6		
LV wall thickness	12.4 ± 0.9	<0.001	8.5 ± 0.7		

Data are presented as the mean ± SD or the number (%) of patients.

[a] Comparison groups are diabetic patients with and without LVH.

[b] There was no difference between controls and diabetic patients with and without LVH.

Table 68.2 Prevalence of mitochondrial DNA variants reported to be associated with DM in the three groups

	1310 12SrRNA C→T	1438 12SrRNA G→A	3290 tRNA[LEU] T→C	3316 ND1 G→A	3394 ND1 T→C	12026 ND4 A→G	15927 tRNA[TR] G→A	16189 Control T→C
Patients with LVH (n = 39)	0 (0%)	1 (3%)	0 (0%)	0 (0%)	0 (0%)	1 (3%)	1 (3%)	18 (55%)*
Patients without LVH (n = 79)	0 (0%)	0 (0%)	1 (1%)	0 (0%)	5 (6%)	1 (1%)	0 (0%)	18 (23%)
Controls (n = 100)	1 (1%)	1 (1%)	0 (0%)	0 (0%)	1 (1%)	3 (3%)	3 (3%)	22 (22%)

* $P<0.005$ compared with diabetic patients without LVH and controls.

np 3243. Among the eight variants reported to be associated with DM, the variant at 16189 was more prevalent in diabetic patients with LVH than in those without LVH and controls (55% vs. 23% and 22%, $P<0.005$) (Table 68.2). The mtDNA sequencing of the nine regions identified a number of nucleotide substitutions in diabetic patients with and without LVH. The variants at 709 and 16217 were also more prevalent in diabetic patients with LVH than without LVH (36% and 21% vs. 15% and 5%, $P<0.025$). However, multivariate analysis revealed that the 16189 variant was significantly associated with LVH independent of hypertension and obesity, but the variants at 709 or 16217 were not. The odds ratio for LVH was 5.6 (95%CI 2.0 to 15.4) for the 16189 variant.

We previously studied the family history of DM and the prevalence of LVH in 834 diabetic patients.[12]

We found that the family history of DM in mothers was an independent factor for LVH, suggesting that some genetic factors of DM may contribute to the development of LVH in DM. Because DM, especially maternally inherited DM, was reported to be associated with mtDNA abnormalities,[1–7] we hypothesized that some mtDNA abnormalities may play a role in the development of LVH in DM. In the present study, we showed the high prevalence of the 16189 variant in diabetic patients with LVH. The 16189 variant was an independent factor associated with LVH in diabetic patients.

The 16189 variant was recently reported to be associated with dilated cardiomyopathy (DCM).[10] Among the mtDNA abnormalities reported to be associated with DM, the 3243 mutation and the variants at 3316 and 15927 were reported in patients with hypertrophic cardiomyopathy (HCM).[7–10]

However, the 3243 mutation was also reported in some patients with DCM.[13] In cardiomyopathy associated with mtDNA abnormalities, mitochondrial metabolic alterations are considered to cause cellular hypertrophy due to markedly increased mitochondria, which leads to LVH-like HCM.[14] Although no association between the 16189 variant and HCM has yet been elucidated, it seems reasonable to think that the 16189 variant could contribute to the development of LVH. The 16189 variant is in the noncoding Control region that contains many control elements for transcription and replication and that is an important area of interaction of mtDNA with nuclear-encoded proteins. The T-to-C transition at np 16189 generates an uninterrupted homopolymeric C-tract that is highly unstable and causes heteroplasmic length variation of mtDNA by replication slippage.[15] The length variation in repetitive sequences within Control region can generate changes in expression of gene products and promote evolutionary flexibility.[16]

In conclusion, a common mtDNA variant at 16189 was found to be associated with LVH in patients with type 2 DM. The 16189 variant may play a role in the development of LVH in DM.

References

1 Otabe S, Sakura H, Shimokawa K *et al.* The high prevalence of the diabetic patients with a mutation in the mitochondrial gene in Japan. *J Clin Endocrinol Metab* 1994; **79**: 768–71.

2 Tawata M, Ohtaka M, Iwase E *et al.* New mitochondrial DNA homoplasmic mutations associated with Japanese patients with type 2 diabetes. *Diabetes* 1998; **47**: 276–7.

3 McCarthy M, Cassell P, Tran T *et al.* Evaluation of the importance of maternal history of diabetes and of mitochondrial variation in the development of NIDDM. *Diabetic Med* 1996; **13**: 420–8.

4 Nakagawa Y, Ikegami H, Yamato E *et al.* A new mitochondrial DNA mutation associated with non-insulin-dependent diabetes mellitus. *Biochem Biophys Res Commun* 1995; **209**: 664–8.

5 Hirai M, Suzuki S, Onoda M *et al.* Mitochondrial DNA 3394 mutation in NADH dehydrogenase subunit 1 associated with non-insulin-dependent diabetes mellitus. *Biochem Biophys Res Commun* 1996; **219**: 951–5.

6 Poulton J, Brown MS, Cooper A *et al.* A common mitochondrial DNA variant is associated with insulin resistance in adult life. *Diabetologia* 1998; **41**: 54–8.

7 Thomas AW, Edwards A, Sherratt EJ *et al.* Molecular scanning of candidate mitochondrial tRNA genes in type 2 (non-insulin dependent) diabetes mellitus. *J Med Genet* 1996; **33**: 253–5.

8 Yoshida R, Ishida Y, Hozumi T *et al.* Congestive heart failure in mitochondrial diabetes mellitus. *Lancet* 1994; **344**: 1375–5.

9 Odawara M, Yamashita K. Mitochondrial DNA abnormalities in hypertrophic cardiomyopathy. *Lancet* 1999; **353**: 150.

10 Khogali SS, Mayosi BM, Beattie JM *et al.* A common mitochondrial DNA variant associated with susceptibility to dilated cardiomyopathy in two different populations. *Lancet* 2001; **357**: 1265–7.

11 Lee M, Gardin JM, Lynch JC *et al.* Diabetes mellitus and echocardiographic left ventricular function in free-living elderly men and women: The Cardiovascular Health Study. *Am Heart J* 1997; **133**: 36–43.

12 Momiyama Y, Suzuki Y, Ohsuzu F *et al.* Maternally transmitted susceptibility to non-insulin-dependent diabetes mellitus and left ventricular hypertrophy. *J Am Coll Cardiol* 1999; **33**: 1372–8.

13 Kitaoka H, Kameoka K, Suzuki Y *et al.* A patient with diabetes mellitus, cardiomyopathy, and a mitochondrial gene mutation: confirmation of a gene mutation in cardiac muscle. *Diabetes Res Clin Pract* 1995; **29**: 207–12.

14 van Ekeren GJ, Stadhouders AM, Egberink GJM *et al.* Hereditary mitochondrial hypertrophic cardiomyopathy with mitochondrial myopathy of skeletal muscle, congenital cataract and lactic acidosis. *Virchows Arch A* 1987; **412**: 47–52.

15 Bendall KE, Sykes BC. Length heteroplasmy in the first hypervariable segment of the human mtDNA control region. *Am J Hum Genet* 1995; **57**: 248–256.

16 Moxon ER, Rainey PB, Novak MA *et al.* Adaptive evolution of highly mutable loci in pathogenic bacteria. *Curr Biol.* 1994; **4**: 24–33.

CHAPTER 69

Mutation analysis of *BMPR2* and other genes in Japanese patients with pediatric primary pulmonary hypertension

Maya Fujiwara, Tsutomu Saji, Tomotaka Nakayama, Kaoru Akimoto, Michiko Furutani, Shinichiro Imamura, Atsuyoshi Takao, Makoto Nakazawa, Rumiko Matsuoka

Primary pulmonary hypertension (PPH) is a rare (annual incidence 1–2 per 10^6) and potentially refractory disorder, characterized by sustained elevation of pulmonary artery pressure above 25 mmHg at rest and 30 mmHg during exercise, without a demonstrable cause.[1] It has been suggested that familial PPH accounts for at least 6% of all PPH patients, and its pattern of inheritance is autosomal dominant disorder disease with a risk of clinical expression of about 10–20%.[2,3] In both familial and sporadic PPH, the disease occurs 1.7–2.0 times more often in females than in males,[4] and symptoms typically develop during the third decade of life, although the disease may occur at any age. On the other hand, in children, PPH occurs at the same rate in females as in males.

In 2000, mutations of the bone morphogenetic protein (BMP) receptor II gene (*BMPR2*) on 2q33 were detected in PPH families.[5] The *BMPR2* encoding a receptor for a member of the transforming growth factor beta (TGF-beta) superfamily, is organized in 13 exons, 3871 bp in total length. Mutations of this gene have been reported in Caucasians: 45% in familial PPH,[6] but only 26% in sporadic PPH.[7]

We have made a genomic study of Japanese patients with pediatric PPH, including *BMPR2* and other genes, which could be candidate genes in the

BMP-signaling pathway (ex. *BMPR1B*), and polymorphism of the angiotensin-converting enzyme (ACE) gene, related to proliferation of vascular smooth muscle cells.[8]

Twenty unrelated Japanese children (males $n = 9$, females $n = 11$) were recruited with clinical symptoms and diagnosed as having PPH after 1 year of age. They were diagnosed at 4–17 years old (median: 10 years old). It was speculated from their clinical symptoms that the age at onset was between 3 months and 3 years before the diagnosis. Four different *BMPR2* mutations were identified in the 20 patients. There were three patients with sporadic PPH and one patient with familial PPH. Thus, mutations of BMPR2 were identified in 17.6% (3/17) of sporadic PPH, and 33.3% (1/3) of familial PPH in Japanese patients. The clinical features of the patients with the *BMPR2* mutations are summarized in Table 69.1. In the clinical course, for example, age at onset, and with or without syncope, PPH patients with *BMPR2* mutation did not differ from those without the mutation. The patients from Familial 4 had the same *BMPR2* mutation and were diagnosed with PPH, but there was variation in the age at onset and clinical symptoms.

We have reported *BMPR2* mutations, i.e. three nonsense mutations and one missense mutation, in-

Table 69.1 PPH patients with the BMPR2 mutation

		Gender	Age at diagnosis (years)	Age at onset (years)	Initial symptom; syncope	Mutation: exon	Amino acid	
Sporadic	1	F	10	9	(+)	3	C123R	Reported
	2	M	11	9	(−)	3	Y113X	Novel
	3	F	17	14	(+)	2	Q42X	Novel
Familial		F	4	4	(−)			
	4	F	4	4	(+)	9	Q403X	Reported
		M	37	37	(−)			

Table 69.2 PPH and ACE polymorphism

	PPH	Control
DD	3	14
DI	9	41
II	8	45 $P = 0.91$

D/I alleles: 0.6/0.53 odds ratio 1.13.

cluding two novel mutations. It has been reported that missense mutations of the *BMPR2* in PPH patients occurred in the ligand-binding protein or in the serin-threonine kinase protein. In our study, the missense mutation of *BMPR2* in PPH was in the ligand binding protein, as previous report. Functional analysis of *BMPR2* showed that *BMPR2* with the missense mutation in the ligand-binding protein caused a severe deterioration of function, as with the nonsense mutation. Each patient in our study showed severe features whether the mutation was of the nonsense or missense type. We investigated the PPH patients based on their clinical data, which showed no correlation between the type of *BMPR2* mutation.

In this study, the *BMPR2* mutation was not found in about 80% of the PPH patients, and so we also studied *BMPR1B* as another candidate gene in the BMP-signaling pathway and ACE I/D polymorphism. Mutations of *BMPR1B* were not found in the other 14 sporadic PPH patients and two PPH families. The distribution of ACE genotypes did not differ between Japanese PPH patients and controls (Table 69.2). We came to the reluctant conclusion that *BMPR1B* and ACE polymorphism were unrelated to PPH.

In conclusion, in sporadic PPH, genetic abnormalities seem to play an important role in children as well as in adults. *BMPR2* is suggested to be only one of the factors which lead to the development of pulmonary hypertension, and pulmonary hypertension only develops when an additional factor, e.g. fenfluramine, or even another genetic factor, such as a molecular gene, become involved. These factors, which may be associated with the development of PPH, remain to be investigated.

Methods

Japanese patients with PPH diagnosed after 1 year of age were screened for mutations of *BMPR2*, *BMPR1B* and polymorphism of ACE, because it is difficult to distinguish between patients with PPH diagnosed before 1 years old and persistent pulmonary hypertension of the newborn (PPHN). Informed consent for genomic examinations was obtained from all patients and/or their families by pediatric cardiologists at each hospital. The diagnosis of primary pulmonary hypertension was made after echocardiography, cardiac catheterization and angiography, lung perfusion scintigraphy, and pulmonary function testing, excluded secondary causes of pulmonary hypertension.

We collected venous blood samples, and extracted DNA from peripheral lymphocytes. The *BMPR2* and *BMPR1B* gene was amplified by PCR, and performed direct sequencing with ABI PRISM dye terminator cycle sequencing kit (Perkin-Elmer), in reference to previous reports or designed by us. When the mutation is detected, we confirmed that these mutations were not observed in 100 Japanese normal controls by single-strand conformational polymorphism (SSCP) analysis or direct sequencing.

The ACE I/D polymorphism was genotyped, using the published primer set as previously described.

References

1 Rubin LJ. Current concepts: primary pulmonary hypertension. *N Engl J Med* 1997; **336**: 111–17.

2 Rich S, Dantzker DR, Ayres SM *et al.* Primary pulmonary hypertension. A national prospective study. *Ann Intern Med* 1987; **107**: 216–23.

3 Gaine S, Rubin LJ. Primary pulmonary hypertension. *Lancet* 1998; **352**: 719–25.

4 Barst RJ. Primary pulmonary hypertension in children. In: Rubin LJ, Rich S, eds. *Primary Pulmonary Hypertension* (Lung Biology in Health and Disease). New York, NY: Dekker, 1996: 99, 179–225.

5 Lane KB, Machado RD, Pauciulo MW *et al.* for the International PPH Consortium. Heterozygous germline mutations in BMPR-II are the cause of familial primary pulmonary hypertension. *Nat Genet* 2000; **26**: 81–4.

6 Machado RD, Pauciulo MW, Thomson JR *et al.* BMPR2 haploinsufficiency as the inherited molecular mechanism for primary pulmonary hypertension. *Am J Hum Genet* 2001; **68(1)**: 92–102.

7 Thomson JR, Machado RD, Pauciulo MW *et al.* Sporadic primary pulmonary hypertension is associated with germline mutations of the gene encoding BMPR-II, a receptor member of the TGF-β family. *J Med Genet* 2000; **37**: 741–5.

8 Rigat B, Hubert C, Corvol P *et al.* PCR detection of the insertion/deletion polymorphism of the human angiotensin converting enzyme gene (DCP1) (dipeptidyl carboxy peptidase 1). *Nucleic Acids Res* 1992; **20**: 1433.

9 Nishihara A, Watabe T, Imamura T, Miyazano K. Functional heterogeneity of bone morphogenetic protein receptor-II mutants found in patients with primary pulmonary hypertension. *Mol Biol Cell* 2002; **13**: 3055–63.

CHAPTER 70

Pathophysiology of Williams syndrome arteriopathy

Damien Bonnet

Williams syndrome is a developmental disorder associated with interstitial deletion of chromosome 7q23 encompassing the elastin gene locus. Hypertension is a common feature of Williams syndrome (WS) and has been attributed to impaired compliance of the arterial tree associated with diffuse hypertrophy of the media.[1] Both *in vitro* and *in vivo* studies demonstrated that increased arterial wall thickness is a common phenotypic trait of the Williams syndrome.[2,3] However, arterial wall hypertrophy in hypertensive subjects is not necessarily associated with reduced distensibility.[4–6] In adult Williams syndrome patients, hypertension can cause remodeling of the conductance arteries overriding primitive alterations of their mechanical properties related to elastin hemizygosity. Here we show that the mechanical properties of the conductance arteries in WS are characterized by normal compliance and low elastic modulus. In addition, we found an activation of various metalloproteases in the aortic wall of WS patients indicating an active remodeling of the arterial wall. We hypothesized that this active remodeling is an adaptive process aiming to normalize the wall stress.

To determine if arterial wall hypertrophy of the elastic arteries was associated with alteration of their mechanical properties in young WS patients, we performed noninvasive analyses of the mechanical properties of the conductance arteries in WS patients. Systolic and diastolic blood pressures were higher in WS patients (125/66 vs. 113/60 mmHg, $P<0.05$). The intima-media thickness was increased in WS patients (0.6 ± 0.07 vs. 0.5 ± 0.03 mm; $P<0.001$). Normotensive WS patients had a lower circumferential wall stress (2.1 ± 0.5 vs. 3 ± 0.7

mmHg, $P<0.01$), a higher distensibility (1.1 ± 0.3 vs. 0.8 ± 0.3 mmHg^{-1}.10^{-2}, $P<0.01$), similar cross-sectional compliance (0.14 ± 0.04 vs. 0.15 ± 0.05 mm^2.mmHg^{-1}, $P>0.05$) and lower incremental elastic modulus (7.4 ± 2 vs. 14 ± 5 mmHg.10^2; $P<0.001$). The compliance of the large elastic arteries is not modified in WS syndrome, even though increased intima-media thickness and lower arterial stiffness are consistent features. Further evidence for the role of disruption of elastin in producing thickening of the arterial wall has been recently proposed in light of a mouse model that lacks elastin.[7,8] The obstructive arterial disease of these mice results in a compensatory increase in the number of rings of elastic lamellae and intimal smooth muscle proliferation and reorganisation. These morphologic changes were independent of the hemodynamic stress as they also occur in arteries that were isolated in organ culture.[7] Although elastin mRNA and protein were reduced by 50% in elastin +/– mice, arterial compliance at physiologic pressures was nearly normal.[8] Consequently, elastin has not only a structural role in the extracellular matrix but also controls smooth muscle proliferation during arterial development. A quantitative change in biosynthesis alters the organization of the various medial elements during development as the knock-out of the elastin gene suggested in mouse. In addition, pathologic observations in Williams patients also showed thick irregular elastic fibers, swirling collagen, and hypertrophied smooth muscle cells. This abnormal deposition of elastin in the media could modify the distribution of the load throughout the arterial wall and shift the load bearing to structures with a low elastic modulus. The above reasons suggest that qualitative changes of elastin, or more specifically changes in the orientation of the elastic fibers might explain the alterations of the mechanical performance of the common carotid artery in Williams syndrome. Therefore, systemic hypertension cannot be attributed to impaired compliance of the arterial tree in this condition.[9]

We then sought to relate the alterations of the extracellular matrix turnover with altered viscoelastic properties of the elastic arteries in elastin related disorders. Morphology of the aortic lamellae obtained at surgery was analyzed by computerized morphometric system. Metalloproteinases (MMP1, MMP2, MMP3, MMP7, MMP9, and TIMPs) expression in the aortic wall was studied by zymographic analysis, Western detection, quantified by image analysis and compared to controls. Morphologic studies showed an increased number of fragmented elastic lamellae with extensive deposition of collagen III. MMP2 and MMP7 (elastases) were strongly expressed in patients with SVAS compared to controls. MMP1 and MMP9 were also present but at a lower level. Activation of metalloproteinases promotes aneurysms formation. In elastin defects, arterial wall hypertrophy is constitutive and not subject to hemodynamic stress. Activation of metalloproteinases leading to an accelerated turn-over of the extra-cellular matrix may be an adaptive process aiming to normalize wall stress by attempting to dilate and/or thin elastic arteries.

Finally, we tested the hypothesis that loss of medial elastin affects the discharge of baroreceptors and consequently the baroreflex sensitivity (BRS). Eight untreated patients with WS (14.8 ± 2.4 years, m ± SEM) were compared to eight healthy subjects (15.1 ± 2.3 years). Blood pressure (BP) was recorded using a Finapres® in the supine position. Systolic BP (SBP) levels were 117.8 ± 4.4 mmHg in WS compared to 110.9 ± 5.7 in controls (NS). HR was higher in the WS (89.8 ± 1.0 vs. 76.8 ± 3.4 beats/min in controls, $P<0.01$). The amplitude of the high frequency (HF, respiratory) PI component (modulus) was reduced in WS (5.7 ± 0.9 vs. 22.4 ± 4.3 ms, $P < 0.01$). The gain of the SBP-PI transfer function was diminished in the low frequency (LF, 0.1 Hz) and the HF range as well (5.9 ± 0.6 vs. 13.8 ± 2.1 ms/mmHg for LF, $P < 0.01$ and 6.0 ± 1.1 vs. 23.7 ± 4.2 ms/mmHg for

HF, $P < 0.01$). The BRS obtained with the sequence technique was also reduced in WS (8.2 ± 0.9 vs. 21.5 ± 2.9 ms/mmHg in controls, $P<0.001$). The per cent of beats involved in baroreflex sequences observed in WS was also diminished to 20% compared to 48% in controls ($P < 0.001$). In conclusion, qualitative changes of elastin might explain the alterations in the mechanical performances of the large arteries involved in baroreceptor discharges.[10] This trait could underlie the BRS reduction and HR elevation observed in WS. The pathophysiology of the WS arteriopathy is complex and today, the precise links between loss of elastin and morphological or hemodynamic features of WS remain unclear.

References

1 Rein AJ, Preminger TJ, Perry SB, Lock JE, Sanders SP. Generalized arteriopathy in Williams syndrome: an intravascular ultrasound study. *J Am Coll Cardiol* 1993; **21**: 1727–30.

2 Sadler LS, Gingell R, Martin DJ. Carotid ultrasound examination in Williams syndrome. *J Pediatr* 1998; **132**: 354–6.

3 O'Connor WN, Davis JB Jr, Geissler R, Cottrill CM, Noonan JA, Todd EP. Supravalvular aortic stenosis. Clinical and pathologic observations in six patients. *Arch Pathol Lab Med* 1985; **109**: 179–85.

4 Hayoz D, Rutschmann B, Perret F *et al.* Conduit artery compliance and distensibility are not necessarily reduced in hypertension. *Hypertension* 1992; **20**: 1–6.

5 Laurent S, Caviezel B, Beck L *et al.* Carotid artery distensibility and distending pressure in hypertensive humans. *Hypertension* 1994; **23(6 Pt 2)**: 878–83.

6 Laurent S, Girerd X, Mourad JJ *et al.* Elastic modulus of the radial artery wall material is not increased in patients with essential hypertension. *Arterioscler Thromb* 1994; **14**: 1223–31.

7 Li DY, Brooke B, Davis EC *et al.* Elastin is an essential determinant of arterial morphogenesis. *Nature* 1998; **393**: 276–80.

8 Li DY, Faury G, Taylor DG *et al.* Novel arterial pathology in mice and humans hemizygous for elastin. *J Clin Invest* 1998; **102**: 1783–7.

9 Aggoun Y, Sidi D, Levy BI, Lyonnet S, Kachaner J, Bonnet D. Mechanical properties of the common carotid artery in Williams syndrome. *Heart* 2000; **84**: 290–3.

10 Girard A, Sidi D, Aggoun Y, Laude D, Bonnet D, Elghozi JL. Elastin mutation is associated with a reduced gain of the baroreceptor–heart rate reflex in patients with Williams syndrome. *Clin Auton Res* 2002; **12**: 72–7.

Index

Page numbers in **bold** type refer to tables; those in *italics* to figures

287